Unseen Enemy

Unseen Enemy: The English, Disease, and Medicine in Colonial Bengal, 1617 – 1847

By

Sudip Bhattacharya

CAMBRIDGE SCHOLARS

PUBLISHING

Unseen Enemy:
The English, Disease, and Medicine in Colonial Bengal, 1617 – 1847,
by Sudip Bhattacharya

This book first published 2014

Cambridge Scholars Publishing

12 Back Chapman Street, Newcastle upon Tyne, NE6 2XX, UK

British Library Cataloguing in Publication Data
A catalogue record for this book is available from the British Library

ISBN (10): 1-4438-6135-9, ISBN (13): 978-1-4438-6135-9

AND THIS ONE TOO IS FOR

SARANYA

CONTENTS

ACKNOWLEDGEMENTS

I thank Cambridge Scholars Publishing for bringing out this book. Thanks are also due to Mr Ranajoy Bose, Executive Member, Christian Burial Board, Kolkata, for allowing me access to the cemeteries under his supervision. This is the second book to emerge from my wanderings in these cemeteries through the last 5 years. Mr Bose takes great interest in my work. We have spent many hours walking along the boulevards of South Park Street cemetery, discussing its various aspects. Bose has unfortunately received little recognition for his assiduousness in preserving this heritage landmark.

Swami Shastrajnananda, Principal, Ramakrishna Mission Vidyamandira, Belur Math, has always been interested in my work. Dr Swarup Ray, Associate Professor and Head, Department of English, and my other departmental colleagues, have taken in good spirit my obsession with death, medicine, and cemeteries. I would like to thank them all for their indulgence and encouragement.

Then there is my family, my father, Major General (Retired) Sujit R Bhattacharya, MD; my mother, Snigdha; my wife, Anindita; and my daughter, Saranya, who have similarly and patiently borne my frequently irritating passion for death and disease.

I must also thank Dr Basujit Gangopadhyay, Consultant Cardiologist, who read several chapters of this book, and provided medical insights.

PREFACE

This is not the story of Tropical medicine. That has been related by others elsewhere. It is also not an attempt to understand and analyse medical practices in the light of our present day knowledge. In this book, we follow the tale of the arrival and settlement of the English in Bengal, in terms of the diseases they suffered here, and how they treated them. In the early phase of the colony, English doctors were willing to observe local medical practices, and learn from them. As time passed, in medicine, as in everything else, attitudes hardened. After 1857, the British medical establishment in India did not consider it important to learn anything from the land to which they considered themselves and their people exiled. While it might have made sense for me to cover the entire span of the British medical experience in India, the sheer volume of writing that this would require kept me from it. It made more sense to focus on the early colonial medical experience, which included several interesting aspects, like the local practice of inoculation for smallpox, as reported by Holwell, and Esdaile's mesmeric surgery, which effectively bracket the period under consideration. Similarly, Balfour's indigenous sol-lunar theory was for long popular and contentious. Other outstanding figures in this history include that of Twining, who migrated from Nova Scotia to England, became a surgeon, joined the army, served in the Peninsular War, and at Waterloo, and then settled to practice in Calcutta, where he died in an accident. Frederick Harrington Brett, an accomplished army surgeon specialised in ophthalmic procedures and author, left service after 18 years in Bengal, and after long travels, probably died in great obscurity far from home. In the same way, John Peter Wade, a brilliant doctor, has lived on in popular memory not because of his exceptional professional aptitude but due to his pioneering history of Assam, where he served several years. The English gained much political influence due to their doctors' proficiency, as proved by Boughton, and Hamilton. Doctors suffered much during political tussles with local rulers, as exemplified by the horrific experiences of the 3 surgeons at Patna.

My aim, as always, has only been to retell the stories noted and mainly published by these medical men, which relate to their experiences in Bengal. Their times were vastly different from ours, and all attempts at interpretation in terms of our world will fail to do them justice. They worked with the medicines and surgical techniques known and available to them, in terms of such scientific knowledge as they had learnt. To their credit, they added to this corpus of knowledge by observing the 'new' diseases they came across in Bengal, and how indigenous medical and home practices were used to treat these conditions. Back home in England, however, their professional colleagues were not greatly enthused by their writings or their findings. James Johnson was, in this regard, unusual, for he spent 3 years in and around Bengal. In any case, he had already gained some reputation in England, and his tome was more acceptable than those written by doctors like Balfour. Balfour's was a sad case, even though Johnson corroborated his theory from personal experience. Eminent English medical men like James Lind, who had never lived in India, found it easy to dismiss Balfour's sol-lunar theory. Other theories impacted medical practice in Bengal, like the Brunonian theory. Based on the complex but rather idiosyncratic concepts of Dr John Brown, one is amazed to find doctors in eighteenth-century Calcutta applying it, with the intention of correcting its inherent errors.

Death was the constant companion of the European in early colonial India. Death came suddenly, and at times, claimed entire families, sometimes in sad order, with the father following the mother and the children into the grave within weeks. Often the demise of the head of a family, in a male-dominated society, meant catastrophe for the bereaved. Many children were orphaned suddenly, and sent back home to relatives they had never seen, in the company of people they hardly knew. Still more tragically, many children died, their ailments not always clear to physicians and surgeons, who simply reduced for them the doses of the same medicines that they used for adults. Since the voyage itself was long and hard, adults and children died on the way out, as they did on the way in. Shipwrecks often occurred, and sometimes ships simply disappeared, and were presumed wrecked with loss of all on board. In such a scenario, Europeans joining service with the East India Company wanted to know about their chances of survival in India. This led to considerably detailed statistical analyses, which seemed to prove that death did not visit as frequently as popularly supposed. However, when one reads that the South Park Street cemetery was opened for burials in 1767 and closed in 1790, one wonders if the statistical findings were correct. This view is strengthened by the fact that at the end of what is Park Street today (and known then as Burial Ground Road), there existed a huge cemetery complex, in addition to other cemeteries in Calcutta, like the French burial ground. Considering that all these cemeteries were full by the middle of the nineteenth century, when another enormous cemetery, the Lower Circular Road burial ground, was established, one is quite certain that life in Bengal took high toll of Europeans who lived here. Of course, they came here to shake the pagoda tree, but this is has nothing to do with their early deaths, or those of their wives and children.

Strolling through the short boulevards of South Park Street cemetery, and reading the sorrowful inscriptions on the tombs, one understands the humane reason for doctors like Balfour to seek out theories that seem amazingly unscientific today. One also understands why Esdaile had to be given the chance to run a Mesmeric Hospital, without his request to do so being dismissed peremptorily. If a hypothesis that claimed to treat disease better if the phases of the moon were observed or a technique like hypnosis could be used to treat disease as painlessly as possible and lower mortality, they were welcome. However, there were doctors who swore by venesection, like James Johnson and William Twining, and surgeons like Brett, whose surgical techniques, imbibed from his teacher, Robert Liston, famous for entering the operation theatre, crying out 'Time me, gentlemen!' horrify one. At the end of it all, it only remains for us to read about these early doctors in Bengal, and form our own thoughts.

INTRODUCTION

DEATH AND DISEASE AMONG EUROPEANS IN COLONIAL BENGAL

Death was not the great leveller among Europeans in colonial Bengal. The wealthy could afford architecturally-designed tombs three stories high, while the humble were interred in ordinary tombs. As a visit to the South Park Street cemetery in Kolkata will show, the intricately-decorated mausoleums of the rich have survived the ravage of time, while humbler graves have mainly disappeared. Wandering among the tombs, one sees the dates of the dead, and realises that they mainly died young: quite certainly so by today's standards. Only a handful of graves hold the remains of elderly persons.

In colonial Bengal, death came suddenly and insidiously to the European. Irrespective of rank and status in society, disease struck without warning, and killed European men, women, and children, even as doctors strove to employ a limited pharmacopoeia to save lives. In colonial Bengal, therefore, disease, and not death, was the great leveller. Sir William Jones was a Justice of the Supreme Court of Judicature, and a renowned scholar of language and culture. He sent his wife home early in 1794, as she had been weakened by local ailments, and needed a change. Within a month of her departure, Sir William discovered that he had developed a tumour 'as big as his fist' in the right side of his abdomen, which he did not bother about, thinking that it would go as innocuously as it had come. Instead, Sir William had exercised himself more than before, frequently walking before his carriage all the way from the courts to his home at Garden Reach, a distance of more than 4 miles. He remained in considerable pain due to the tumour but did not consult any physician, preferring to follow the classical ideal of not allowing the mind to succumb to bodily ache. Around 17 April 1794, Sir William began suffering a bilious fever, possibly accompanied by delirium. Dr David Hare attended Sir William, and discovered the tumour. The usual limited curatives were employed, and by the night of Saturday, 26 April, it was held that Sir William was responding to treatment and would soon be well enough to consider returning to Europe aboard a ship sailing from Botany Bay. The following morning, Sir William's *khansamah* ran into Sir John Shore's presence and proclaimed that his master had gone mad. Sir John, accompanied by General Sir Robert Abercrombie, went to Sir William's house, only to be greeted with news from other servants that soon after the *khansamah* had left, Sir William had asked for some tea, and having had it, died. Sir John and General Sir Robert confirmed this, finding Sir William on his couch, quite dead.

William Hickey, the social gadfly and memoirist of Calcutta, had met Charlotte Barry in England in 1781, and was smitten. She became his mistress soon, and around the end of the year, so Hickey wrote in his *Memoirs*, he offered her marriage, which she refused. Since she was only 21 when she died 2 years later, she must have been 19 at the time she became 'Mrs Hickey'. Recalling the moment when Charlotte declined to marry him on the grounds that should he at some time in future regret his marriage it would break her heart, Hickey wrote over 40 years later that from then on, he considered himself her husband as much as 'the strictest forms and ceremonies of the Church' could have made him. His dissipated lifestyle having impoverished them, William and Charlotte decided to sail to India. Failing to get a ship from England, they sailed to Lisbon early in 1782, whence they availed of a ship to India in June. In between, Charlotte had been seriously ill, and was sent back to Falmouth under medical advice. Hickey often wrote of her general weakness but Charlotte refused to be separated from William, and she returned to Lisbon. The couple reached India at a bad time, when the British and the French were at war. After their ship had been captured by the French, the Hickeys were well-treated by Admiral Suffren at Trincomalee, and they reached Madras in March 1783. Following a brief but interesting sojourn there, during which they met an old family friend, the 'famous' Paul Benfield, the Hickeys sailed aboard a Royal Navy ship to Bengal, landing at Budge-Budge towards the end of June 1783. Of the sinister manner in which disease, unknown and unpredictable, struck, is exemplified by the manner in which Emily, the mistress of Hickey's friend, Robert Potts, was carried off. Robert and Emily had sailed from Madras for Calcutta in May 1782. Given the time of year, when the weather is hot and humid, Emily soon began suffering from 'the prickly heat', 'a sort of rash or eruption upon the skin, very prevalent in hot countries, especially in Asia'. The rash makes the skin extremely sensitive, and the sufferer finds it difficult to endure lying down. Hickey wrote that the prickly heat was common among newcomers, and was caused by 'the superior richness or nicer susceptibility of the blood and general system'. While drinking cold fluids eased the discomfort, this also greatly increased the rash. Hickey's opinion, which was the general medical opinion of the time, classified the prickly heat as 'a sign of vigorous health'. Sufferers did not die of it, and tolerating the discomfort brought future immunity. Emily, however, drank tumblers of cold milk diluted with water. She downed 2 such glassfuls when their ship came in sight of Kulpi, and at once complained of feeling very sick and faint. Within moments, she was comatose, and soon died. Her prickly heat was seen to have disappeared entirely.

Hickey's arrival at Calcutta on 30 June 1783 was not a happy one. His name as attorney had been struck off the rolls at the Supreme Court. Despite the fact that he had occasionally made some money at Madras by providing legal advice to acquaintances, Hickey was in great financial trouble, having incurred vast debts in England, Lisbon, and Madras, at interests varying between 10 and 12 per cent. Illness changed people, and Hickey wad amazed to find among his former friends in Calcutta, Ulysses Brown, of the Horse Guards, who had just passed through a long and dangerous ailment, 'which had so altered and reduced him that except from the voice I should not have recognised him'. Nonetheless, with Potts' help, and Sir Elijah Impey's friendship, Hickey's name was soon enrolled once more as an attorney. Moreover, June was probably the wrong time to arrive in Calcutta, given that this was the beginning of the monsoon. Renewing past friendships, Hickey found that many of those he had known in Calcutta during his previous visit were dead of bilious fevers and similar mysterious ailments. Having spent three months at his friend Potts' garden-house, often travelling to the city on work since many of his former clients had returned to him, Hickey moved to a conveniently situated rented house in Calcutta on 1 September 1783. However, Charlotte was ill. At Potts' Gardens she had often complained of 'sudden and violent pains in her breast', which were medically dismissed as being 'nervous' attacks, curable through 'change of weather'. In Calcutta, Charlotte fell ill more frequently. Recollecting decades later, William said that 'The seeds of a fatal disease were nevertheless then lurking about her, the progress of which was hastened by the uninterrupted course of entertainments she was engaged in'. European social life in early colonial Calcutta was hectic, and they kept late hours, drank much wine, and ate heavy meals, which took their toll on their minds and bodies, given the climate. In November, the weather became pleasant, and balls became common. Charlotte attended these, and was in great demand, for she loved to dance. By the end of November, William noticed in her 'daily increased weakness and languor'. He called in Dr James Stark, the 'favourite practitioner of Calcutta'. Dr Stark advised rest and quiet for a while. This did not have the necessary effect. On Charlotte's health further declining, Hickey called in Drs James Wilson and Stark. They now advised a 'change of air' through a river cruise. William took Charlotte on 7 December 1783 to Budge-Budge, where Major Mestayer, a friend, lived. Briefly revived, Charlotte soon relapsed and begged William to take her back to Calcutta. The doctors remained convinced that there was nothing seriously wrong with Charlotte. But William saw her sinking daily, and even his appointment as Under-Sheriff of Calcutta failed to draw him from Charlotte's side. On 19 December Dr Stark declared Charlotte to be mortally ill. He warned William to be ready for her death, which was fast approaching. She was stricken with a 'painful disease', William wrote, which she bore uncomplainingly, probably because she had been prescribed heavy doses of laudanum. He had his public duties, and although his fellow Englishmen were sympathetic and helpful, he daily rushed home, expecting the worst. She lingered until Christmas Day, 1783. That morning she slept uneasily for 3 hours under the influence of probably still heavier doses of laudanum. Awaking, she spoke to William, and fainted. The doctors made a dramatic appearance at that moment, and proclaimed that she was gone. William was taken away from the house, and the doctors kept watch over Charlotte, who was comatose. She died at 10 pm 'with a gentle sigh'. She was buried the following day, and William, devastated, accepted an invitation from Potts to go and stay with him at Burdwan, where the latter was in charge of the district. William stayed there until 10 January 1784, when he returned to Calcutta and, in his loneliness, commenced a fast life, going to bed drunk every night, and caring nothing for his mounting debts even as he earned great sums from his practice.

Mrs Charles Lushington, when leaving Calcutta in 1827 for England by the overland route, noted that her life in Bengal had been driven by 'a resignation similar to that of the sufferers in Dante's Purgatory'. 'To return to England was the incessant yearning of my heart', she wrote, this attitude having been formed by her experience of 'frequent illness, from witnessing the generally dreadful devastation of the climate, or from loss of friends'. The English cemeteries in India were 'particularly melancholy', she said, since a visit to any one of them would reveal that these 'well-tenanted burying grounds of the cities' contained little more than 'the graves of the youthful, who have been cut off by some violent disease amid the buoyancy of health, or the tombs of those of middle age arrested by death when just about to reap the fruit of long toil and privation in a return to their native land'. Consequently, among Europeans in India there were 'scarcely any old persons' as nearly everybody was 'a temporary resident'. The European widow's fate was worse in India because in England she had at least a protective family circle for herself and the children. When disease carried off the head of the family, its sole earning member, the European widow in India was dispossessed of her home within weeks, the family movables either packed or auctioned off to meet debts, and she hurried aboard a ship to England with the children, 'almost ignorant of the spot where her husband's remains are deposited'. Little remained to help her remind her children of their father, other than the information that he lay buried in a distant land, and his tomb was inaccessible to them.

The Company, however, took care to see that the family of a deceased employee was not deprived of its rightful dues. The wills of their dead servants were placed for the consideration of the council, who examined their legal veracity, questioned the witnesses, and had the testaments meticulously noted in their consultations diary, a copy of which was sent to England at the end of each calendar year. The case of Paul Graton is a random but relevant example. Graton was presumably a sailor of French descent in the Company's service, since, following his death, 'the French Director' at Hooghly sent his effects to the council at Calcutta in March 1714. The French had sent Graton's effects to the English because Graton's widow had married an Englishman, John Castle. Paul Graton also left behind an infant son, Gabriel. The Calcutta council, despite being absorbed then with their hectic preparation for the Surman embassy to Delhi, examined Graton's effects, and gave John Castle 'Particulars amounting to 92 rupees 12 annas … to be reckoned to him as part of his Wife's share of her late Husband Paul Graton's Estate' on 12 March 1714. On 9 April, they provided a full account of Paul Graton's estate, 'and division of it between his Widow and Infant Son'. The gross amount was 5353 rupees. From this, the cost of 'his Wife's diet and Lodging in Hooghly whilst he was at sea', 103 rupees, was deducted, and the amount to be divided assessed at 5250 rupees. Of this, Graton's widow, 'now the wife of John Castle', was given 1750 rupees, 'her dividend being one third' of her late husband's estate. John Castle was given a written acknowledgement that the remainder, 3500 rupees, 'remains in the Honourable Company's Cash at Interest for the use and Account of Gabriel Graton the infant son of Paul Graton'. On 11 April 1715, the council paid to John Castle 520 rupees as interest when John Castle demanded it 'to defray the charge of maintaining the Child'. The final entry in this matter may be found in a council decision dated 3 December 1716, when John Castle demanded an advance of 500 rupees to send

Gabriel Graton to England to be educated. The council agreed to this payment, and the child was to voyage aboard the *Prince Frederick.*

The problem with leaving India was that England offered few similar advantages of life, particularly the easy extravagance, power, and chance to make a fortune. Decisions to leave India therefore brought 'sobered anticipations of the future' to Mrs Lushington, such that she did not wonder at those who decided to remain 'one year more'. However, she also noted that this determination proved fatal to many. An example of this fatal determination is Major General the Hon Sir William Casement, KCB, of the Bengal Army, and also Member of the Supreme Council of India, who, after 47 and a half years' distinguished service, 'was swayed by a sense of duty to accede to the pressing instance of the Governor General in Council to deter his departure from India, a step which exposed him to the fatal malady which terminated his valuable life' (Inscription on his tomb, at the Lower Circular Road Cemetery, Calcutta). General Casement died on 16 April 1844, aged 61.

Since few could choose to leave India before they had completed their tenures, it became essential to study local disease alongside traditional treatment. Disease came suddenly to the European in India, disparaged the rudimentary medical resistance offered, and took quick toll of life, leaving in its wake graves with piteous inscriptions of lamentation. Disease did not discriminate, but took young and old, men and women, irrespective of status. Even doctors were prey to ailments. James Kerr, Surgeon in the service of the East India Company upon the Bengal Establishment, 'distinguished as well by his Medical knowledge as by his improving the arts and enriching science by his discoveries in India' died in Calcutta on 17 September 1782, aged 44. Dr Rowland Jackson, MRCP (London) died aged 63 on 29 March 1784. Some of the other medical men interred in the South Park Street cemetery include James Arthur, Surgeon, who died on 22 May 1786, aged 49, Edmund Bengough, MD, who died aged 55 on 10 January 1787, and John Campbell, MD, 'Assistant Surgeon in the service of the Honourable East India Company, who was carried off by a fever, at the General Hospital, Presidency', on 19 November 1803, aged 24.

The Honourable East India Company offered its employees statistics on life-expectancy so that they would know the odds for and against their survival in India. *A General Register of the Hon'ble East India Company's Civil Servants of the Bengal Establishment from 1790 to 1842* (1844), compiled by Ramchunder Doss, under the direction of H T Prinsep, gives us the necessary figures. Adjusting variables to suit conditions of appointment, travel, arrival, and joining service in Bengal, the *Register* informs us that between 1790 and 1836, 90 out of 1525 civilians died between the ages of 20 and 25 or, up to 5 years' service. This is only 1.98% of the total number of civil servants employed by the Company. Between 5 and 10 years' service, the number of civilians is placed at 3454.5 (after adjustments), and the number of deaths is 72. The risk rises marginally during this period to 2%. Between 10 and 15 years' service, the numbers are 2469.5 civilians against 41 deaths, which drop the risk factor to 1.66%. As a number of retirements took place between 15 and 20 years' service, in this period there were 1879 civilians on the rolls, and 44 deaths, raising the risk to 2.34%. Many more retirements and resignations from service taking place between 20 and 25 years' service, the number of civilians included in this group was 1214.5, with 43 deaths, pushing up the risk to 3.54%. Against this higher risk, there were 33 retirements during this period, showing that the increase was inflated. Fewer civilians stayed to serve up to 30 years, 660.5 against 24 deaths and 31 retirements, which pushed up the risk still higher to 3.63%. At the end of 35 years' service, 299 civilians continued in employment, of whom 16 died and 20 retired, pushing up the risk to 5.35%. Few remained in service after 35 years in Bengal, 109 against 3 deaths and 8 retirements, a risk of 2.75%. Only 25 civilians remained on the Company's rolls with 40 to 45 years' service, and of these, 2 died and 2 retired, raising the risk to 8%. In another table, Prinsep demonstrates that during the same period, most deaths took place during the 2nd, 8th, and 9th years of residence in Bengal, peaking briefly again in the 17th, falling thereafter, to 2 in the 30th year of service. It was presumed that the newly appointed Writer was aged 20, which leads us to the conclusion that most deaths occurred at the ages of 22, 28, 29, and 37.

Prinsep's calculations were in response to an article published in *Gleanings in Science*, September 1831, titled 'On the Duration of Life in the Bengal Civil Service'. While admitting that the subject of the article in *Gleanings* 'is of first rate interest', Prinsep says that the conclusions of this paper 'are too startling to be admitted without a strict examination of the data, which are the basis of calculation'. The results are indeed startling, for the author shows that between 1790 and 1799, 217 Writers were appointed, of whom 79 left the service, 84 died, and 54 remained. During the period 1790 and 1800, 246 were appointed, 85 left service, 93 died, and 68 remained. The figures are worst for 1790-1802, when 289 were appointed, 91 left service for some reason or other including dismissal, 100 died, and 98 remained. During 1790-1808, the corresponding numbers are 436 appointees, against 75 resignations or dismissals, 109 deaths, and 252 survivals. Further analysis showed that by age 23, the annual decrement of life for the newly appointed Writer rose to 4%. This is in keeping with the two-monsoon rule of thumb that determined the survival rate of a European in India. The annual decrement of life fell thereafter, peaking again at the ages of 40, 44, 45, 47, and 49, when it hovered around 10%. More adjustments for periodicity and averages show that the ages between 40 and 50 are most dangerous for the Bengal civilian. The author of the article concluded that the article showed the influence of the Indian climate on European constitutions that 'it induces premature old age', even under 'the most favourable circumstances'. 'Arriving in the country at the most advantageous age, subject to little exposure', the Bengal civilians 'with incomes sufficient to command all the comforts of life, and for facilities for renovating impaired health by temporary removal to another climate', it was astounding that the high mortality rate among them was in fact many times better than 'any other class of residents in the country'. Considering that the Company had recently allowed a 3-year absentee allowance to those compelled to retire to England due to illness, furlough allowance for 3 years to those who had spent 10 years in India, and a pension of £1000 to those completing 25 years' service, the author held that in terms of the life tables, these measures would 'probably lessen the mortality, from the ages of 20 to 40; increase it from 40 to 45, by the inducement they will hold out to endanger a broken constitution, for a few more years, in hopes of obtaining the pension; and materially lessen it subsequently to the age of 45'. The figures in all these studies deal only with the lives of men, and do not venture to analyse the survival statistics for women and children.

The editor of *Gleanings* acknowledged the importance of the article as well as the fact that the figures and tables needed thorough analysis, while agreeing that the ages ranging from 40-50 were the most hazardous period for the Bengal civilian. After pointing out the need for certain adjustments to the author's calculations, the editor writes that the paper seemed to conclude that the results were 'far too favourable for the chances of life during the first few years of residence, and perhaps a little too unfavourable towards the close of his series'. This aberration arose, the editor felt, from the contributor's lack of precise information about 'deaths in the service, each to its proper year, reckoned from the arrival of the individual, which seems to be the only way to ascertain the influence of the climate upon his constitution'. The reason why everyone found this study of interest and importance was because sickness nearly always meant death, and death speeded up the possibility of promotion along a slow, time-bound system where seniority (and hence survival) alone mattered. Even if it did not kill outright, sickness often removed a man from the system, forcing him home with his family, on medical certificate.

Sir James Ranald Martin presents in his book, *The Influence of Tropical Climates in Producing the Acute Endemic Diseases of Europeans* (1855, first edition; 1861, second edition), two 20-year lists of deaths, between, compiled from the vestry records of the Protestant burial ground in Calcutta. The first list covered the years between 1796 and 1815, and the second, between 1818 and 1838. These lists are both fascinating and tragic. During these 40 years, 1036 European children aged below 5, and 6750 Europeans aged more than 5, died in Calcutta. The worst months during 1818 and 1838 were May, and the period between August and January. For 1796 – 1815, most deaths took place between August and December, with a significant peak in November. In both lists, February was the healthiest month. A further study of the returns of patients from the Presidency General Hospital in Calcutta showed that during 12 years, 15,293 Europeans were admitted, of whom 1704 died. Martin concluded that this showed a ratio of 1 death to 9 admissions. "From the 'Medical Board's Table of Seasons'", Martin continued, "it appears that the most healthy months comparatively are February, March, April, and May; that from June to January the admissions range high, these also being by far the most fatal months'. Remittent fevers, hepatitis, dysentery, and diarrhoea, he writes, were worst during October to January, while intermittent fevers were most common in September.

Another table, found by Martin in 'the records of the Committee for the Improvement of Calcutta', studied mortality in Calcutta during 1817 and 1836, again using burial records. This table shows that 5065 Protestants died during the period concerned, as did 240 Scots (in the Scottish burial ground), and over 8000 Catholics, followed by 24 Greeks, and 315 Armenians. Further analysis showed that the mortality rates for the English worked out to less than 1 in 28 per annum, as compared to 1 in 36 for the locals, since the latter added up to nearly 60,000 persons. The mortality rate for Armenians was almost the same as that for the English, since it stood at 1 in 25 for the former.

The Medical Board to the Committee for the Improvement of Calcutta stated that during 1 January 1808 to 31 December 1837, the number of Europeans admitted to the Presidency General Hospital was 35119, of whom 3607 died, leading Martin to conclude that the mortality rate for admissions for this 30-year period stood at 10.27%. Looking at the mortality of civil servants during 1790 – 1836, he found that per thousand, 48.6% of those aged over 50, and with 30 years of service, died; for those aged 40-50, with 25-30 years' service, this figure was 36.4%; for those aged 40-45, and 20-25 years' service, at 35.4%; for those aged 35-40 and 15-20 years' service, at 23.4%; for those aged 30-35, and 10-15 years' service, at 16.6%; for those aged 25-30, and 5-10 years' service, at 20.8%, and for those aged 20-25, with 1-5 years' service, at 19.9%. The mortality percentage for civil servants aged 20-35 was nearly the same. However, the figure was lower for the next stage because, as Martin reminds us, civil servants were allowed to go home on 3 years' leave on the completion of 10 years' service. This added to longevity, and detracted from the mortality percentage for that age and service seniority. 'The official results in regard to the mortality at each age among the military officers and civil servants of the Bengal Presidency, afford a convincing proof that in the East Indies', Martin wrote, 'no advantage has hitherto been derived from length of residence'. This statement is supported by a comparative study of mortality among European troops in other tropical locations. In Jamaica, for example, mortality was around 128% for all ages. Similarly, it was high in Ceylon (86.4% for age-group 33-40; 126% for those aged 40-50). The mortality rates were nearly the same for all age-groups in Mauritius, Bombay, and Bengal. Of these, Bombay was statistically the healthiest. Writing in 1855, Sir James Ranald Martin took up the most obvious question, 'do we not live under an improved climate, and is not the mortality of Europeans greatly diminished of late years?' Answering this question, which every European in Bengal wanted to ask, Martin stated that it was not easy to arrive at a conclusion, 'owing to the absence of older statistical record'. However, it had to be admitted that 'the climate of the actual site of Calcutta is improved to a certain extent … and that European general mortality is likewise diminished, amongst the better classes especially'. A return of the figures relevant to European officers, soldiers, and their families, in the Bengal Presidency shows that between 1 April 1850 and 31 March 1854, mortality among children stood at the horrifying figure of 84.1 per 1000.

The *East India Sketchbook*, by an anonymous writer, was published in 1832-33, in 2 volumes. The second volume contains a short story titled 'The Sick Certificate', whose theme is the politics of sickness in the Company's service. Captain Darnley, the protagonist, has been ill with 'some severe malady'. At the beginning of the story Darnley and his wife sit together, contemplating their future. Darnley fears that he does not improve, and Anne, his wife, thinks the same but will not concede it. Darnley looks at his vest, and tells his wife that not so long ago it fitted him so closely but now was obviously loose on a wasted frame. Anne assures him that this is typical of India: 'You know in this country how soon one is pulled down! And then recovery is always so slow!' Darnley would not be thus put off, and he wanted to be told what the doctor had recommended. "He said, 'India will not do for Darnley, he must go home'", his wife told him. The doctor, Assistant Surgeon Thompson, is presented as a 30-year old man with black hair worn long, red eyes, and a 'burly-looking' yet deceptive face. His excessive kindness of manner is belied by shifty eyes whose sideward glances 'could be translated only into a looking-out keenly after his own interest'. The writer goes on to note Thompson's ability in 'quickly discovering the good qualities of any officer who happened to have influential connexions, and commendably prudent in eschewing the society of such refractory youths as ventured to canvass the doings of their betters'. He had little direct interest in Captain Darnley, for Darnley had nothing more than his career, pay, and debts. To Thompson's surprise, Darnley had no interest in India beyond his profession, where he was a popular officer. Unlike other officers, Darnley preferred his domestic life, and 'economised to the utmost'. Consequently, Darnley was not a favourite of his commanding officer, Lieutenant Colonel Bore.

When asked by Anne when he was going to issue Darnley a sick certificate, which would allow him to sail home, Thompson was evasive: 'of course, I should be unwilling to send him away, except in a case of absolute necessity, for his own sake', he said, adding that furlough 'adds so much to an officer's term of slavery', indicating the minimum period Darnley would have to serve in order to settle his debts. Anne disagreed with Thompson, and he riposted by stating that in his professional opinion, Anne rather than Darnley needed to travel home immediately. Offended, Anne refused, and asked Thompson for permission to Darnley to travel to the presidency headquarters and 'see whether the medical gentlemen there disagree with you – whence we shall call on you for a statement of Darnley's case and your mode of treatment', she thundered. His 'naturally red face' glowing purple under this rebuke, Thompson strove to smoothen things by saying that he would, if necessary, issue the sick certificate. However, Anne remained obdurate and told Thompson that if the following day Darnley's symptoms did not improve, he would apply for leave to the presidency headquarters, for the review of his case. Thompson quitted the Darnleys' presence and after he had left, Anne called him 'a base and time-serving wretch'.

Later, out in the garden, Darnley overheard Thompson's conversation with another officer from the same regiment, Captain Ashton. Ashton was unfazed by Thompson's fear of Anne's rage. 'To let Darnley once quit these shores without first getting fairly out of my way, will be actual destruction to my prospects', Ashton said. Darnley was Ashton's sole obstacle for promotion to Major. Ensigns and Lieutenants waited in queue for a vacancy to occur. Ashton reminded Thompson that he owed it to them all to keep Darnley in India 'until he is fairly sickened', and only then to allow him to go home 'conditionally', or with the caveat that he would resign his commission. In return, Thompson wanted Ashton, who obviously had considerable influence, to put in a word for him at the Adjutant General's office for his appointment as chief of the 'Zillah of Bopore'. A civil appointment would get Thompson a higher salary and far brighter prospects than time-bound service as an army doctor. Unable to restrain his passion, Darnley stepped out of concealment and calling Ashton and Thompson scoundrels and cowards, challenged the former to a duel as soon as his health was restored. Ordered off the premises by Ashton, Darnley left after having warned them of dire consequences for conspiring against him.

This excitement led to Darnley's relapse. Soon after he had recovered, he was visited by the Adjutant, who placed him under arrest by order of Colonel Bore who, in connivance with Ashton and Thompson, had laid three charges for court-martial against Darnley. Under the general charge of conduct unbecoming an officer and gentleman, Darnley was accused of forcing himself into Ashton's presence, of having challenged him to a duel without provocation, and of having called Ashton 'liar and coward'. The court-martial would as surely remove Darnley from Ashton's path as sickness and resignation, for, if the charges were proved, the sentence would be dismissal from service. Meanwhile, even as Darnley recuperated slowly, his wife wrote to the commander-in-chief of the presidency, giving all the details of his sickness, of the manner in which Darnley had been baited by Bore and Ashton, and of Thompson's involvement, contrary to the rules of his profession.

The court-martial was conducted by the Judge Advocate General, and at its conclusion all, including Darnley, expected the sentence to be the worst possible for a career officer. The court sent its findings for confirmation by the commander-in-chief, who soon replied, ordering all European officers to attend the announcement at the Division Headquarters. While agreeing that Darnley had been intemperate in behaviour, the commander-in-chief commented that the provocation had been extreme, and Darnley's character was borne by the testimony of the majority of his fellow officers. He was released from arrest and restored to duty. The next day's orders removed Colonel Bore from command, and placed Ashton and Thompson under arrest pending court-martial at the presidency headquarters. Ashton and Thompson were dismissed the service, Darnley having testified at their trial. However, 'Darnley and his wife felt no triumph when they knew that their adversaries were disgraced and ruined'.

Instead, they travelled home, where Darnley obtained employment and built himself a beautiful home by the sea in one of the southern counties.

In viewing life for the European in India as 'a skeleton dressed in glittering robes' Darnley and his wife were echoing the same sentiments as Mrs Lushington. Philip Meadows Taylor, newly appointed to a commission in the army of the Nizam of Hyderabad, travelled from Bombay to Aurangabad in November 1824. The Western Ghats delighted Taylor: 'Deep glens and ravines, bounded by tremendous precipices; trees and flowers all new to me; fresh and invigorating air, so cold and bracing, and so like, so I thought, to dear old England!' However, when called up on active service during the monsoon the following year, Taylor soon fell ill with 'very severe jungle fever'. He recovered, suffered a relapse at Aurangabad, and was conveyed to Ahmednagar, which did not help. From Ahmednagar he was removed to Poona, where his life was again despaired of, and he was despatched thence to Bombay, where 'the pure sea-air' helped his recovery.

In addition to sickness, the European in Bengal (as in the rest of India) had also to contend with medical incompetence. One of the best contemporary pictures of everyday life for the European in India, is to be found in Captain G F Atkinson's *Curry and Rice (On Forty Plates) or, The Ingredients of Social Life at 'Our' Station in India* (1859). In the preface, Atkinson distinguishes between the classes among the English in India, the 'Qui Hyes' of Bengal, the 'Mulls' of Madras, and the 'Ducks' of Bombay, who 'adhere to, and defend their own customs with jealous warmth of feeling'. Atkinson's imaginary station is the village of Kabob, which is situated in the great plains of Dekchy, in the province of Bobarchy, within the presidency of Bengal. Kabob 'is bounded in the north and east by a mountainous range – of flaming brick-kilns, whilst on the south and west it is embraced in the tortuous sinousities of a circumambient ravine populous with pigs'. Consisting of mud cottages and houses, Kabob is open to the vicissitudes of the harsh weather. There are 4 doctors in Kabob: Dr Goley, the Civil Surgeon, lives in the Civil Lines; Dr De Why attends to the soldiers of the artillery and the staff; Dr McGhee is Kabob's consulting physician and general practitioner; 'and all three repose beneath the superintending and vigilant glance of the great Dr Fogrum, whose responsible and arduous duties consist in permanently sitting as president of a standing committee to provide for the sick and needy in their affliction, by the administering of medical certificates, which enable the then joyful recipients to escape for a while from their exile in the shadeless plains'. Dr McGhee is 'of an acquisitive and accumulative turn of mind, which resolves itself into performances that afford food for the amusement of the young blood of Kabob and the enlivenment of the coffee-shop'. Medicine and surgery no longer hold any interest for McGhee. In fact, the popular impression about him is so bad that 'the really sick ... are never admitted to his destructive powers'. Consequently, the 'Great Plague of Kabob' occupies his time 'in a more genial way, by devotion to the business of the Kabob Bank'. This is because Dr McGhee is a director of the bank, having established and originated it. Instead of looking to patients, McGhee 'does funny things in that quiet bank parlour', like 'cancelling shares in a peculiarly acquisitive, and not altogether unprofitable manner, and performing other delicate but lucrative operations, which augment and develop the resources of his individual purse'. In addition to his banking operations, Dr McGhee also has many other investments, including the *Kabob Chronicle*, which he solely owns. In between all his financial preoccupations, the doctor finds time to visit the hospital. However, Dr McGhee does not have the time to greet anyone, for "his thoughts are too much occupied with rupees and with what he can do to turn a penny out of someone at 'Our Station'".

Not all doctors were thus. The English owed the imperial *firman* allotting them landowners' rights to the villages constituent of, and territories around, Calcutta, to the skill of their surgeon, William Hamilton. Hamilton sailed as ship's surgeon aboard the East Indiaman *Sherborne* in 1709. The ship's captain, Henry Cornwall, was tyrannical and detested by his crew. After many problems between captain and sailors, the ship reached Calcutta late in the year 1710. Like his shipmates, Hamilton too must have suffered Cornwall's temper until he could bear it no more. Hamilton left ship on 3 May 1711, while it was at Fort St David. Thence he travelled to Madras. Cornwall applied to the council at Fort St George to have his surgeon returned. Hamilton disobeyed the council's order and proceeded to Calcutta, where he was appointed Second Surgeon on 27 December 1711.

The Mughal emperor, Farrukhsiyar, was cured of a lingering ailment by Hamilton in 1715, upon which he decided to keep Hamilton with him as his attending physician. However, due to Hamilton's fervent plea to be allowed to return to his wife and children in England, the emperor released him on the condition that Hamilton would resume his position at the imperial court immediately on his return. Hamilton and the rest of the English party returned to Calcutta in 1717, having finally obtained the elusive *firman* in June of that year. Hamilton neither went back to England, nor to the imperial court, for he died at Calcutta on 4 December 1717. Buried in the small cemetery that now adjoins St John's Church,

Hamilton's tombstone was rediscovered when the foundations for the church were being dug in Warren Hastings' time.

This was the second time in the history of the English in India that an English surgeon had obtained special privileges from the Mughal emperor. In 'the year of the Hegira 1046' [1636? 1644?], Jahanara, Emperor Shah Jahan's favourite daughter, was 'dreadfully burnt, by her clothes catching fire'. An English doctor was sought on the advice of the vizier, Asad Khan, and the council in Surat recommended Gabriel Boughton [Thomas Bowrey calls him 'Bowden'], the surgeon of the Company's ship *Hopewell*, 'a very Eminent Doctor of Phisick'. Boughton seems to have studied at Guy's Hospital, and according to legend, he travelled to the Emperor's camp in the Deccan, and succeeded in bringing about the princess's recovery. Thus began the tale of Boughton's success in Bengal. When asked by the overjoyed and magnanimous Emperor to name his reward, Boughton 'with that liberality which characterises Britons', sought nothing for himself. Rather, he asked that 'his nation might have liberty to trade, free of all duties, to Bengal, and to establish factories in that country'. A *firman* to this effect was soon granted, and Boughton proceeded to Pipli in Bengal.

Pipli is situated at the mouth of the river Ichamati, and its port had been used by the English since 1634. The first English factory on the east coast was established by Ralph Cartwright in 1633. When a ship from England reached Pipli 2 years later, its cargo was unloaded without the payment of any duties, thanks to Boughton's imperial permit. Boughton's tale does not end here. Shah Shuja (1616-1661), the Emperor's second son, became the governor of Bengal in 1641, and he would not have looked kindly upon Boughton's special permission, despite its being issued in his father's name, had fate not intervened. On Shah Shuja's assumption of the governorship, Gabriel Boughton went to pay him his respects at the provincial capital, Rajmahal. Just then, a lady of the governor's harem fell seriously ill 'with a complaint in her side'. Boughton was consulted, and he successfully treated the malady. This raised him immensely in the governor's esteem. Soon the *Lyoness* arrived from England, bringing on board James Bridgeman of the Company, who had been assigned to 'advance and increase the trade' in Bengal. London had received news of Boughton's imperial influence and permission, but his particular sway over the provincial durbar helped Bridgeman establish a factory at Hooghly in 1650-51. Little is known about Boughton after this, and he seems to have died around 1652. There are many inconsistencies in Gabriel Boughton's tale in the form in which it is related by various authors, and many think that he was sent to Agra not to attend to any emergency but only because English doctors were much in demand, and Asad Khan felt one ought to be in attendance at the Imperial capital. In any case, Boughton's professional service certainly helped the English receive trade concessions in Bengal.

Medicines do not figure in the list of goods prescribed by Sir Thomas Roe as suitable gifts for the imperial court, and the emperor. Roe's advice was to give presents to the emperor as behove his position, such as Arras cloth, of silk and gold, rich stones, caparison and saddle per Indian designs, embroidered satin coats, or perhaps a crown set with small stones. While gifts undoubtedly helped obtain concessions, it was medicine that provided greater aid. Sir Thomas Roe was continually afflicted with various ailments throughout his stay in India, and this made him state, 'all my actions have been mingled with crosses and rubs that I might say I wrestled then walked towards my grave'.

Disease and death often resulted in seriously troubled minds. An example of this was Robert Needham Cust (1821-1909). Cust was an Orientalist, a formidable scholar, proficient in many languages, author of several books, and renowned lecturer. He had been to Eton and thence to Trinity College with the intention of taking a degree and being called to the Bar. However in 1840 he was offered a place at the East India College in Haileybury. Just as he had excelled at Eton, Cust left Haileybury as 'Senior', 'with gold medals and scores of volumes as prizes'. Cust titled the part of his autobiography that deals with his experience in India, 'Exile in India'. In Calcutta Cust became proficient in Bengali, Urdu, Persian, and Sanskrit, as a result of which he earned monetary rewards. He had a fine career and in 1855 he decided to use his entitlement of 3 years' furlough to go and see his father, who was ailing. This saved him from the worst effects of the mutiny but like all other Company officers he was ordered to India in 1857.

Writing with hindsight, Cust noted in his memoirs, 'This year, 1856, was the last happy year of my life: troubles gathered around me, from which I have never escaped'. His first wife, Marie Adelaide Hobart and their daughter came out to join him at Lahore in 1859. The following year his daughter fell so seriously ill that her life was despaired of, and he came to the conclusion that his family, which now included an infant son as well, had to leave for England at once if they were to live. He put them aboard a ship for home in November 1860. Exactly a year later, Marie Cust returned to India to re-join Robert, with their third child, an infant son. In June 1862 cholera struck the Punjab and Cust was tired with his work: 'I used to talk with my wife of what we would do when we got back to England, for I was weary of India'. His memoirs thereafter list deaths and premonitions of final partings.

In 1863 Cust took stock of his achievements: 'I had attained some of the highest posts of the State, and had prospects of still higher ones before my eyes, but my ambition was quite gone'. This was written in retrospect. On 17 January 1864, soon after the birth of their fifth child, his wife died. He left India with his children in February: 'My career was finished, and I took leave of India, never intending or wishing to return'. However, at home he found himself quite unemployed, and seized an offer by Lord Lawrence to become a Member of the Legislative Council of India. He assumed this post in November 1864, and served for 3 months as Home Secretary. Suddenly he decided to leave India again, and this he did in April 1865, receiving at Cairo the news of his youngest child's death. Again he soon found no professional openings for him in England, and again he accepted Lawrence's offer of the post of Member, Board of Revenue, North West Provinces. He married his second wife, Emma Carlyon, in November 1865. With her he set off for India the following year. En route, his wife fell ill with a fever and she was landed in Calcutta in a serious condition and even though Cust was 'in a state of great despondency', she recovered and they went to Allahabad, where he was to stay. His wife was 'weak and poorly' and it was April, the beginning of the hottest season of the year. Cust was tormented by doubts: 'How I wished that I had not returned to India!' On 13 July 1867, in her second summer in India, Emma Cust suffered 'a shiver', following which 'the evil commenced' and she died on 10 August, despite 'a month of careful nursing and the most devoted attention on the part of the medical men'. In fact, the doctors had told Cust on 15 July that there was no hope. Cholera was raging in Allahabad and his wife, who had been pregnant, delivered a girl prematurely.

Cust's grief was too deep for words. He blamed himself: 'I had been the cause of a second sweet young woman leaving her home to die in India, only to die: a grave in each of the Capitals of the two great Provinces, at Lahore and Allahabad, records my unhappy destiny'. He laboured on for he had his little girl to look after, though he was probably not quite normal, for he admitted: 'I used to peep through the garden fences, and see my happy neighbours, husbands and wives, parents and little children, and I used to ask why I was thus tortured'. He feared he was becoming suicidal: 'In the solitude of an Indian bungalow, after the business of the day had been despatched, in my excited state of feelings, and with my overtaxed brain, and excitable temperament, I might be tempted to some rash action'. In November 1866 Cust obtained a medical certificate to travel to England with his three-month old daughter. However, no matter where he looked, he saw disease and death take their terrible toll. During the interval of his arrival at Calcutta, and his departure, Cust received a letter from a former college friend, who begged his company, for his wife was dying. Cust responded at once, 'I went and found her just passing away, and sat by the side of the distracted husband the whole night'. The day before he left, Cust also consoled a very young lady, who had been widowed and left penniless. Her passage home had been arranged by friends. Cust found himself coming across 'other widows and widowers' on board the ship. Death seemed to follow him. In Cairo Cust asked after his cousin, posted in Egypt at the time, only to be told that the cousin had died the previous day in Alexandria. Cust's depression worsened: 'I felt keenly that with blasted hopes, ruined fortunes, legitimate ambitions crushed, opportunities of usefulness gone, I was creeping home like a cur, which had been flogged, or like a soldier, who had been cashiered, with one poor motherless child to add to add to the four other motherless children already in England'. At the age of 47, he had the alternative, so he wrote, of either dying or making a new life for himself in a new environment.

Cust listed the pros and cons of this new environment. Against official appointments and arrivals and departures by steamer, there were the new problems of 'reduced income, choice of residence, worry of a family'. Most of all 'The horror surrounding a Death in India is gone forever'. In saying this, Cust gave voice to the greatest concern of the European sojourner in India. Death had not been defied; it would come quietly, and "no telegraphic communications will disturb a party of young children at their tea, that 'Father is dead'". Writing his memoirs at the age of 80, Cust could exult that he was alive while a son of one of the Lieutenant Governors (probably a contemporary of Cust in the Company's service) was writing his father's life, a father whom he had never seen or known. There were others, like his former colleagues, Arthur Roberts and Cuthbert Thornhill, whose 'domestic happiness' Cust used to envy. They both died in 1868, even as Lawrence once more offered Cust a lucrative post in India, and he had only 9 months left to serve to secure his full pension of £1,000 a year. Roberts and Thornhill 'had served their time, which secured their pensions, were happy in the company of the wives of their youth and their children, *and both died* in India' [Cust's emphasis]. His Haileybury friend, Bellasis, had only a month to serve for full pension, and he went out to Bombay to complete this formality but died there. Yet money remained a problem, for in 1868 Cust resigned the service under medical certificate, and was awarded a pension of £450 a year. He underwent a bitter struggle to decide this but finally realised that 'Life, Health, and an English home' were all that he wanted most. Sir Herbert Edwardes too died in 1868, not having reached the age of 50. Cust went on to list at least 25 eminent persons who had made great names for themselves as administrators or soldiers but were dead by 1867. Many, like Sir Herbert, had died before they were 50. 'I indeed have reason to be thankful for the last thirty blessed years', Cust concluded. This lesson was driven home by the fate of the former Lieutenant Governor of Punjab, Sir Donald McLeod. McLeod too had lost his wife within a few months of marriage but he had worked on in India, achieved great honours, only to be killed in a grisly manner while trying to board a moving train at the Kensington Underground station. 'I followed the remains to the hospital', Cust wrote, 'and saw them in four separate parcels, and attended the Coroner's Inquest'. Death continued to pursue Cust; his eldest son died in February 1871. This was the last of his personal tragedies for though his younger son fell ill with typhoid in 1878 Cust spared no expense to bring him the best medical care, as a result of which he recovered. Cust found new interest in language studies and soon became a regular on the lecture circuit.

CHAPTER ONE

JOHN WOODALL AND HIS *SURGEON'S CHEST*

The Fellowship of Surgeons was united to the Company of Barbers by an Act of Parliament, 3 Henry VIII cap 42, in 1540. Subsequently, a coat of arms was granted to the Company of Barber-Surgeons in 1569. As one peruses the lists of Masters and Wardens of the Company from 1308 on, scanning names that sometimes are suffixed by initials like KB (King's Barber), KS (King's Surgeon), and SS (Sergeant-Surgeon), one comes across John Woodall, who was Warden in 1625 and 1627, and Master in 1633. Since the 12th century, barbers had helped monks in minor medical and surgical procedures such as venesection, tooth-drawing, cauterisation, and the preparation of medical baths. Clergymen were not supposed to be engaged in surgical work, particularly after they were thus prohibited by an edict issued in 1163 by Pope Alexander II. This edict, called the Edict of Tours, allowed clerics to pursue medical treatment but barred them from surgery since it required the shedding of blood. Therefore, surgery became the exclusive work of the barbers.

In December 1308, Richard le Barber was recognised as the first Master of the Company of Barbers, then only a guild, by the Court of Aldermen of London. He promised, under oath, to ensure to 'make scrutiny throughout the whole of his trade' and remove or punish members of his profession, who actions were scandalous to the trade. By 1310, barbers were appointed keepers of the City gates, for their specialised medical and surgical knowledge would allow them to screen visitors and keep out those afflicted with leprosy and others suffering from similar ailments. By 1376 there were so many quacks in practice that the guild was forced to appoint 2 Masters each year to superintend the trade. One such quack, discovered, tried, and convicted in 1382, was sentenced to be turned out of the City on an unsaddled horse, with his magical parchment that was promised to cure fevers, a whetstone and a urinal hung around his neck, and an additional urinal upon his back. Despite their royal sanction, the Royal College of Physicians (Chartered 1518) was unwilling to see the barber-surgeons as medical men. Even the Royal College of Surgeons wanted to disengage from their association with the barbers. They succeeded in this in 1745. The physicians, had long been averse to sharing their medical practice with surgeons, or allowing the latter the same social status as theirs.

John Woodall (1556?-1643) wrote what might be considered the first textbook of medicine meant for the instruction of, and use by, surgeons in the employ of the East India Company. Woodall was apprenticed at a very young age, gained practical knowledge through experience in war and peace, and rose to become Surgeon General in 1612 of the newly chartered East India Company. His effective use of his nostrum, *aurum vitae*, during the London plague of 1603 established his reputation. He had seen active service as an army surgeon and lived for 7 years on the Continent, which added to his medical training. There seems to be no recorded reference to his surgeon-generalship, since Court Minute books of the East India Company between January 1610 and January 1614 are missing. In 1612 John Woodall seems to have also been a member of the Drapers' Company, since he is listed in the fourth volume of the Revd A H Johnson's *History of the Worshipful Company of the Drapers of London* (1922) as having invested £37 in the 'Companies of Virginia, Somers Isles, and North West Passage'. His profession is given as 'a surgeon in the army in 1612'. This was a substantial amount then, and shows that Woodall was wealthy. In the *Calendar of State Papers* 1553-1616, there are some references to Woodall. On 23 September 1614, as Surgeon-General, he appears to have been ordered to provide 'Surgeons' chests with good drugs'. The same day, Dr John Burgis, 'professing great skill in the cure of the scurvy', was 'admitted gratis' to the Company.

The court minutes for 20 June 1615 note 'Great abuses by Wooddall the surgeon'. This was due to a letter, which had arrived in England on 24 November 1615, aboard the East Indiaman *Hope*. In this letter, dated 20 June 1615, Richard Baker, agent at Saldania, had furiously complained against the inadequacy of the surgeons' chests supplied by Woodall, as well as the inexperience of the surgeons sent aboard. Baker wrote of 'Mr Woodall's great abuses in the chirurgeon's chest, putting divers boxes of one simple, whereas he writeth in superscriptions their diverse; drugs rotten, unguents made of kitchen stuff'. Woodall had sent out 'Boys that have no skill thrust into place of chirurgeons'. Thus Woodall alone was 'to be accounted guilty of so many men as perish through his default'. Like most other complaints of this nature, this one too was soon passed over, for we come across a note on 27 August of the same year, stating 'Payment to Wooddall for supplying the surgeons' chests for the last eight ships'. This is followed by a brief and cryptic statement, 'remarks on his proceedings and the system adopted by the Hollanders'. Dutch doctors were probably better equipped for the East. It does not take much acuity to conclude that Woodall had been lining his pocket by selling inadequate surgical chests and drugs to the Company, even as he was making money by sending out as ships' surgeons youths with insufficient knowledge and little skill. In any case, medical practice at the time was crude, and to this was added the vagaries of tropical ailments. Woodall could not be held directly responsible for high mortality in the Company's trading posts. However, there clearly ensued much criticism since Woodall was compelled to write a textbook on the subject of medical and surgical practice. Woodall continued to be esteemed, for he became Surgeon at St Bartholomew's Hospital in January 1616, and the Court Minutes for 26-27 March 1618 confirm the raise in Woodall's salary to £30 a year, 'for his services as surgeon'.

Nevertheless, Woodall's corruption continued to claim lives in the East. On 15 October 1620, the factors in Jakarta, Edward Meade, John Goninge, William Moore, and Thomas Johnson, complained to the Company about the uselessness of the surgeons in the fleet at Bantam: 'The surgeons' mates in the fleet, and the master surgeon in the Bear, good for nothing; neither understand anything belonging to surgery'. Considering the lives lost to this ineptitude, the factors wrote, 'Woodall wrongs the Company by entertaining insufficient men, never trained up in that faculty, who claim they are bound to give him two thirds of their wages'. This letter was received from a Dutch ship, the *Walkeron*, on 12 June 1621, long before which Woodall's absolute control on the medical matters of the Company had started to loosen. At the meeting of the general Court on 3 July 1619, a motion for the recruitment of 'surgeons of skill provided for the voyage chosen with the approbation of the Surgeons' Hall' was placed but defeated. Woodall's monopoly was eroding. In February 1620, Woodall got into trouble with one Mr Mellyn, whose ill behaviour had previously been noted in the Court minutes. On 4 February, Sir John Wolstenholme had opined on Mellyn's 'seditious and scandalous conduct'. This was followed on 7 February by the complaint of one Mr Wiech 'against Mellyn for scandalous speeches against himself and his son at a General Court'. Two days later Wiech urged the Company to give him redress for 'Mellyn's speeches against himself and his son'. Wolstenholme again stated that he considered Mellyn to be of 'a mutinous disposition, and unworthy to be admitted into any civil company'. Then the minutes enigmatically state that Mellyn had also complained against Woodall. This is still more mysteriously followed by the decision to discover 'Some punishment to be inflicted answerable to the quality of Mellyn's offence'. A minute recorded on 11 February reads 'Woodall's counter charges against Mellyn, referred'. This was followed 3 days later by an enquiry into Mellyn's charges against Woodall, on the same day on which, very interestingly, 'All the surgeons' chests' were 'viewed by the Master and Wardens of the Surgeons and the Master and Wardens of the Apothecaries'. Woodall seemed to be losing ground fast, for this was succeeded on 16 February by the decision that 'The surgeons' chests to be more carefully looked to hereafter'. Woodall and an apothecary were appointed 'to provide the surgery', while Dr Atkins, a physician and 'one of the Company, a very honest and sufficient gentleman and great adventurer', was to look after 'physical things'. Woodall was further ordered to examine 'the chests at Gravesend', where the ships for Surat had gathered. On 18 February 1620 the Company decided that 'Things provided by Woodall for the surgeons' chests' were 'to be shown to Drs Torye and Raven and, if approved, to be sent down to Gravesend. On 10 March the Master and Wardens of the Surgeons' Hall again reported to the Company 'on the state of the surgeons' chests now prepared [by Woodall] for the Indies'. The quarrel between Mellyn and Woodall seems to have been settled, though Mellyn continued to be castigated by the Court for his misbehaviour, his 'arrogance' being noted on 28 March. On 4 April, Mellyn's 'violent and factious behaviour' resulted in his dismissal from the Court. Woodall probably wished to clear himself of the odium of defalcation, since an entry in the Court's minutes for 13 July 1621 reads, 'Woodall the surgeon's account to be audited; his desire to answer any complaints against him in open court'.

On 26 November 1621, the Company decided that several committees were to look after the provisioning of the ships being then readied for Surat at Deptford, Woodbridge, and Blackwall. In the case of medical preparations, the decision was, 'all samples to be bought of one apothecary to be named by the Company'. This decision was passed again the following day, 27 November: 'Drugs and samples to be bought of the apothecary appointed by the Company'. The surgeons' chests provided by Woodall continued to be the subject of discussion at the Court at the end of December 1621, while his selection and appointment of surgeons came up for criticism during 25-26 February 1622, when Edward Charley of the East Indiaman *Blessing* was replaced by Thomas Parkes, a veteran of 5 voyages, and obviously one of Woodall's men. On 27 February Thomas Parkes was examined 'in the presence of Dr Winston and Mr Fenton and others'. He was found 'grossly ignorant and incompetent' and discharged the service. Charley was reappointed to his post. The Court decided that thenceforth all surgeons were to be examined before being engaged, for which purpose Dr Winston offered his free service. Dr Winston soon became Woodall's nemesis. On 17 May 1622 the doctor's said to the Court that 'the last surgeon's chest sent to Surat had a much greater provision than was necessary'. The reason for this is amazing because it represents a state of mind that lasted less than 200 years. By the second decade of the 18th century, western medicine, even though unable to cope with Indian ailments, had become steeped in its isolated sense of superiority. Dr Winston's reason was that 'the Indies hath drugs in far greater plenty and perfection than here'. However, Woodall's fears about being elbowed out were ended by another Court decision the same day: 'Woodall's salary of £30 for the providing of surgeon's chests, on account of his services to be continued until Midsummer'.

Matters appear to have worsened during the year, for on 9 July 1623, the Court was not sympathetic to Woodall when it admitted his petition 'against any other being allowed to provide the chest for the Charles'. The *Charles*, rated at over 900 tonnes, had a successful record of voyages to the East Indies. In 1622 it was being very carefully provisioned for its third journey. She was 'a ship of great charge', and because she would sail alone, her master, Richard Swann, was chosen reluctantly, since the Court 'took distaste to Mr Swann's peremptory demands, yet because they had experience of his honesty and sufficiency, he is to be once more spoken with, and if he shall continue with his resolution the Company will never treat with him again'. As things turned out, Richard Swann sailed the *Charles* on a very successful journey during 1623-26. Since the Court was much concerned about the ship, it worried about her sailors and their health. Hence, following Woodall's petition, the Court resolved on debate that 'a trial medicine chest for 100 men, with the prices, be provided by those that will undertake it'. Woodall's monopoly had ended.

Nevertheless, Woodall continued to wrest the situation to his advantage. He approved the candidature of John Hedlow (or Headly) as 'master surgeon' of the *Charles*. The Court took care to ask 'Doctors Atkins and Winston to make proof of and report on his proficiency'. Woodall had chosen carefully this time, and on 16 July 1623 the Court acknowledged the 'Certificate of Doctors Atkins and Winston that of three surgeons examined by them, John Headly is the most sufficient'. As the time for the *Charles* to sail approached, the issue of the surgeon's chests became the focal point for the control of the Company's considerable medical matters. Woodall had provided chests for the ship, as had Doctors Atkins and Winston. The Court, forced to choose, noted on 5 September that 'Mr Woodall, against whom objections are made', would not be deprived, since 'the Company do not hold it just to displace an old servant before they have heard him'. The matter would be settled with the competing chests being 'viewed by the master and wardens of the apothecaries, the master and wardens of the surgeons, and certain physicians, who are to give their judgements on both chests'. On 10 September, the Court minutes record that 'Doctors Atkins and Winston, having had their surgeon's chest viewed and allowed by the College of Physicians, will not come into contestation by surgeons, as a thing ill becoming their calling'. Since the doctors were members of the College of Physicians, this was their trump card. However the Court disagreed with them and resolved "to view both it and Woodall's". Two days later, the Court issued its notice on this, asking the competing chests to be inspected by 'Drs Mountsford, Mayerme, and Hudson, and the master and warden of the Apothecaries and Surgeons, and such of the surgeons now returned (from the Indies) as can be found'. An interesting digression is that Woodall's medical services to the Company were expensive, as may be seen in the charge for £4 19s 4d for curing 'John Martin, who fell from the main-yard of the *Charles* and broke his leg'. The report on Woodall's surgeon's chest was noted in the Court minutes of 5 December 1623. Probably the report was not satisfactory, since the minutes note nothing to this effect. Instead, the Company took a conciliatory tone for it did not want to be the cause of animosity between surgeons and physicians. Thus the Court ordered 'that Woodall receive £40 by way of imprest for that service [the provision of the chest], and that the committees crave the help of both surgeons and physicians to view the things proper to their several faculties'.

No reconciliation having been effected, the matter of the surgeon's chests came up again for discussion in Court on 3 February 1624. In addition to Atkins and Winston, one Dr Wheatley had also provided a chest for examination, which was viewed alongside Woodall's. To make matters equable, the Court decided to add Sir William Pady and Dr Raven to the board of examiners, of which Atkins and Winston were already members. This board was to examine surgeons seeking employment aboard the Company's ships. However, 'To the motion that surgeons entertained be examined, it was answered that the surgeons of this fleet are all experienced men, who have been in the Indies long, have performed extraordinary cures, and are men approved for their sufficiency in their profession, and such as will scorn to be examined'. One presumes that this answer was made by Woodall, the Surgeon-General, who undoubtedly had a deep personal interest in the matter; the Court agreed, saying that 'such surgeons as come home well approved from the Indies and proceed again shall not be subject to examination', which would apply to 'new unknown' applicants. This too was contrary to Woodall's interests. Suddenly on 9 February the Court took cognisance of Woodall's having 'suppressed' Dr

Atkins' order to the surgeons appointed to the fleet then readying for voyage, to attend him. The Deputy Governor of the Company went on record to note that he had 'spoken with a learned physician, who wondered that physicians should take it upon them to set down surgeons' proportions, the same not being proper to their art, save only for matter of physic'. It was determined 'that in matters of physic they [the Company] consult with physicians, and for matters of surgery the surgeons give satisfaction to the committees'. Just as the Company's merchants and factors in the Indies were engaged in private trade, those like Woodall with access to ships and the possibility of fleecing the Company, used such access to great effect. On 13 October 1624 Woodall was summoned to the Court and charged 'with seeking his own gain by thrusting his servants upon the Company'. Woodall admitted that he had 7 apprentices then in the Indies as surgeon's mates. He had previously had 20 in the Company's service but these were dead. They were 'set out at his great charge' and his profit was 'their two months' pay yearly'. Woodall self-righteously asserted that 'such as live to return prove the ablest for that employment by reason of their practice, as will appear upon examination of skilful surgeons to whom he refers'. Strangely, the Court was satisfied with this explanation despite that fact that the next item for debate on the agenda was a case in Chancery against Woodall by one John Parker and his wife, Barbara, for having detained the goods of Francis Moore, who had died in the Indies. Moore was probably one of Woodall's apprentices, and his belongings were withheld in lieu of his 2 months' pay due to Woodall. The Governor of the Company personally intervened on 15 October in the matter between the Parkers and Woodall, 'with the liking of both parties'. The reason for the Court's satisfaction was an order passed in December 1619, which allowed Woodall to claim 2 months' salary a year from those he appointed.

Woodall was soon involved in a grave problem. Early in 1625 he had a writ issued to Sir Thomas Merry, a member of the King's household, for his failure to repay a debt. Instead Woodall was arrested by order of the Lord Steward and imprisoned. Woodall appealed to the Company to secure his release, which was done. The Court minutes for 28 January 1625 note that the Governor had applied to the Lord Steward for Woodall's release. The Lord Steward had asked 'if no other man could serve the Company's turn but that one', and sought time to consider this request, saying 'how unsufferable a thing it is that the King's servants be served with process in the King's house'. Woodall was released but only for 10 or 12 days, for on 31 January he acknowledged the Company's favour in helping him. The Company wanted him freed so that he could get the surgeon's chests for that year's outward bound spring fleet ready. This was profitable business for Woodall too, as is evidenced by the payment of £100 to him on 7 February. Woodall was imprisoned at the order of the Lord Steward for the second time that month, 'to the hazard of his utter undoing'. A Court minute of 23 February notes that Sir Humphrey Handford urged the Company to once more plead for his release, which was agreed to, provided he used 'his own best means first' to be set free. This imprisonment seemed to have arisen due to the machinations of Woodall's 'private enemies'. He was presumably soon freed. His name thereafter appears occasionally in the minutes, for payments due to him. On 5 January 1627 Woodall petitioned the Company 'for recompense for his many good services in recovering divers of their maimed and hurt servants; the Court having given him no gratuity these three years, deferred until those then in cure were recovered'. He had been in the service of the Company for 15 years. 10 days after this petition, Bartholomew Simonds, appointed surgeon for his 5th voyage on one of the East Indiamen, complained to the Court that he was 'being opposed by Woodall only through malice and some differences of 20 years' standing'. The Court decided the summon Woodall to be warned at its next meeting. On 17 January 1627 Woodall, summoned to Court, charged Simonds 'to his face' with 'drunkenness, insufficiency in his art, and bad and dissolute behaviour, besides having stabbed two men'. Simonds 'not being able to clear himself of all these imputations, he was absolutely dismissed'.

On 9 February 1627 Woodall was castigated by the Court for having omitted to see to the provisioning of lemon juice aboard ships, 'the want of which might endanger the whole fleet'. Woodall was "much blamed 'for not speaking more timely'". Woodall and another surgeon, Ralph Harris of the *Mary*, recommended to the Court on 7 March the stocking of red wine on board ships, since it was "very useful and 'physical' for men sick of the flux". The Company at once ordered the purchase of 3 hogsheads for medical use. Despite this, Woodall had to petition for professional recompense 'that formerly he had been allowed a labourers pay in Blackwall Yard and 2d per month out of every workman's wages there for curing and healing those hurt, which had both been detained these three years past'. He was ordered to be paid £30 'in full recompense of all charges and pains to that day'. Woodall was a conscientious surgeon, as is evidenced by a Court minute of 27 July 1627, whereby Andrew Anderson, who had been hurt in the Company's service, and paid £11 4s as compensation, requested that the amount be given to Woodall instead, since he had spent that amount on Anderson's care. The Company rewarded its faithful Surgeon-General by confirming on 5 October 1627 the order of 1619, which allowed him 'to have two months' pay yearly of all his servants' wages in the Indies'.

Scarcely had the year turned, when Woodall was again ordered to attend Court in January 1628 'to answer a great complaint of Capt Christopher Browne, James Slade and others of the insufficiency of all the surgeons in that fleet'. Nothing further seems to have come of this matter. In any case, the Company was going through hard times, and was dismissing persons in its employ. On 2 May 'The great charge of the Company's servants was taken into serious consideration'. The Governor read out the name of every man on its list of employees: 'in the counting house, the auditors, secretary's office, mariner's office, husband's office, clerks of the spice and indigo warehouses, officers at Blackwall, the surgeon, solicitor, porter, beadle, powder maker, clerk of the powder, and, lastly the Amboyna pensioners'. 4 of these were discharged, while many of the rest, mainly those drawing higher pay, underwent cuts in salary. Woodall's annual pay fell from £30 to £20. The scrimping intensified, probably to Woodall's benefit, for on 25 February 1629, the surgeon travelling out on the *London* reported that the surgeon's chest was 'exceeding good', which made the Court decide that they might 'save the charge they were wont to give to these doctors and surgeons, whose pains they entreated in this behalf, and … resolved to rely on the honesty of Mr Woodall and the Surgeon that hath examined them'. In other words, the Company did not want to pay consultation fees, as it previously had, to other physicians and surgeons to examine the chests. Surgeon's chests provisioned by Woodall had been criticised as insufficient but to the Company saving money was important, ensuring its sailors' health was not. The Company's dependence on Woodall is proved on 13 October 1630 by the additional payment of £100 'over and above' £100 already paid him for providing surgeon's chests.

Woodall was probably not keeping good health when he asked the Court on 10 December 1630 that the Company grant him a weekly allowance of 8 shillings to appoint a surgeon 'to live at Blackwall and give attendance in the yard and ships'. He also petitioned 'for some satisfaction for almost three years during which he has cured many hurt in their service'. 5 days later the Court ordered 'Gratuity of £20 to Mr Woodall, surgeon, for 2 ½ years' extraordinary service in curing divers of the Company's servants hurt aboard ship or in the yard, and for boat hire, etc'. On 19 January 1631, Sheriff Abdy complained to the Court that 'contrary to their orders and custom Mr Woodall, their surgeon, had sent away the surgeons chests for the Mary, Exchange, and Speedwell without being viewed'. Woodall's excuse was that he was short of time, and 'that he would be more careful hereafter'. Nonetheless, Woodall's influence was waning. On 12 December 1632 the Court 'utterly' deemed as 'superfluous' his recommendation 'for an increase of stores for surgery to be sent on shore as well as to the southwards as northwards'. Woodall reported to the Court on 26 April 1633 that the saltpetre refiners were falling ill 'occasioned by their coming fasting in a morning to their work'. He urged the Court to 'allow them some hot caudles to eat before they fell to their work, to keep out the steam and smoke, which otherwise will get into their stomachs and in a short time kill them, their bodies being already sunk and much impaired'. The Court directed Woodall to see to the preparation of such breakfasts for these workers as would restore their health and 'prevent their sickness for a month or two' while the Company decided whether it was worth the cost to have saltpetre refined or to sell it unrefined.

The increasing trade activities of the Company alongside high mortality in the factories increased the demand for surgeons. On 20 November 1633 the Court ordered, 'on information of the great want of Chirurgeons and Chirurgery to the southwards, that Woodall send an experienced man to Bantam and another to Jambi, and make ready two sets of Chirurgery ware besides the ship's provisions, taking care they be wholesome and orderly packed'. 2 months later, the Court reversed this decision, noting that Surat and Persia 'afford many provisions in this kind', while the southern ports, when given additional supplies, 'they were lavishly spent and given away, more upon natives than their own servants'. On 4 February 1635 the Court turned around once more and noted the want of surgeons in Surat and Persia, and directed Woodall 'to prepare two small chests of all kinds of chirurgery beyond the proportion usually sent, to be brought to the East India House by the 10th of March', and also to appoint 2 experienced surgeons besides the ship's, for service at those places.

Woodall again petitioned the Court for a gratuity in December 1633, 'showing that it is near three years since he received any gratuity for healing their servants, since which time he hath cured above 50 persons, many of great diseases, as broken legs and arms, broken sculls [*sic*], bones out of joint, and other great wounds and bruises, and disbursed money for their diets, paid women to attend them and otherwise put to charge by water and land and carrying them to hospitals and curing them there'. The Court immediately ordered 'the Company's Chirurgeon' paid £30, 'which he thankfully accepted'. Even though he continued to be paid for his services directly, Woodall was struck off the Company's list of salaried employees as part of a cost-cutting measure in December 1635. On 8 May

1640 Woodall appealed to the Court for his wages, "representing that he has cured above fifty people since then and written 'a booke of chirurgery for the good of the East India voyage'". The Court awarded his £60 as settlement of his demands. Woodall continued to exercise considerable influence in the appointment of surgeons in the Company's service, as is proved by a Court minute of 7 January 1642: "John Sleeman is entertained as surgeon in the *Blessing*, but Nicholas Welch, who had been chosen as surgeon's mate on that ship, is discharged, Mr Woodall having reported him to be 'a meere barbor'". By this time Woodall was being paid £250 for providing surgeons' chests to the Company's ships. Nonetheless Woodall was not above providing substandard drugs for the Company's ships. On 9 November 1642, Woodall was called into the Court and asked whether "he did not 'new boyle the salves againe' and so make the Company pay for them twice". Woodall had previously been permitted to buy back the old chirurgery chests at cost price, whose contents he recycled when asked to provide chests for outward bound vessels. Complaints against this must have arisen, following which the Court had refused to resell the chests to him. Woodall denied that he reused the surgeon's chests 'on his reputacion' but contradicted himself and confessed that he had used them at "Christ's [St Bartholomew's?] Hospital 'for the cureing of poor people'". He was forgiven, and allowed to buy the old chests back again.

By this time John Woodall had had a long and extraordinary career, having served the Company for over 30 years. On 16 May 1643, Woodall submitted to the Court that he was 'very sick and weak and unable to serve the Company any more'. In his place, undoubtedly on his recommendation, his nephew, Henry Boone was appointed, though not as Surgeon-General but the Company's surgeon. However, this was not the end of the Company's dealings with Woodall. On 23 June 1643, the Court of committees heard an appeal from him, "for something towards 'the repayre of his languishing necessities and his better support' as he was old and bed-ridden and his grown-up children 'lying very heavy upon him' which with his many losses and misfortunes" compelled him to seek the Company's favour. The Court rejected this appeal, 'some of the Committees having inquired and found that he is not in need and has a sufficient estate'. Richard Smyth's *Obituary* notes that 'Old Mr Woodhall [*sic*], ye surgeon, died' on 28 August 1643.

Woodall's book, *The Surgeon's Mate*, was published in 1617. The subtitle of this book explains its purpose, which was to provide the lonely ship's or factory doctor with the necessary guidance: *A Treatise Discovering Faithfully and Plainly the due contents of the Surgeon's*

Chest, and the Uses of the Instrument, the virtues and operations of the Medicines, the cures of the most frequent diseases at Sea. Alongside discussions on the uses of sal volatile, sulphur, and mercury, this book focused on the treatment of wounds, ulcers, fistulae, fractures, dislocations, amputation, fluxes of the belly, and scurvy. Woodall had been made Surgeon General at the behest of Sir Thomas Smith (1558-1625). Sir Thomas was the first governor of the East India Company, although he held this office very briefly in 1600, and then continuously, with only a year's break, between 1603 and 1621. Hence, Woodall dedicated his book to Sir Thomas, 'The far renowned, virtuous and worthy Knight … my singular good Patron'. As Ulysses had been shielded by Ajax, so Woodall sought to be protected from the 'envy of malicious detractors' by Sir Thomas. Fawning upon his patron, Woodall wrote that his book was inspired by Sir Thomas' 'especial providence and great care for the health and preservation of such as have been or hereafter may be, employed' by the East India Company. To this end, Woodall was only discharging his duty, to which he had been appointed, and granted an annual stipend, in writing this book. His own experience had been that the Company employed many young surgeons, who due to youth and lack of practice had 'not attained to that perfection of knowledge, that were requisite' for long journeys and alien lands. Woodall's book was intended for the 'weaker sort of such Surgeons'. In his preface to the reader, Woodall writes, 'I held it a charitable work, however the world taketh it, to instruct such young men as were employed to the East Indies the best I could'. Hitherto he had provided instructions in writing to every ship, 'and being wearied with writing for every ship the same instructions anew, I held it my best course to put these in print'. The plea to Sir Thomas for protection from detractors is clarified when Woodall states that 'Some have already accused me to have lost time in writing of the cures of diverse diseases, far better written of by others, which I cannot deny, yet say if each Surgeon's mate had a library, and inducement to use it, my labour I confess were idle'.

Woodall begins his treatise with a dissertation upon the duties of the surgeon's mate. The first duty is unto God, and the second to the assistance and service of the chief surgeon, whose assistant the mate is. The first error of many surgeons is to neglect the first, as a result of which they are soon given to 'boasting and brave phrases, censuring others in many things, but not feeling their own wretchedness at all'. Many are so 'given and dedicated to the pot and Tobacco-pipe … that thereby they become in themselves base'.

He then proceeds to a list of the contents of the surgeon's and his mate's chests, which are strange to the modern reader. The surgical instruments are listed and diagrammatically presented. They look barbarous. For this reason Woodall advises the surgeon 'to be very careful to hide his sharp instruments ever as much as is possible from the sight of the Patient, for many reasons too long to recite here'. Surgical knives were to be clean, 'sharp, and fitly ground, and not too thin-edged'. As a surgeon with much experience, Woodall counsels young surgeons to 'be practising often with the worst of his knives and Lancets, till he be able to make them serviceable'. Other necessities include 'the dismembering Saw', a 'great and terrible instrument only ordained for amputation or dismembering'. Another unique instrument was the *speculum ani*, 'belonging only to the *ano* or the fundament, to open the same as occasion shall be offered'. The use of the instrument would be clear to the surgeon, though Woodall cautioned against using it unless really necessary: 'For if … without it he can cure the Patient, it is much better to do so, and much easier to the Patient than to use the instrument'. The reason was that patients did not often have the power of 'giving way to the safe use of this instrument'. Forcing the instrument would cause bruised muscles, which would only worsen the patient's condition.

Other horrors in the surgeon's chest include the cauterising irons, which 'The ancient Chirurgeons of former ages used far more than these in our times'. Though very useful, they were no longer popular 'by reason the terror thereof to the patient' being great. Besides cauterising 'any vein or Artery in strong fluxes of blood which otherwise cannot be stayed', these were handy in dealing with epilepsy, the 'falling sickness', apoplexy, and 'Lethargie', 'And surely they are far better in my judgement for the good of the patient in many Apostumes than the Lancet'. Yet even Woodall would fain use them to open apostumes or abscesses because of the fear they put into patients. This notwithstanding, Woodall recommended the inclusion of 'divers sorts of them' in the surgeon's chest, if money allowed it.

The next set of instruments read more like a plumber's list than a surgeon's, consisting of 'Stork's Bill, Ravens Bill, Crows Bill, Goose Bill, and the Terebellum'. These were valuable in helping the surgeon 'to draw out bullets, arrow heads, broken bones, or whatsoever else unnatural things are gotten into any part of man[s] body'. To the lonely surgeon dealing with an emergency on ship or shore, Woodall imparts practical advice. Should a bone or bullet be 'merely loose, it is best to take it out the first dressing; if it be loose at one end only, and fast at the other, except thou without flux of blood or danger of the member canst remove it, forbear and give nature leave to do her office, and have patience'. Should the young surgeon continue to have doubts either about the use of these instruments, the surgical method, or the prognosis, more sage advice followed: 'since experience and reason maketh an Art, if thou have reason be careful to ask counsel both of God and man, that thou mayst answer both here and in the world to come, for the subject of thy Art is the most precious of God's creatures'.

Woodall also warned the surgeon against instruments that had no practical use, like the 'Incision Shears'. These were there because some things were to be had 'for form and order's sake'. These shears 'are generally desired, but scarce once in a man's life worth usage'. The shears were applied for enlarging incisions or wounds, for which Woodall recommended the incision knife. Having named this fearsome surgical tool Woodall stated that he would apply no 'persuasive words to urge the use of it'. By contrast, the Probe, which is next on Woodall's list, is presented as a tool that can 'in no way be forborne in the Surgeon's chest, for no chirurgical work is well and artificially effected without some occasion of the use thereof'. While the probes were very useful in cleaning wounds using lint dipped in oil, lotion, or liquor, inexperienced, 'unconscionable or ignorant' surgeons needed to beware of doing their patients great harm by 'forcing too far the Probe, thereby to make the grief appear deeper'. Some surgeons 'are so wise in their own conceits' that they use 'the longer sort of probes with eyes like needles' to draw a linen cloth through a wound and leave it there as a dressing, which Woodall disliked, 'for I know in all wounds nature striveth to make unison of the parts divided, for who so keepeth asunder the parts by such courses it shall repent him, except he be graceless'. He had dealt with wounds that had pierced the entire body or limb by being content 'with putting to each orifice a short and easy tent, which I commonly make from *emplastrum stipticum Paracelsi*, or some other good plaster spread on a cloth and rolled gently tent wise, and so applied dipped in balm, the tent being but of half an inch or an inch long at the most'.

Spatulas or 'splatters' come next, being 'the most needful instrument to spread unguent, and emplasters withal, and also to stir about, and the better to compound, any medicine on the fire'. The first of this species of surgical instruments was the '*Spatula mundani*', devised by Woodall himself: 'to serve upon any occasion of extreme continence, which often happeneth to seamen, so that no purging medicine, neither upward nor downward, administered or taken will work'. In such cases that fearful instrument, the speculum ani was used to open the fundament, and the hard excrements drawn out using the spoon end of Woodall's spatula.

'This disease killeth many', he wrote, 'this grief cometh now and then to men which have the scurvy'. Extreme pain and discomfort, followed by 'hard excrement after which followeth a most extreme and painful flux of blood', killing most. Woodall's instrument had the advantage in that it could be used without the speculum. The spatula would be 'anointed, greased, and first warmed a little', and used effectively, 'that the party being in time diligently attended (by God his mercy) may have comfort and remedy for once'.

The surgeon's work included dentistry, and as dental problems could easily turn life-threatening at sea, the surgeon's chest needed to have adequate implements. These included 'Pacis, Pullicans, Punches or Forcers, Crow's Bill, Stems, Grazers and files for teeth'. These 'cannot be well forborne for the drawing of teeth, as also for the cleansing of the teeth and gums, and the letting of the gums blood are often o small things for keeping men in health'. Often the lack of instruments resulted in either an apostume 'under a rotten or hollow tooth for want of drawing of the same', or 'by undiscreet drawing of a tooth either the jaw is broken or some other bad accident is provoked'. Hence, Woodall wrote, 'I hold none worthy to go for a Surgeons Mate to sea, who is ignorant of tooth-drawing; and I esteem him an unworthy Surgeon, how high so ever he bears his head, that can draw a tooth well, but will upon need at sea scorn or deny to do it'. Describing briefly the use of each instrument, Woodall provides some general directions for properly drawing teeth: 'Wherefore for one general rule ere you draw a tooth, forget not to thrust down your instrument as low as you can possibly towards the root of the tooth, and that you grip it steady and fast, that as you seem somewhat to wrench your hand, that you may more intend to pluck the tooth upward according to the situation of the tooth, for saving the jaw'. Another cardinal rule to prevent dislocated jaws was that at the same time 'you must with your other hand take hold and stay the jaw'. 'Be not too sudden or rash in raising or drawing the tooth', he warned, for he himself had suffered the pain of ill-drawn teeth 'in my own head twice'. The surgeon had 'pinched off the heads of two of my own teeth, and left the roots behind, which maketh me the more commiserate others in that behalf'. The wound could be cleaned using vinegar and liquors but again Woodall shared his experience, 'but vinegar I utterly mislike: I never use other thing but salt betwixt my fingers thrust into the place where the tooth stood, and then with my fingers close again the gum easily together'.

For minor emergencies like a particle in the eye, or in the ear, Woodall recommended the bundle of small instruments of German make, which contained 'at the least 20 small instruments of strange form'.

The Glister Syringe was a special device meant for ailments 'not only in the East Indies, but also all hot countries'. In these places there were 'two principal and capital evils which chiefly hasten the ends of many of our loving Countrymen at sea', the 'first and principal' being 'an extreme looseness and weakness of the stomach, and internals causing a flux of the belly', and the other its opposite, 'extreme continence'. Given the importance of the syringe for successful treatment in these cases, the surgeon was urged to care for it, 'that when you have used it you wipe it clean, and hang it up in your Cabin in two parts being drawn out, namely the staff and the barrel, each by itself, for if it be kept close it will be musty and the tow rotten'. The surgeon in the tropics would do as well to have 'in readiness a crooked neck much like an elbow, belonging to the same instrument, that how crooked so ever the patient may lie, the medicine may be administered to him'. If the surgeon himself fell ill, this crooked neck could be used, for it allowed 'any man to give himself a Glister very easily without the help of another'. The entire method of administration was highly uncomfortable, and irrespective of what Woodall had to say, demanded considerable expertise on the part of the surgeon and the cooperation of the patient. After anointing 'the head of it with some fat substance', the syringe having been filled with the necessary glister, was thrust up 'to the head … laying the firing in an even position if it may be', and emptied 'till all be in the gut'. After this the patient was to 'turn himself on his back, forcing himself by all possible means to retain the medicine given him for one hour if he can'. Other subtle tricks, like the use of a thin oily cloth in the syringe, were explained to the surgeon, if the hardness of excrement or its clammy nature prevented satisfactory administration. In cases of extreme resistance to the insertion of the syringe, the surgeon was to apply first the *speculum mundani* to clear the passage. Often the patient was too ill and weak to cooperate, and in such cases Woodall admonished the surgeon to use a cloth or some such material to hold it in. To those who were 'fine fingered, squeamish, or disdainful', Woodall told the surgeon to be 'full of humanity and Christian commiseration', and 'consider your brother by yourself'. The technique could only be mastered through experience, and so 'the young practitioner must as I have done before him, either by reading, inquiring, or practicing, find it out, and if he know more than myself, thank God for it, and let him impart some to others, and not scorn for this'.

Unlike the Glister Syringe, the 'small syringe' was mostly used for the cure of gonorrhoea. Thus Woodall asks, 'for what Barber's boy is not practiced in the use of the small syringe?' The surgeon needed to care for this syringe as well, 'let it be clean; that it be smooth at the end … that it go not by jumps nor too stiff, and that you carry a steady and even hand in delivering it'. This injection too was embarrassing and uncomfortable, requiring greater skill that the Glister Syringe for administration, and proportionately greater assistance from the patient. The aim was to send the medicine up the urethra to the bladder, ensuring that it went to the bladder. The surgeon was told to 'assure thyself the water will never come at the neck of the bladder, nor further than the pipe is put in; whereas often the defect is in the neck of the bladder, and thy medicine commeth not there'. The medicine was to be neither too hot, nor cold, but at the right temperature, 'so hot as piss is the true temper'. Considering the time he was writing, one is surprised to find Woodall cautioning against the use of '*Mercurial lotions*, I mean any which have *Mercury Sublimate Precipitate*'. Though they were effective against gonorrhoea, 'they are upon my knowledge and experience dangerous, used by way of injection into the yard, for they will utterly alter and overthrow the natural faculty of the yard … and so calcine the same that it will become impotent to his natural work'.

The next important implement listed is the lancet, which was essential for the vital task of venesection or bloodletting. Since venesection was an important, almost inevitable, part of treatment, Woodall wrote, 'First therefore methinks it is not amiss to advise him [the surgeon's mate], that he carry with him at least six of the best sort, besides six more common ones, for an East Indie voyage'. These were to be carefully tended, oiled or anointed with axungia [soft animal or bird fat], and wrapped in 'oily clothes'. The surgeon's mate must also take along a band to tie the arm, one of 'worsted gartering' being the best, for wool and linen ones would slip. Bloodletting could kill if too much was drawn, so the phlebotomist should always remember that 'in the blood consisteth the life of man'. At sea 'fresh food of good nourishment' not being available, 'it is good to be sparing in the quantity of blood to be taken away'. Should the surgeon diagnose 'idleness in the head' due to 'distemper of the blood' at sea, Woodall advised the use of 'cooling broths' rather than bloodletting. For cases wherein bloodletting was inevitable, Woodall informed the surgeon and his assistant that 'The veins commonly opened, are six in number … one in the forehead, one under the tongue, three in the arm, and one in the foot'.

During his second journey to the East, Tavernier travelled as far as Golconda. On 2 October 1640 he reached the home of a Dutch surgeon, Peter de Lan, 4 leagues from the city of Golconda, having already noted that there were hardly any physicians in the principalities of Golconda and Bijapur, save those attending princes and other rich persons, to look to the ailments of the common people. This Dutch surgeon had been posted there 'at the King's earnest entreaty'. The Nawab suffered from constant headache, and though the physicians had decided that 'he should be let blood in four places under the tongue', none dared undertake this task because they had no practical surgical experience. In addition, should something go awry, their lives would be at stake. So Peter de Lan, being then present, was asked if he could blood the Nawab, and he answered, so Tavernier relates, that 'there was nothing so easy in Chirurgery'. This confident answer decided the Nawab, who sent for de Lan and told him to proceed, with the proviso that 'he should take a care of not drawing away above eight ounces'. The next day de Lan went to durbar, where he was received by some old women and eunuchs, led to a bath, washed, 'especially his hands', rubbed down with 'Aromatick-drugs', and dressed in a robe in the 'fashion of the Country'. Then he was taken to the Nawab's chamber, where his personal physicians waited with 'four little Porringers of Gold', which they had already weighed. Peter de Lan completed his work, and when the blood drawn was weighed, it was 'but bare eight ounces'. The Nawab was pleased and he gave the surgeon 300 pagodas. Following this success, the 'Young-Queen and the Queen-Mother' both 'resolved to be let-blood too'. This de Lan again did well, though differently. The ladies stretched their arms through curtains, and were bled. De Lan's rewards were 50 pagodas from the queen and 30 from the queen-mother. While the Nawab's physicians used gold porringers to measure the amount of blood drawn from his highness, Woodall's surgeon made do with porringers made of ordinary metal, which would hold 3 ounces each.

Considering that William Harvey was the physician in charge of St Bartholomew's Hospital, and so Woodall's colleague, one is surprised to come across Woodall's dictum to the surgeon that if a patient was being bled to relieve the liver, any vein would do, 'for thou must know that all veins have their original in the liver'. Bloodletting would continue to dominate medical and surgical practice for 200 years more. In the first volume of the *Cyclopaedia of Practical Medicine* (1833), bloodletting is presented as 'of all our remedies, the most powerful'. By 1833 the art of venesection had been refined into 'general' and 'local' bloodletting. The former involved the use of the lancet, while the latter depended on the use of leeches and cupping glasses. Some of the most important contents of the surgeon's chest were the cupping glasses. These, Woodall said, could be used to cure pains, aches, lethargy, and 'divers more griefs'. There were 3 types of cups, depending on size. The largest were 'fittest on the thighs, the lesser on the arms, and the least for the hands or feet'. Still smaller cups were applied, so the *Cyclopaedia* tells us, to the 'nape of the neck, behind the ears, to the temples'. The aim of cupping was to draw away the humours, particularly blood and choler. Woodall described the process of cupping for the young surgeon. One cannot think of a more painful procedure for the patient. Interestingly, in the *Cyclopaedia*, cupping was considered 'a more efficient remedy than leeching'. Woodall's method begins with the selection of the place on the patient's body for cupping. The spot would be wetted, and rubbed well with a sponge dipped in hot water. Next, Woodall placed 'a great candle' close to the spot. The cupping glass, also wet, would be briefly heated in the flame, and clapped 'quickly on the place whilst yet the steam of the light is in it'. The surgeon would wait until he saw that the cup had 'drawn well, which by the blackness and rising of the skin you may easily see'. The agony of patient can only be barely imagined. After this the surgeon could remove the cup, scarify the blistered place, and reapply the cup, forcing the blood to flow, 'drawing as much blood as you see good, and when no more blood will come … which is known by a yellow water which cometh at the last'. The place was then to be cleansed with 'fair water', and dried with a sponge or cloth. The place was to be anointed with *unguentum album* only once. This unguent was made of olive oil, white wax, and spermaceti. Woodall warned the surgeon against scarifying too deep.

The issue of venesection was a serious one, since drawing too much blood from a morbid patient meant the sufferer's death. Hence, Woodall urged the surgeon to use the 3-ounce porringers rather than the brass basin, to measure the amount of blood drawn, 'except he be of good judgement indeed'. Woodall's own practice was to draw at most 2 ½ porringers from a patient who came to him either of his own accord or on a physician's advice, to be bled. 'I will rather offend in too little, than in too much taking of blood away'. A strong body, with enough nourishment afterwards, would soon make good up to '7 or 8 ounces … without harm' but 'if you grow to ten ounces, you may [in] many ways do harm in the body, except your warrant be good'.

Woodall's dry humour appears in his dismissal of the brass basin. This was included in the surgeon's chest. Woodall declared, 'I have nothing to write concerning it, but that at least the Surgeon's Mate have one if not two, and if he find no use for it let him sell it for good liquor at *Bantam* as a Surgeon's Mate lately did one of mine'. Similarly, while discussing the 'Diet Pot' Woodall digresses into the recipe for a cooling drink for a patient afflicted with 'an unnatural hot fever at Sea'. This was to be made of 3 ounces of French barley, easily substituted by ordinary barley or wheat flour, 2 gallons of fresh water, 1 ounce liquorice (or ½ ounce of liquorice juice), and a dozen cloves. This was to be boiled down to 4 or 5 quarts, cleared, and stored in an earthen or glass vessel. If the fever should have robbed the patient of taste, the concoction could be flavoured by adding oil or spirit of vitriol 'as will a little change the taste sourish, but not too tart in any wise'. The taste could be bettered by adding 1 spoonful each of rose water, rose vinegar, wine vinegar, and cinnamon water. 4 ounces of the syrup or juice of lemon could be added too. If the surgeon should have prescribed this drink to one 'which is loose in his belly', a common disorder in the East, Woodall recommended the addition of *succus acatiae*, the juice of acacia. William Lewis notes in his work, *The New Dispensatory* (1753), that gums and mucilage, like the juice of acacia, were used in cases 'where the natural mucus of the intestine is abraded'. Woodall however calls it a 'foreign medicine', which 'doth refrigerate, bind, and repel; it stayeth all fluxes of the belly, healeth excoriations of the entrails, strengtheneth much the stomach'.

Discussions on the loose belly lead to those on the 'close-stool'. Woodall writes that he knows beforehand he will undergo many 'witty and eloquent' jabs from 'young gallants of my own profession' for mentioning so 'base' an object as the close-stool as essential to the surgeon. Nonetheless, on this subject 'neither can my book blush, neither myself I hope shall have cause'. This is because he did not hesitate to recommend at least one of these toilets aboard each ship going to the East Indies 'by reason of the bloody or other fluxes, being so dangerous diseases, and so deadly amongst our men'. The 'poor weak man in his extremities' was not to be expected 'continually to go to the shrouds or beakhead to ease himself, nor be noisome to his fellows, but might through the help of his Mate find comfort in his most pitiful distress'. The surgeon was warned, in God's name, not to be 'fine-fingered, slothful, or scornful' in dealing with this 'fearful disease', the flux.

One way in which the close-stool could be used was by placing a hot brick in the pail, 'which hot brick with wine and vinegar or any other like fitting medicine of experience may be sprinkled to comfort the part aggrieved withal'. This treatment, accompanied by rest, supplemented by the use of three or four grains of laudanum and a 'good regiment of diet', could cure this otherwise fatal illness.

Though Woodall does not refer to Harvey while discussing veins and bloodletting, he does so later on, while discussing the 'newly found' purgative from the East Indies, *Cambogiae or Guttigambe*. This is the fruit of the plant *Garcinia gummi-gata*, or *Garcinia cambogia*, also known as the 'Malabar tamarind', which is rich in citric acid and is also believed to have antibacterial properties. Woodall says that this medicine 'is already in use by diverse reverend Physicians, among which Doctor Harvy [*sic*] useth it in St Bartholomew's Hospital, and calleth it *Crocus purgans*'. Woodall recommended this medicine, on the basis that it 'purgeth well the head', was 'good to open obstructions', worked well against 'the yellow Jaundice', and also 'openeth well' the spleen and liver. While Harvey administered this drug in pills, Woodall 'mixed it with pills for the head', the dose being 12 grains. Woodall obviously differed with Harvey, since this new drug was obviously very different from the original '*Crocus* or Saffron', which was 'good for the brain, quickeneth the senses, cheereth the heart, causeth digestion, helpeth the diseases of the breast, lung, and liver, it mollifieth all hardness, and ripeneth all tumours'.

After a reasonably comprehensive survey of the pharmacopeia available to the surgeon, Woodall moves on to common medical emergencies and their treatment. For surgeons aboard ships and ashore in foreign lands, the commonest emergency is the wound. Woodall defines this as 'a recent solution of continuity; or a division which was knit together without putrefaction; and common as well to the soft and organic parts as to the harder'. The cause for a wound could be 'internal … as the malice of bad humours' or, more commonly, from an external cause, 'by the violence of some instrument'. The means of curing wounds were 2, by nature, in which case the surgeon was saved from labour, and by medicine. In the latter case, the surgeon had to remember that 'The first intention in curing of wounds is to take away whatsoever is besides nature, as iron, wood, lead, or aught else with fit instruments, and that without pain, if it may be, to the diseased, that consolidation may be the better affected'. This was to be accompanied by 'The universal regiment', which 'consisteth in purging medicines, as potions, glisters, a sober and frugal diet, abstinence from wine, venery, and all kinds of meats which may move or attenuate humours, and moderate use of good, nourishing sustenance, all which helps the poor Seaman is not capable of in long voyages'.

The wound may be accompanied by palpitation, swooning, convulsions, and fever. The last is 'a heat in the heart more than natural, infused and dispersed through the whole body, whose cure is by purging, bleeding, and good government'. Convulsions were symptoms of 'a dangerous disease of the brain', and were often 'a forerunner or messenger of death'. Alongside wounds and injuries of various kinds, including burns, Woodall informs the surgeon how to deal with other emergencies such as animal bites, fractures, dislocations, and, most importantly, amputations. 'Amputation or dismembering is the most lamentable part of chirurgery', Woodall confesses in his book. It therefore behove the surgeon 'never to use dismembering at all if it were possible for him to heal all he undertook'. Since such drastic surgery was then accompanied by certain death, Woodall's advice to the surgeon was to preserve his honour: 'If you be constrained to use your Saw, let first your Patient be well informed of the imminent danger of death by the use whereof; proscribe him no certainty of life, and let the work be done with his own free will, and request'. The patient was to 'prepare his soul as a ready sacrifice to the Lord by earnest prayers, craving mercy and help unfeignedly'. The surgeon too was to pray, 'For it is no small presumption to Dismember the Image of God'.

The other illnesses addressed by Woodall include scurvy, and 'Fluxes of the belly'. Both were ailments common to the long sea voyages to the East Indies. The types of flux included lientery, diarrhoea, and dysentery. The first, lientery, 'either passeth the sustenance taken, wholly undigested, and that without any blood at all, and without great pain, or as it were, half-digested', due to the 'imbecility and weakness of the stomach' caused by the weakening of the 'virtue retentive'. It also occurs when 'the stomach reserving apostumation is wholly weakened, and cold and broken, or sometimes by crude humidities is oppressed, and must be strengthened, both inwardly and outwardly, by things that corroborate and warm the same'. The cure involved administering emetics, and keeping the patient from food. Laudanum was advised to give the patient adequate rest. Diarrhoea, on the other hand, 'is a Flux of the belly which is either merely waterish, or with humours and with slime mixed'. The surgeon was advised to do nothing to stop it if he saw that the patient was strong, 'for that it is many times a benefit of Nature, whereby she avoideth the superfluous, or venomous, or otherwise vicious and offensive humours'. Later Woodall provides the rule that 'No flux of the belly before the fourth day of the patient be strong, is to be restrained'. Medical intervention became necessary only if diarrhoea persisted over several days and weakened the patient. The surgeon was then to administer powdered rhubarb in an infusion of wine or fresh water, along with 3 or 4 grains of laudanum. If fever accompanied diarrhoea, the laudanum was to be given first.

Other precautions included warm covering for the patient, the aim of treatment being to 'refrain and resist as much as is possible the motions', 'not to strain or force the body being at stool', 'not to sit long' there, and to rest. While diarrhoea was speedily cured in Europe, 'in the Indies it is very hardly cured' due to 'the great wilfulness and disorder of the Patient' and the ignorance of the surgeon. Dysentery too occurred mainly in the hot countries, and was seen among soldiers and seamen, 'chiefly when after short and hard allowances, they shall happen on the sudden to get a great store of raw fruit, fresh meat, flesh or fish or any other great change of pleasant diet'. Dysentery was a major cause of death among soldiers and sailors, as well as those of the Company's service then living in Bantam. Depending on an entirely ineffective pharmacopoeia, Woodall recommended most emphatically doses of laudanum, which 'exceedeth all other medicines in fluxes, for that assuageth all pains and causeth quiet sleep, which often even alone is the true perfection of the cure'. To help the sick recover, the surgeon should give a diet 'that may warm and comfort the stomach' such as the 'Brothe of Chickings'. Should all attempts fail, and the disease show itself 'to proceed from any contagiousness of the air', then both surgeon and patient should cast their lot into God's hands, 'when therefore the air that we are forced to receive in our bodies shall threaten us'. Woodall suspected, as many who saw dysentery at work, that 'the breath and excrements of the sick man may easily infect a sick man', the cause for this being the 'infectious vapours' from 'putrefied and diseased bowels', that 'ascend and descend'. Coming from so experienced a surgeon, younger surgeons may be scared to visit the sick for fear of contracting dysentery. Woodall declared for all such to 'take that rule from me, in the fear of God, I hold no disease infectious to me, in that I have a lawful calling, and I am therefore bound to visit the diseased, which who so neglecteth, God will find him out with that disease or a worse'. Woodall had other tips for the inexperienced surgeon, such as the place of pain in flux: 'The higher towards the stomach the disease hath its beginning the more dangerous it may be adjudged'. This was because 'If this disease proceed from a former great obstruction of the Liver, of the Lungs, or the Spleen, there is small hope of life to be had'. Death was also imminent if the flux was accompanied by hiccups, vomiting, and convulsions. Another sign of approaching death was a 'black or bluish spot … behind the left ear of the sick'. Nonetheless the most important aspect of treating the flux, as in all other treatment, was the surgeon's judgement, 'first let him have good consideration, whether it be convenient to use any such medicine, or no, for where easier remedies will cure never attempt greater'. This, Woodall said, was not for 'grave Artists' but written out 'of love only to children in Art'.

The flux was a dreaded ailment, sometimes spreading fast among a ship's crew or a factory garrison. Woodall provided the young surgeon with the symptoms of flux: 'Pain and torture of the intestines, or ventricles'. This pain would be 'above or below the navel', the former making the patient bring forth 'A painful slow expulsion of the excrements of the belly, with small fragments bloody and fatty', which should inform the surgeon that the higher intestines were involved, while the latter would bring 'much fatness with fragments', which would be 'more gross and less mingled with the excrements'. In all cases, flux of the belly accompanied by 'weakness of the appetite, inconsistence of the mind, heaviness in sleep, imbecility of the legs, a hoarse and barking voice, a weak pulse, beating often, pains over the whole body, chiefly about the belly, blackness of the face, … and coldness in all extreme parts' foretold death.

Moving on to the qualities and kinds of salt, Woodall includes a poem in praise of salt for the young surgeon, followed by one in praise of sulphur, another of quicksilver or mercury, The fount of poetry having begun spouting, Woodall follows it all up with 'Certain Chemical Verses, or Goodwill to Young Artists from the Author': 'Some verses plain at vacant times / I framed and laid aside: / Intending youths which leisure have / Might view what I have tried'. This poem runs through pages until one comes to interesting stanzas like this one: 'A noise domestic shrill I hear / And I dare stay no longer: / Good friends adieu till further time / I must obey the stronger'. Woodall indeed stayed no longer, for he wound up his book in rather an abrupt and unprofessional manner by listing the alchemical terms he had listed in his poem.

Woodall's book represents the beginning of western medicine's tryst with the East Indies. Had Woodall himself completed a voyage or two, his book would have been enriched by direct experience. As it was, Woodall wrote through his own understanding of how medicine was to be adapted to the East. Other than the information that ailments contracted in the East were worsened by the hot climate, neither he nor his contemporaries had anything more to offer the young ship's surgeon. The basics of medicine would remain the same for 200 years to come, including the use of purgatives, emetics, and opiates, phlebotomy, and barbarous surgery with very high mortality. Woodall hardly discusses fevers, which will feature prominently in later texts. The reason for this seems to be his own limited experience, and general ignorance of the physician's work. The ship's surgeon was meant to attend to emergencies, medical and dental, but not to follow prolonged illnesses through to their resolution. Hence Woodall and his apprentices were more concerned with gunshot wounds, injuries, amputations, scurvy, tooth-drawing, and fluxes. Woodall himself gained knowledge through practice, and though he was Surgeon at St Bartholomew's, he claimed no degrees unlike his physician colleague, William Harvey. Harvey not only held a baccalaureate degree from Caius College, Cambridge, but also was an MD of the University of Padua. Soon after Woodall's appointment as Surgeon-General to the East India Company, Harvey became Physician Extraordinary to King James. In 1602 Harvey was awarded an MD by the University of Cambridge, and in

1607 was made a Fellow of the College of Physicians. He later became Physician-in-Ordinary to King Charles I. Woodall never moved in such exalted society. Nonetheless, while Harvey lectured and wrote his classic work on the circulation of blood, Woodall appointed surgeons to ships and provisioned them with surgeon's chests that would commence English medical interaction with India, and particularly Bengal. To help them deal with emergencies he wrote a textbook of practical medicine, which started a theoretical interaction that would continue for the next 300 years.

CHAPTER TWO

MEDICINE AND THE ARRIVAL AND SETTLEMENT OF THE ENGLISH IN BENGAL

The first European settlers in Bengal seem to have been Portuguese, who joined the service of local princes by offering their maritime expertise. They usefulness was soon evident and their employers rewarded them with high posts and much land. The Portuguese adventurers established their estates in the Arakan and around Chittagong. Before long they became involved in local politics and a source of trouble to the Raja of the Arakan, who was compelled to attack them in 1607. Several of the Portuguese were killed, and the rest dispersed. Those who escaped settled in the islands at the estuary of the Ganges, and made them bases of piracy. Their depredations on local shipping forced the Mughal garrison commander on the island of Sandwip, Fateh Khan, to arrest and kill all the Portuguese there. He then set out to destroy the Portuguese pirate flotilla but was killed in action. The Portuguese returned to Sandwip and put to death the entire Mughal garrison. Soon an independent Portuguese state ruled by Sebastian Gonzales Tibao came into being. It consisted of a number of islands, and was defended by a Portuguese force of 1000 Portuguese soldiers, 2000 Indians, and 80 vessels of various sizes, well-armed with cannon. The security provided by Gonzales caused merchants to trade under his protection, which yielded much money to the Portuguese. Gonzales had established himself at Sandwip without any formal sanction from the Portuguese Governor at Goa.

Sebastian Gonzales Tibao was a pirate, and he entered into various nefarious engagements with local princes, especially his former enemy, the Raja of Arakan. Without any compunction, he turned, in 1613, upon the Raja and plundered his fleet and several coastal towns. The climate of Sandwip in particular and of the estuary in general, was unhealthy for Europeans. Finding himself in need of European troops, Gonzales wrote to the Governor at Goa, offering the wealth of the Arakan in return for official recognition. The Governor agreed to a joint conquest and sent a considerable fleet from Goa under Don Francis de Menezes. The joint attack took place on 15 November 1615, and the Portuguese were defeated because the Raja of Arakan had managed to secure the assistance of a number of Dutch ships that were then in harbour. Don Francis was killed in action, and his fleet returned to Goa, taking with them a number of the Portuguese from Sandwip, who were unwilling to live there anymore. On receiving information of Gonzales's weakened force, the Raja of Arakan soon attacked Sandwip, defeated Gonzales, and took over his territory.

The Portuguese again appeared on the scene around 1630, when the Governor of Bengal, Nawab Kasim Khan, was offended by their ravages around the town of Hooghly, where they had established themselves as traders. Rather than behaving as merchants, the Portuguese had fortified the town, and begun taxing all vessels passing their fort. Consequently, the port was avoided by merchants to the detriment of local commerce. The Mughal attack was carefully planned over a considerable period of time, and carried out with precision in 1632. Hooghly fell in October 1632, and a large number of Portuguese were killed, while many others, including women and children, were taken prisoner. Soon after this, Kasim Khan died, and was replaced by Nawab Azim Khan. It was during Azim Khan's governorship that the English received the Imperial firman to trade in Bengal. However, the local Mughal administration, drawing on their several recent ill experiences with the Portuguese, did not allow the English ships further than Pipli, where the English set up a factory in 1634. Gabriel Boughton, whose tale had already been told, entered the story soon after this and secured a firman, reportedly from Emperor Shah Jahan but actually probably only from Shah Shuja, the Governor of Bengal, favouring the Company's trade in Bengal.

By the end of the first governorship of Nawab Shaista Khan (1663-1677), English trade had grown vastly in Bengal. They had factories in Balasore (1642), Hooghly (1651), Patna (1659), Cossimbazar (1658), Dacca (1668), and Malda (1676). Shaista Khan gave the English permission in 1672 to trade freely throughout the province. Consequently by the time of his removal to Agra, the English were exporting, among other goods, around 1000 tonnes of saltpetre, and importing £110,000 worth of bullion annually. Despite this, there were complaints that the Nawab's officers were often making forcible exactions. It was also during this time that in addition to the Portuguese, the Dutch, and the English, the Danes and the French set up their trading posts in Bengal. European curios and medicine were always welcome, as were bullion, gunpowder, artillery, arms, and gunners.

Francois Tavernier's contemporary description of Bengal in his *Travels* is necessary at this point. He twice visited Bengal, and in preference to Egypt, called it 'the finest and most fruitful country in the world'. Rice was abundantly grown and exported, as was sugar. Wheat, though not a local staple, was nonetheless cultivated enough to provide the Dutch, English, and Portuguese, with 'excellent and cheap sea-biscuits'. Animals and fowl being also plentiful, 'This meat is salted at a cheap rate by the Dutch and English, for the supply of their vessels'. Tavernier found Bengal to be 'the common storehouse' of cotton and silk, which were available in great quantity. The Dutch exported Bengal cotton cloth 'of every sort, fine and coarse, white and coloured', to Japan and Europe. Bengal silk, though not in Tavernier's opinion as fine as that from Persia and Syria, was cheaper, and hence much in demand. 'The Dutch have', writes Tavernier, 'sometimes seven or eight hundred natives employed in their silk factory' at Cossimbazar, while the English employ 'a proportionate number'. Saltpetre was another major item of export, 'carried down the Ganges with great facility' from Patna and shipped by the Dutch and the English to Europe. Other items for export included wax, opium, lac, and 'various drugs'. Nonetheless, Tavernier noted that 'strangers [viz. Europeans] seldom find the air salubrious, particularly near the sea'. Tavernier tells us that when they had first settled in Bengal, there was 'a great mortality' among them. Over time, Europeans learned to 'live with more caution', which had diminished the mortality. Tavernier was a physician, and he gave it as his opinion that 'those who live carefully need not be sick, nor will the mortality be greater among them than with the rest of the world'.

Shaista Khan's second governorship (1679-88) was more important in terms of the consolidation of English power and trade. By 1680 the Company's trade interests in Bengal had increased enough to warrant its independence from Fort St George. As a result, William Hedges (1632-1701) was appointed Chief of the Bengal Agency of the Company on 14 November 1681. He reached Hooghly, his headquarters, on 24 July 1682, and assumed charge. To maintain the dignity of his office, Hedges had been allowed a guard of 20 European soldiers commanded by a corporal. In keeping with usual practice, Hedges was to be assisted by a council comprising Job Charnock, John Beard, John Richard, Francis Ellis, Joseph Dodd, and William Johnson.

Job Charnock was the chief of the Cossimbazar factory at the time, an irascible but experienced merchant faithful to the Company, who according to legend had defied local custom in 1677 by saving a young woman from becoming a Sati, and wedding her. They had several children, and he remained devoted to her all his life, going to extent to sacrificing a cock on her grave on every anniversary of her death for so long as he lived. Soon Hedges began receiving complaints against Charnock, who, as second in council, was the next most important Company official in Bengal. This set Charnock against Hedges.

In the meantime, Hedges, pursuing zealously his instructions to stamp out private trade and interloping, became disagreeable to the Company's officials in Bengal. John Beard, the third in council, wrote a private letter in January 1683 to Sir Josiah Child, the Director, complaining against Hedges and his wife. Hedges apprehended the letter, and held it back, determining to take up the matter in council with Beard. However, he failed in this and thus became the subject of suspicion. Through April 1683 Hedges followed up complaints against persons alleged to be in the private employ of Job Charnock, and engaged in trade for the interlopers. Nonetheless Hedges never brought any allegations directly against either Charnock or Beard. In any case, Charnock was sure of victory and boasted that the next ship from home would bring Hedges' dismissal. On 17 July 1684, a ship from Fort St George brought news of Hedges' removal, and the appointment of John Beard as chief in Hooghly, subordinate to the governor at Fort St George. Hedges left Bengal on 31 December 1684, reaching England on 4 April 1687, after a long, deliberate, and dangerous overland journey. Local merchants had complained to the civil judge at Cossimbazar that Job Charnock owed them 43,000 rupees. The judge found against Charnock, and the judgement was ratified by the Nawab, Shaista Khan, who summoned Charnock to Dacca. However, Charnock managed to keep to the factory premises, and finally escaped to Hooghly, where he became the chief.

In Bengal, during Hedges' time, there had arisen a quarrel between the English, who refused to pay a cess of 3 ½ per cent on all imports, and Shaista Khan. The English claimed a waiver deriving from their imperial firman, which only required them to pay an annual sum of 3000 rupees, while Shaista Khan refused to recognise this claim. On 10 October 1682, William Hedges travelled to Dacca to meet the Nawab and obtain permission for the waiver but failed to move him. This issue was exacerbated by the English demand for the Nawab's permission to fortify Hijili to keep out the Interlopers, who had become a menace to the Company's monopoly. This place would soon become very important to the English. Charles Stewart described Hijili thus in his *History of Bengal* (1813): 'Injelee [*sic*] is an island in the mouth of the river Ganges, but separated from the western bank by only a narrow stream; the greater part of it is covered with long grass, the habitation of tigers; nor does it produce a drop of good water'. This is an incorrect representation. Hijili was well-populated then as now, with a fort and batteries. Shaista Khan did not acquiesce. The Mughals had learnt a lesson from the Portuguese at Hooghly and elsewhere that they would not forget soon. In England, preparations soon began for war to protect the trade in Bengal, and a fleet of 10 ships under Vice-Admiral Nicholson was prepared. A regiment of 600 soldiers were to sail aboard this fleet, and Nicholson was to reduce Chittagong, and make it the equivalent, on the eastern coast, of Fort St George. To this end he was instructed to seek the alliance of local rulers unhappy with the Mughals, including the Raja of Arakan. With Chittagong as his base, the Admiral was to evict the Nawab from his capital, Dacca, which would become vulnerable with the loss of Chittagong. However, the Admiral was also given letters to the Nawab and his master, the Emperor Aurangzeb, informing them of the injustices done to the English, whose remedy would result in the avoidance of hostilities. While such preparations were praiseworthy in terms of keeping up stockholders' confidence, in effect, the fleet was delayed by contrary winds, and then scattered, due to which only some ships, the flagship, the *Beaufort*, the *Rochester*, and the *Nathaniel*, each accompanied by a frigate, sailed up to Hooghly rather than Chittagong. Meanwhile, Fort St George had sent 400 soldiers to Bengal, and had instructed Charnock to recruit a company from among the Portuguese, in charge of Company's officers. Shaista Khan was alarmed by these warlike preparations and stationed his troops close to Hooghly.

Too many troops had gathered around Hooghly, the conflagration needed only a spark, which was provided on 28 October 1686 by a bazaar brawl between the Company's and the Nawab's soldiers. This spread to a battle temporarily halted by an armistice between the local commander and Job Charnock, the latter's interest being in transporting goods from the factory to the ships to prevent damage. The local commander agreed to allow the English their former rights until a clarification was obtained on the firman from the imperial court. However Shaista Khan ordered the seizure of the English factories at Patna, Malda, Cossimbazar, and Dacca, and sent a larger reinforcement to battle the English force at Hooghly. Charnock considered defence untenable at Hooghly, and he decided to move on 20 December to Sutanuti, one of the 3 settlements that later formed Calcutta, where he would be directly under naval protection. O'Malley, in his *Bengal District Gazetteer: 24 Parganas* (1914) informs us that 4 families of Bysakhs and 1 of Seths had settled the village of Gobindapur, close to Sutanuti, the cotton market. Armenians also settled there, as proved by a tombstone that recorded a death in 1630, that of the wife of 'the charitable Sookeas'.

Shaista Khan sent arbitrators late in December 1686 with the seeming intention to settle a draft treaty with the English. The discussions proceeded through January 1687 but early in the next month the Nawab's forces suddenly concentrated on Hooghly to drive out the English. Charnock decided to retreat from Sutanuti to Hijili, sacking en route the fort at Thana, the Nawab's granaries, and seizing some of his vessels. Nicholson and Charnock occupied and fortified the island of Hijili and anchored the *Beaufort*, her frigate, and several of the Company's sloops midstream, thereby stopping all possible means of access. Meanwhile, a force accompanied by the *Rochester,* and the *Nathaniel* attacked and pillaged Balasore, after which it re-joined Charnock at Hijili. However, the English erred, for their real enemy was living with them. The Nawab's forces were content to stay on mainland, while the English were decimated by disease, mainly malaria, heat, and insufficient food. Within months the English force was reduced to half its strength. In their letter dated 10 September 1687 Job Charnock and Francis Ellis wrote to Sir John Child, 'The Mortality this Year hath been Very Great, but more Especially at that place of Hidgley [*sic*], which was not only in respect of what died there but great Numbers Died afterwards through the Disease they contracted there, in so much that we have buried the Last Year from the Ships and the Military nigh 500 men, amongst which are 14 of the Right Honourable Company's Servants and 6 women'. Again peace was broached and accepted hurriedly by Charnock even though he had received a reinforcement of 70 men, since Hijili had already claimed so many lives. In return, Shaista Khan issued orders on 2 July and 16 August 1687, blaming the English for the recent atrocity but allowing them to build a dock at Uluberia, and to return to their factories in Bengal, which had been seized. The Nawab stated that he would await the Emperor's orders on such outstanding issues as exemption from the cess of 3 ½ per cent, establishment of a mint at Hooghly, and compensation for the recent fighting. Charnock remained convinced that the war was far from over.

Around this time, the English had also been fighting with the Mughal governor of Surat, due to which the chief there, Sir John Child, was forced to flee to Bombay. Soon the Emperor Aurangzeb intervened in the matter, and urged peace in the interest of commerce, in Surat and Bengal. Charnock occupied Uluberia, found it equally unhealthy and returned to Sutanuti in September 1687, determined to make his headquarters there. However, peace was short, for English pugnacity found unfortunate expression in the Company's determination to continue the war against the Mughal Empire, since it was felt in London that the highly profitable trade with Bengal needed protection through the establishment of a fort, surrounded by an adequate territory with right to coin money. This had been successfully achieved at Fort St George, and although its utility had been doubted when first settled and fortified, that place served as a model for trade in Bengal. This idea had gathered support in England during the preceding 3 years. While dismissing Hedges, the Court had discussed the recommendation by several officials including Hedges, 'to mend our condition … by seizing and fortifying one of those pleasant islands in the Ganges'. Despite the considerable time lapses in the passage of news from India to England, by 1686, this cry for the militaristic enforcement of trade had been accepted by the Company. Most members of the Court of Directors had never been to India, and knew nothing of the Ganges, Bengal, and the Mughal Empire. As C R Walker writes, 'They did not very well know where Chittagong was, and appear to have thought it would be found some way up the Ganges, but they were sure it was the right place for the English settlement in Bengal'.

So the English ignorantly initiated the next round of hostilities, having decided that Chittagong had to be taken and fortified. They were so impressed, Walker writes, by the 'swaggering and boasting' of Captain William Heath that they thought they had found the right leader to conduct their affairs in Bengal. They had been confused by Charnock's apparent spinelessness in accepting the commands of the local governor instead to moving decisively against him, they did not understand why Charnock so willingly seized chances at arriving at treaties instead of fighting it out to the death, and they mistook Heath's swagger for actual ability in dealing with the Mughal Empire and its representatives. In their letter dated 27 August 1688 they informed Charnock, 'It was not your wit or contrivance, but God Almighty's good providence' that had allowed him to survive Hijili and gain permission to resume trade. Hence the Court directed Captain Heath to assume command of a fleet of 10 ships and sail with a troop of 160 soldiers to take Chittagong and turn it into an English stronghold like Fort St George. This Heath did early in 1688. At the same time in Bengal, Charnock and his countrymen were desperately trying to hold on to Sutanuti. They lived in huts, until brick buildings could be constructed, suffered, and succumbed to the heat, humidity, and fevers. Charnock dealt as craftily as he could with the Nawab, seeking permission for a permanent settlement there.

Heath's arrival at Calcutta on 20 September 1688 must have been as much a blow to Charnock as the Nawab's conclusion on the basis of reports that fighting between the English and the Mughals had recommenced on the Malabar Coast. Shaista Khan at once ordered the English back to Hooghly. They were not to construct any dwellings of brick or stone at Sutanuti. They were to provide adequate compensation for damages incurred during the recent fighting in and around Hijili and Balasore. Charnock sent to Dacca Eyre and Braddyll to negotiate with the Nawab for acquiescence to buy enough land from locals at Sutanuti, to set up a factory there, in view of the proximity and navigability of the river. In the letter of 27 August 1687, the Company had urged Charnock to look to the settling of Uluberia: 'We hope you may so manage that place or Town of Ullabarreah [*sic*], which you have articled for, that it may in time become a famous and well-governed English Colony'. The Court's letter to Fort St George on Heath's enterprise was confused. While Heath, as commander-in-chief of the Company's forces, was expected to carry Chittagong by surprise, should the place Charnock 'may have already settled and fortified upon will in any measure answer our known purpose … we would have you proceed to strengthen that place already settled, and to forbear proceeding against Chittegam [*sic*] until you receive further orders from us'. Heath met Charnock and his council, and told them that matters as he found them made him conclude that they would have to wind up their affairs at Calcutta by 10 November 1688, and leave aboard the ships pending an attack on Chittagong, unless some news arrived from the two councillors, Eyre and Braddyll, then at Dacca. On 1 November news came that the factory at Balasore had been seized and the English there imprisoned by the new Nawab, Bahadur Khan. At the same time Eyre and Braddyll seem to have been successful in dealing with the Nawab, since he sent Malik Barkhurdar to negotiate with the English. However, Heath refused to believe in Malik Barkhurdar, since he had been the source of the previous false treaties. Instead, he advanced the date for departure by 2 days and sailed away on 8 November. Surprised, Malik Barkhurdar sent messages after the ships, which were ignored, as were the possible fates of Eyre, Braddyll, and other English people elsewhere in Bengal. When Charnock and Heath reached Balasore Roads on 17 November, they found no supplies available; instead they were told that in return for the release of their countrymen, they were to help the Nawab gratis to take the Arakan.

After attempting to reduce Balasore in vain, Heath and his fleet reached Chittagong on 24 December, and sent out news under flag of truce that they had come to assist the Nawab in taking the Arakan. Before this Heath had sent away 2 ships to the Arakan, telling the Raja that the English were willing to help him fight their common enemy, the Nawab. For all his trouble, Heath received the answer of the Raja of Arakan that the Raja would provision the English if they took Chittagong but he had no troops to spare. With this humiliation to hand, Heath and his fleet, the sailors 'much distempered with the scurvy', made for Fort St George on 17 February 1689. In the meantime, the English left behind in Bengal were incarcerated at the orders of Nawab Bahadur Khan.

At the end of this wild goose chase, Job Charnock lived at Fort St George until Aurangzeb, aware that hostility with the English was leading nowhere but affecting commerce, wrote to Nawab Ibrahim Khan, who had replaced Bahadur Khan, at Dacca, informing him that the English had been sufficiently chastised; that they were to be thenceforth allowed on his orders to resume trade as before. Ibrahim Khan had already ordered the release of the English captives. Now he sent to Fort St George, requesting the English to return. Charnock was chary, and asked for an Imperial warrant assuring their security. Ibrahim Khan forwarded his message to the Imperial court. Charnock and his councillors escorted by 30 soldiers, reached Calcutta on 24 August 1690 for the final time. However, of their former residences, they found little left: 'nothing being left for our present accommodation and the rain falling day and night'. Consequently, they were forced to shelter aboard ship until some accommodation became available. On 10 January 1691 an Imperial firman was issued, allowing the English to trade as before, with an annual payment of 3000 rupees. The old buildings had been plundered, burnt, and left to the ravages of nature, and none of the new arrivals had a high opinion of the place. It remained as filled with illness as before. Sometime later Charnock's people protested vehemently against staying on in Calcutta rather than returning to the comfort of Hooghly. On 25 May 1691 the council of Fort St George wrote to the Court that 'They (in Bengal) could dispose of little, nor have they safe godowns to secure them from damage, and the truth is they live in a wild, unsettled condition at Chuttinuttee [*sic*], neither fortified houses nor godowns, only Tents, huts, and boats'. Charnock's obduracy to live on in Calcutta in inhospitable and unhealthy conditions was incomprehensible, as this letter stated, 'he continues there, contrary to all reason, or consent of the Government, who will neither permit building or Factory, nor Merchants to settle or trade with them, but offer a more convenient place for it, two miles below the Hughley [*sic*] but that he will not hear of'. This obduracy derived, so it was guessed, from his 'fears of being seized by some of the Government, his irreconcilable enemies'.

A consultation at Sutanuti on 28 August 1690 gives us a list of planned buildings for that place, to be built with mud walls and thatched roofs. These include a warehouse, a dining room, a room to sort cloth in, an apartment for the Company's servants, and a guardhouse. Buildings listed for repair included the secretary's office, and Charnock's house, which were only partly standing. Francis Ellis's residence had been 'totally demolished', and a new one was sanctioned.

On 31 July 1691, 4 'Victualling Houses' were permitted in Calcutta, for which the owners would pay the Company 50 rupees for the first year, and renew the licences annually. These Victualling Houses were to have 'such houses and accommodations as shall be convenient'.

Job Charnock died in Calcutta on 10 January 1693, aged 63, and the Company's letter to Bengal dated 3 January 1694 carried the bare statement, 'we hear of the death of our good Agent Mr Charnock, for which we are very sorry, but we must all submit to God's will'. In his place they appointed Francis Ellis, who had long been in Bengal, and with Charnock. In a letter to Fort St George of the same date, the Court referred to 'the deceased Agent Charnock, who was always a faithful man to the Company'. A consultation for 19 December 1694 records that at 11 the previous night Job Charnock's home was burnt down 'through the Peons making a large Fire under a thatched wall adjoining'.

Through the next decade Calcutta grew into a thriving trade centre with a substantial European population reconciled to sudden death. In some years the grim reaper claimed as many as 400 lives, and it became usual to rhyme Calcutta with Golgotha. Charnock left behind him a temporary settlement, which his successor, Francis Ellis, did little to improve. Sir John Goldsborough sailed from Vishakhapatnam in July 1693 and reached Calcutta the following month. He found things in disorder there, for Charnock's death and Ellis's promotion had only worsened things. Writing to the Company in October 1693, Goldsborough referred to Ellis as 'a Man too Easy and weak to stand alone in the head of such an affair as this is'. He led 'too Loose a Life to give any good Example or Govern this place'. Goldsborough discovered that the right man was Charles Eyre, who was given to 'the Country Habits and Customs', but generally well-spoken of. Charnock, strangely had not recommended Eyre for any position of responsibility when he discussed, while on his deathbed, with Captain Dobrill the names of those he intended for posts in Calcutta.

We get a picture of the English settlement in Calcutta from Sir John Goldsborough's letter of 30 September 1693 to Charles Eyre. Since the Agent and Council had not marked a place 'whence to build a factory on … everyone built strangely where and how they pleased'. Some had built on 'the most properest place for a factory', and had dug holes and tanks that would cost the Company money to refill. To settle matters, Goldsborough ordered a suitable piece of land to be enclosed by a mud wall, awaiting permission from the local government to build a factory therein. He also told Eyre of his decision to add, by providing stairs 'to the

2 Terraces 4 Rooms or Chambers' to the Walsh's house [the only brick house there] bring in 'the Accomptants and Secretaries, and the books and papers in their charge, which now Lie ... in thatched houses Liable to the hazard of fire everyday'. Sir John Goldsborough soon succumbed to the same ailments that took such heavy toll of the Europeans, and died in November 1693. Charles Eyre reached Calcutta on 25 January 1694 and took charge of the factory the following day from Francis Ellis.

By 1695 the Company had decided that Calcutta would be the residence of the Company's chief agent in Bengal. By November 1695, the Bengal establishment consisted of the Council (Charles Eyre, John Beard, Roger Braddyll, and Edward Cornell), the doctor, Francis Simson, 6 senior merchants, 3 merchants, 7 factors, and 4 writers. At this point in time, a local rebellion, whose details lie beyond the scope of this book, allowed the English to assist the Mughal administration in Bengal and thus obtain in 1698 permission to rent ample land around Sutanuti and fortify their factory. However, the local landowners contested this claim on the grounds that the firman did not bear the seal of the governor's Dewan. The matter was not settled until January 1700, or until a year had passed since Charles Eyre had handed over charge to John Beard and left for England to recover his health. Eyre recovered his health very soon, being knighted before long and offering further services to the Company. Sir Charles Eyre was appointed President of the Council of Bengal in December 1699. Among Sir Charles's instructions was the completion of the fortifications he had begun, the fort to be named Fort William in honour of the King. Sir Charles reached Calcutta in May 1700 but did little there, having fallen in love with a lady in England. Consequently, he left Bengal for the last time, after a ridiculously brief tenure, in January 1701.

Captain Alexander Hamilton's *A New Account of the East Indies* was published in 1745. Hamilton lived in the East Indies between 1688 and 1723, and his narrative is a vigorous representation of life as it then was. 'The English settled there about the Year 1690', he wrote, meaning Calcutta, 'after the Mogul had pardoned all the Robberies and Murders committed on his Subjects'. Misspelling 'Charnock' as 'Channock', Hamilton noted that though permitted to settle anywhere below Hooghly, Channock chose the present spot 'for the sake of a large shady tree'. In so doing, Channock 'could not have chosen a more unhealthful place on all the River'. 3 miles to the northeast of 'the Company's Colony of Calcutta' is a 'Salt-water Lake that overflows in September and October', when 'prodigious Numbers of fish resort thither'. During November and December when 'the Floods are dissipated' these fish 'are left dry and with their Putrefaction affect the Air with thick stinking Vapours'. These

'Vapours', carried by northeaster winds to Fort William, caused great mortality there. The English population of Calcutta comprised of merchants, Company's employees, military, and seamen from ships anchored off the town. Hamilton relates that one year when he was there, there were 1200 Englishmen in Calcutta in the month of August, of whom 460 had succumbed to disease by the following January. According to Hamilton, Charnock was oblivious to this. In fact, he 'reigned more Absolute than a Rajah, only he wanted much of their Humanity'. Any native who transgressed his laws was ordered to be severely whipped, which was particularly done when Charnock was at dinner, and 'so near his Dining-room that the Groans and Cries of the poor Delinquent served him for Music'.

Not all years claimed so many lives. A general letter from the Court to Bengal dated 16 April 1697 noted, 'We are glad to hear that your Town … increases so exceedingly … and that you have had your healths so extraordinarily well this last two years'. A similar sentiment is found in the general letter from the Court dated 26 January 1698: 'We rejoice to hear Chuttanuttee improves in Healthiness and much more that by a praiseworthy Temperance our People shut up that Door through Diseases and Mortality have broken in upon our Servants in Bengal, as it will do in the most temperate Climate'. One reason for improved health was the draining and filling up of several tanks around the factory wall. The same letter from the Court, dated 20 December 1699, which bore news of the reappointment of Charles Eyre, also carried the Company's guidelines on how Fort William was to be built. The shape prescribed was a pentagon, and the walls built very strongly of brick and lime, and the main timbers of the floor strong enough to bear a heavy gun. The windows were to be designed to act as port holes on necessity. The corners of the building, which the letter confusedly calls a 'factory', were to be built outwards sufficiently to give the impression that they were closets, while their actual purpose was to allow flankers to scour the walls in case of attack. However, as Alexander Hamilton noted, the fort 'was built an irregular Tetragon'. The town was 'built without Order, as the Builders thought most convenient for their own, every one taking in what Ground best pleased them for Gardening, so that in most Houses you must pass through a Garden into the House, the English building near the River's Side, and the natives within Land'. About 50 yards from the fort stood the church, where merchants often had to officiate at services due to the high mortality, which claimed the lives of 'Ministers of the Gospel'. A consultation dated 10 February 1707 noted that the building of this church was incomplete due to the lack of 'Regular Proceedings'.

Most importantly, Hamilton noted that 'The Company has a pretty good Hospital at Calcutta, where many go in to undergo the Penance of Physick, but few come out to give Account of its Operation'. The construction of this hospital found mention in the consultation for 16 October 1707. Since many sailors and soldiers fell sick every year, 'the Doctors representing to us, that for want of an Hospital or Convenient Lodging for them is mostly the occasion of their Sickness', the council decided that 'a Convenient spot of ground near the fort be pitched upon to build an Hospital on', for which 2000 rupees was decided to be paid out of the Company's cash. Additional funds were to be collected from the captains of the ships then in port, and from the European inhabitants. The charge of completing the construction of the hospital was given to Abraham Addams, under the general guidance of the council. Addams was advanced an additional amount of 5000 rupees by a consultation dated 4 October 1707 to complete his task. The 'Doctors' referred to were themselves not above moral turpitude, as Benjamin Adams, the 'sober, virtuous, and learned man' who was appointed Company's Chaplain in Calcutta in November 1699, pointed out. Adams was outraged by the immorality of the Surgeon to the Factory, William Warren. Warren, 'a man of most pernicious principles and debauched manners' seems to have been married, whose wife was then living in England, and quite willing to voyage to Calcutta to join him. However, while in Calcutta, Warren wed the widow Elizabeth Biuns, 'though admonished, advised, and cautioned to the contrary'. Adams' indignation was deepened by the fact that Mrs Biuns knew, as nearly everyone else in Calcutta society did, that Warren had a wife back home. Nonetheless, Warren's medical services were indispensable to the Europeans, and in view of his workload, he was assigned an assistant surgeon in August 1705. A list dated 24 October 1704 shows Warren as the only doctor in the Company's service. The entry against the date of his arrival in India is blank, and he was paid a salary of £36, or 144 rupees every 6 months. Considering that in 1676 the Company had ordained the Surgeon's salary at the factory in Hooghly at 4 rupees per month, Warren's pay was very attractive.

The record goes on to state that William Warren was employed in the 'Old Company's' service, and elected to the United Company's service by 'the Manager's Consultation' on 16 February 1704. The climate took toll on Benjamin Adams too, for on 24 April 1706 he was summoned by the council and counselled to be of a 'more peaceable temper', and 'civil and respectful' to the government after he had kept his servant from arrest for having beaten up one of the Company's Indian employees. Adams resigned his chaplaincy on 7 September 1706. The council was miffed about this, so while they agreed to pay his salary they rejected the following month his application for a gratuity.

The Company had its own garden, which provided the Agent's table with 'Herbage and Fruits'. There were also fish-ponds, 'to serve his Kitchen with good Carp, Calkops, and Mullet'. Irrespective of his position in the Company's hierarchy, the European had equally easy access to 'all sorts of Provisions, both wild and tame, being plentiful, good and cheap' including clothing. Nonetheless, the town and fort were so placed that 'the Afternoon's sun is full in the Fronts of the Houses, and shines hot on the streets that are both above and below the Fort'. The inhabitants of Calcutta around 1705, 'Most Gentlemen and Ladies', were found by Hamilton to 'live both splendidly and pleasantly'. Their daily routine would remain unchanged during the next 200 years. The forenoon was dedicated to business, followed by rest after dinner, 'and in the Evening to recreate themselves in Chaises or *Palankins* in the Fields, or to Gardens, or by Water in their *Budgeroes* … and before Night, they make friendly Visits to one another'. On 26 December 1710, the council ordered the auction of Captain Alexander Hamilton's house to repay his debts. It sold for 2500 rupees.

The building of a ditch around the town and fort at Calcutta had been discussed in London. It was to serve a dual purpose, protect the habitation and drain away excess water. The general letter from the Court dated 4 February 1709 particularly instructs the council, 'Be sure remember to drain the grounds and fill up the Tanks if it be true … which is told us that the Standing Water thereabouts contributes to the unhealthiness of the Place and Subjects People to Agues, fevers, and fluxes, and no wonder for it has the same effect in England in our low Marsh grounds'. The letter went on, 'We are informed the greatest part of the Standing Water thereabouts is occasioned by the Peoples digging the Earth to make their Houses with and then the next rains the Holes are filled with Water which there Stagnates and corrupts'. In any case, the Company urged the council to 'do whatever you think proper to make the Place healthy but with as little charge as may be'. Clean water was a problem, and the council noted on 28 February 1709 that during March and April the river water was brackish and unsuitable. So they ordered the enlarging, deepening, and cleaning of the tank to the east of the fort for use from the following season. At a consultation on 14 August 1710, it was decided to clear the land around the fort of the trees set close around it, 'country thatched houses', and 'standing pools of stinking water', thereby making the place 'wholesome and healthful'. In February 1711, it was agreed that 'The thickness of the trees in Calcutta being injurious to the health of the place, shall thin them and keep them in rows, and cut away all Bamboos'. So bad were the climate and the town sanitation that on 11 January 1711 we find the council discharging the Surgeon to the Factory, Dr James Phillip Richardson and the Assistant Surgeon, Mr John Parney, to give them the chance to recover their health through a change of air. Later that year Dr William James, who had come as ship's surgeon aboard the *Bouverie* in 1710, was appointed Surgeon, and in December 1712, William Hamilton Second Surgeon.

On 3 January 1713, the governor, John Russell, had fallen ill and been advised the usual remedy of a change of air 'as the only means left for the Recovery of his health'. He travelled towards Nadia, accompanied by a doctor and an escort of 50 soldiers commanded by Captain Woodville. This doctor was Richard Harvey, who had arrived in Calcutta in 1712 as the surgeon of the ship *Recovery*. On 17 February Russell returned to Calcutta, much recovered, and happy with the medical knowledge and services of Harvey. In the meanwhile, William James had returned to England, and on 19 February the council appointed Harvey in his place, 'he being a good Physician and offering his services to us'. Governor Russell again fell ill 10 days later, which was attributed to 'the difference between the air of this place and Nuddea'. Hence he was advised to go there again, this time with a guard of 30 soldiers, and 'Several of the Company's Servants who are now Indisposed ... for the Recovery of their Health'. In keeping with the suddenness with which disease fatally struck Europeans in Bengal, Rebecca Russell, the governor's wife, died on 14 April 1713 at Chandernagore, leaving behind their 3 children to be brought up by their father. She died aged 42, and they had been married over 15 years. Her body was brought the next day to Calcutta for internment. John Russell was devastated. He returned, recovered in body but not in mind, from Chandernagore, on 29 May.

The duties of the surgeons extended to medical jurisprudence. William Hall and Jean Suin, a Frenchman, quarrelled and fought after 9 pm on Saturday 25 July, as a result of which Hall was wounded, and died on 30 July 1713. The council asked the doctors to 'give in their opinion in Writing whether he Died of the Wound then received'. On 6 August Doctors Hamilton and Harvey submitted to the council that their autopsy revealed that William Hall 'had received a wound by a Rapier in the lower part of his Belly on the right side Obliquely passing under the Guts wounding the Coats of the Nerves of the Kidneys, Emulgent Arteries, and great Lacteal Veins from which Wounds he received his Death'. The next day Suin was tried, and it was found that he had acted in self-defence when attacked by Hall. Hall's injury was at first not considered serious.

Captain Woodville visited Hall and spoke to him before he died, when Hall admitted that he had first attacked Suin. Suin was acquitted of the charge, and 'discharged without paying any fees to the Guard'.

On 20 August 1713 Doctors Hamilton and Harvey submitted a set of regulations for the hospital, which the council sanctioned. The first required the Company to give the hospital 30 cots and bedding, 20 gowns, and 20 'pieces Gurrahs' [earthen pots], 6 brass pots, 6 saucepans, 12 porringers, and 1 'corge' [score] of pewter plates with 20 spoons. The second rule demanded that every unmarried soldier report to the hospital when sick. This probably had to be enforced because of a number of reasons, from malingering to fear of contemporary medical practice, though the council preferred to believe this was 'by reason the Doctors can Visit them oftener than when they lie at their Lodgings which are far distant from one another' . The third rule contains one of the reasons why soldiers had to be ordered to report to the hospital when sick; all sick soldiers in hospital were to pay 4 annas per day 'for his maintenance', while corporals were to pay 6 annas, and sergeants half a rupee. The fourth rule required a sentry to 'secure the Sick from going abroad till admitted by the Surgeon', and 'to hinder all Strong Liquors being brought in'. The next demand was for the appointment of a steward who would supply all necessary material to those admitted to hospital, for which he would be paid a monthly wage of 30 rupees, 'out of which to pay for fire Wood, oil, etc'. The doctors did not walk to see their patients, as proved by a council decision dated 4 March 1714. The entry reads, 'The hot weather coming in very vehement and it being impossible for our Doctors Mate to perform his duties without a Palankeen to shelter him from the heat and rain', for which the Doctors Mate was allotted 8 rupees per month to pay for 4 bearers to carry him about in his Palankeen.

Another interesting medical incident occurred the same day, 20 August 1713, when several soldiers who had come aboard the *Cardigan*, complained to the council that Dr Kettle, their ship's surgeon, 'did not take due care of them in the Voyage'. The council examined Dr Kettle, and discovered him to be German who spoke 'broken English'. They wrote to the Company whether, given the complaint, Dr Kettle could claim the gratuity of 10 shillings 'a head for this care of those soldiers'. After reviewing the case on 23 November 1713, presumably with the assistance of Hamilton and Harvey, the council came to know that the soldiers who had complained had behaved mutinously during the voyage. Additionally, 'Some other soldiers who had been Sick were called and they attested all necessary care was taken of them'. Therefore, the council agreed to pay Dr Kettle 208 rupees as his gratuity at 10 shillings a head, for 52 soldiers.

The most important decision relating to William Hamilton was taken on 5 January 1714. John Surman was selected to lead the embassy for a firman from the Emperor at Delhi. His party included John Pratt, Edward Stephenson, and since a surgeon was necessary, William Hamilton was chosen. The selection of John Surman caused resentment, since he was a Writer, and they thought a councillor like Frankland was more suited to be the leader of the embassy. This was overruled by the council, and soon John Pratt wrote letters to several friends that he 'Scorns to go inferior to Mr John Surman'. The council decided that those letters 'manifested his Pride and ambition Joined with such a temper as may occasion Quarrels and hazard the ruin of our affairs'. Hence he was replaced as second in the embassy by Edward Stephenson, and John Barker, then at Patna, its secretary. The embassy left Calcutta in May 1714, bearing goods worth 102,472 rupees for Emperor Farrukhsiyar and 108,218 rupees for his courtiers. Additionally, the embassy carried goods worth 29,958 rupees for the personal use of the members of the embassy, besides 47 bales of 'Bengal piece goods' to sell in Delhi on account of the merchants in Bengal. The Emperor, notified over a year earlier of the embassy and its presents for him, had decided to pay the cost of the embassy's carriage from Patna to Delhi, and had issued all necessary permits in this connection. This payment of carriage was useful since the embassy's goods required 100 wagons. This grand procession also included camels and more oxen to pull the guns. A huge retinue of servants accompanied the embassy. It must have been a sight worth beholding.

The embassy officially left Patna on 11 January 1715 but was delayed at Naubatpur, outside Patna, until 7 April. After an arduous though, for the times, safe, journey, the entire cavalcade, goods and ambassadors included, reached Delhi on 4 July 1715. William Hamilton's medical services must have been constantly demanded while on the march. At Delhi too he was soon indispensable. At first he attended to the high steward, whom he found afflicted with an incurable ailment. Then in August 1715, the Emperor fell ill with swellings in the groin, of which Hamilton cured him. In October, Hamilton was sent for by the Empress-Mother, who held through the purdah a long discussion on the Emperor's new complaint, a possible fistula. Hamilton attended the Emperor through the month, and on 20 November, the Emperor was declared cured. While Hamilton was treating the Emperor, he was the subject of considerable suspicion. Monsieur Martin, the Emperor's French doctor, did not care to have an Englishman in medical attendance on his patron, and neither did the local practitioners. In fact, rumours about the Emperor's demise often spread, and on one occasion, Hamilton was struck on the head by a pebble thrown by someone, while he was returning home at night from the fort. On another occasion, a huge mob gathered around the house occupied by the English ambassadors due to a sudden rumour that the English surgeon's ministrations had led to the Emperor's death. The mob was diverted from attacking by the Emperor's showing himself from a gallery of his palace. The Emperor rewarded Hamilton with a jewelled plume, a vest, 2 diamond rings, an elephant, a horse, and 5000 rupees. He ordered gold buttons for a suit of clothes for Hamilton, to be set with diamonds and rubies, and the handles of all his small instruments to be made of gold. The Emperor's mother gave Hamilton a dress of honour, a horse, and 1000 rupees. Still later, after the firman was obtained (10 April 1717) and the English attended court for the final time on 30 May 1717, while Hamilton like the others was invested with a robe of honour, the Emperor ordered him to resume his seat at court while his colleagues were permitted to leave for Calcutta. Hamilton steadfastly refused to serve at the Imperial court under any terms and sought permission to depart. This was granted on 4 June, on condition that on returning from Europe after meeting his family, he would serve at the court. On 16 June Hamilton confirmed this under his own signature. The embassy formally left Delhi on 18 July 1717. They met the monsoon en route, and suffered accordingly. They reached Patna on 21 September, and commenced their journey to Calcutta on 21 October 1717. Hamilton fell ill around this time, and was critical for a while around 27 October, when they were close to Monghyr. He proceeded by boat to Calcutta while the others travelled by road. Hamilton wrote his will while on the boat, which soon brought him to Calcutta and English medical care. However, it was probably too late, or maybe his fellow doctors did not know what afflicted him, and employed the usual debilitating range of drugs. In any case, William Hamilton died on 4 December 1717 in Calcutta and was interred in the old burying ground where Job Charnock's mausoleum stood. John Surman and Edward Stephenson wrote and submitted their last final communication to the council in Calcutta on 14 December 1717. One wonders if no thought about their late companion passed their minds. In fact, William Hamilton was soon forgotten, and his tombstone was rediscovered during the digging of the foundation of St John Church, Calcutta, which, so the story goes, was noticed by Warren Hastings. Hastings wished the tombstone placed at the entrance to the church but it found place in Charnock's mausoleum.

By 1722 the swampy land around Gobindapur had been drained, making available land for new inhabitants, in addition to making Calcutta healthier. Due to the Company's many financial problems, by December

1728, the hospital in Calcutta was found to be in a state of disrepair. The engineers' report by Thomas Snow and John Aloffe, dated 11 May 1730, to the council, disclosed that the beams, and door and window frames were in so rotten a state that they feared the roof would fall in during the next rains unless work to shore up the beams was immediately undertaken. This was presumably done, for the next reference to the hospital is found in the consultation dated 26 March 1735, when it was decided that the hospital needed 'a Couple of upper Rooms' for one of the doctors to live there, 'for the Attendance of the Sick'. At the same time, it was decided to build 'a Shop for the Medicines at one of the Ends of the Hospital'.

In 1749, Holwell, who had come out to Calcutta as surgeon, left for England, whence he would soon return as a covenanted servant, and he was replaced by William Fullerton, who would play a major role in events in Bengal 20 years later. Holwell became assistant surgeon in place of Dr William Lindsay, who had died of a fever on 29 March 1740. By 1745 the city had grown many times, and the drains were insufficient for an increased population. They were often blocked and they stank. On 21 October 1745, Joshua Briggs, the secretary to the council wrote to Bartholomew Plaisted, 'Surveyor of the Company's Works', to 'take a Survey of the Drains and Ditches and report the Condition thereof with an Estimation of the Expense it will cost to put them in good order and keep the Town wholesome and free from the offensive smells therein'. Plaisted did his work and reported on 21 October that many of the drains were blocked since 'Inhabitants had filled up part of the Ditches which were drains to the Town and made Encroachments in the Roads and Streets'. Writing to the Court in January 1746, the council pointed to this as the cause of 'the late great Sickness'. They noted they had ordered this to be corrected. Similarly, a general letter from the Court dated 16 January 1752, ordered the council to thin or cut down 'the Great number of Trees at the South and South East part of the Town', which reportedly 'contribute greatly to the Unhealthiness of the inhabitants in the rainy Seasons, by intercepting and stagnating the Air'. The Court ordered the council to clear the drains and do whatever else 'may be necessary for preserving the Healths of the numerous Inhabitants, although at some Expense to Us'. The council was urged to make 'the Richer Sort' of inhabitants to pay for some of the charges to be incurred in this exercise. On 27 October 1752, Bartholomew Plaisted, visiting the hospital, reported to the council that 'The Doctors are of opinion that Tuckposts for every room, made to takeout at pleasure, will be a great preservation, as all lower rooms are very damp'.

However paternalistic the Company may have been, there was considerable corruption among its servants in Calcutta. Bartholomew Plaisted was suspended from his post and forced to return to England, when he exposed some of this corruption. In England, Plaisted successfully pursued his case, and was reinstated, although he was coldly received in Calcutta when he returned, and even murderously set upon by one Mr McGuire, whom he had implicated. The council, ordered by the Company to enquire into this matter, found for McGuire, and eventually caused Plaisted to be suspended once more under their 'severest Resentment' for insubordination, as a result of which Plaisted returned to England again in November 1755. McGuire too was permitted to return home at the same time 'to vindicate himself from any insinuations Mr Plaisted may there make to his disadvantage'. As events turned out, McGuire's defence was rejected, and given the emergency in Bengal in 1756, Plaisted reappointed once more as Surveyor of the Company's Works on 31 December 1758. Although later transferred to Bombay, he was sent to survey the coast of Chittagong, which he did very efficiently.

By Holwell's estimation, the population of Calcutta in 1752 was 409,000. C R Wilson, in his *Early Annals of Bengal* (1909) considered this too high, and recalculated it to 105,000. The hospital was, by 1754, in an acute state of disrepair. On receiving a report from the doctors in this matter, they sent Paul Richard Pearkes, the Import Warehouse Keeper, to survey it. His report, presented to the council on 25 July 1754, shows the hospital's pathetic condition. It had been struck by lightning, its beams, door and window frames were rotten, 'The Westerly Wall' had 'bellied out two feet', and the 'North East End' of the hospital cracked in many places, which would allow the rain to seep through and separate mud from brick. Despite this survey, action was slow, and soon Calcutta fell to Nawab Siraj-ud-Daulah. This is not the place to analyse the causes of this unfortunate battle, compare its many contemporary accounts, or its aftermath. Suffice it to say that Admiral Watson arrived with a Royal Naval fleet bearing English troops from Madras, most particularly Lieutenant-Colonel Robert Clive, whose decisive military, administrative, and covert actions soon reversed the English defeat. Fearfulness of the Directors had assumed such enormity that the council informed the Court on 7 December 1755 that though they had informed Writers, per the Court's order dated 24 January 1754, that they were not to avail of horses, chairs, or palanquins during their Writership, the violent rains of the monsoon made palanquins a necessity to keep them from sickness during the rainy months. Another paragraph from the same letter, dated 7 December, informs us that the senior surgeon then was Mr George Gray, who had recommended his son to the Company's service. Another step towards improving health was taken on 12 May 1755, when Holwell, then Collector, sought permission to repair the great tank to the south of the fort. He also wanted to 'prohibit the washing of people and horses therein, the latter practice making the tank at times so offensive there is no passing either to the southward or northward'.

Mortality was clearly taking heavy toll of life, since the council wrote to the Company on 22 August 1755, asking for 'three or four expert Gentlemen educated in the branch of Engineering and carrying on in the most regular manner plans of Fortification'. However, the council had learned from experience that 'men's lives advanced to or nigh the age of Forty are very precarious in such a change of climate from their native Country', and wanted younger men, whose youth would hopefully save them for early death.

The summer and monsoon seasons of 1757 and 1758 were particularly unhealthy. In 1757, 707 patients were admitted to the General Hospital, of whom 101 died. On 10 January 1758, the council noted that the previous season had been very sickly, and the European garrison of Calcutta was reduced to '4 or 500 Rank and File', which worried them about how to thwart a possible attack by the French. Of the total number admitted, 147 were ill due to 'putrid fever' and 155 by 'putrid flux'. Hence on 6 September 1759, it was decided at council that the hospital was not large enough 'for Reception of the sick', and 'Dr Gray's House' was purchased for the sum of 'Current Rupees 14000', which was deemed a reasonable price given the urgency of the time, considering that the old hospital was valued at 12,000 rupees in 1757. By 1759, there was a great shortage of houses for writers in Calcutta, and on 29 December 1759, Bartholomew Plaisted was order to build 'slight apartments' with thatched roofs for writers and European troops, which would require fewer bricks, given that there was a shortage of experienced bricklayers in Calcutta. On 7 August 1760, the surgeons of the hospital reported to the council that they were no longer able to 'diet' the military sick on 6 rupees a month, due to which the amount was increased by 2 rupees per head. Around the same time the following year, the surgeons presented a bill for clothing for the sick amounting to 5,358 rupees, which was passed. Not all these surgeons seem to have held proper qualifications. Peter Smith, surgeon's mate to the army at Patna, came down to Calcutta on 11 November 1762 to be examined by surgeons aboard Europe ships, who were required to report to the board whether they considered him qualified to apply for promotion to surgeon. Peter Smith, we are told, was passed by his examiners, and became an army surgeon.

On 11 October 1762, the hospital was again deemed insufficient and in want of 'the Benefit of a free and open Air'. Until the new Fort William was ready, the council decided on a temporary building of trees and thatched roof. The state of the 'Old Hospital Adjoining to the Head Surgeon's house' so worsened, as did the condition of Dr Gray's house, which had been bought to supplement it, that Mr Fortnom, the Civil Architect, recommended to the council on 3 March 1766, that it be taken down to 'prevent its doing mischief'. Since repairs to these buildings were deemed too expensive, on 31 March the council ordered them sold. The sale was nonetheless delayed until February 1769, when it was recorded that the Old Hospital had been entirely brought down by a violent storm. The building had been estimated at 41,554 rupees. Its 'remains' fetched only 414 rupees. By 29 September the need of a good hospital having become acute, the council ordered the Civil Architect 'to point out a proper Spot for a Hospital to be built upon'. This hospital was to be 'a commodious One [to] be erected as soon as possible'. Another significant decision made the same day noted that 'The present Burying-ground situate in the middle of the Town is also very detrimental to the Healths of the Inhabitants and too much confined'. Again, the Civil Architect was told to 'point out a more convenient Situation for one to be made of proper dimensions'. One additional reason for a new hospital and burial ground could have been the fact that the old hospital and cemetery were situated next to each other, which would have been psychologically or physically uplifting.

In the general letter from Bengal to the Court dated 28 November 1766, the council regretted that the Court had denied them permission to build a church until all other essential constructions had been completed, and reported that the new hospital and burial ground had been given precedence. It was easier to find a new cemetery, which the council soon did, noting on 25 August 1767 that 'the New burying Ground near Mr Vansittart's garden now being ready, they desired the clergyman to consecrate it as the sickly season is approaching'. On the same day the new cemetery had its first unfortunate occupant, the body of John Wood, a Writer. Other burials rapidly followed. However, it appears that the new cemetery was not consecrated until May 1768, since the Rev William Parry wrote to the council on 18 May 1768 that if he was to consecrate the new burial ground (and travel thither whenever required), he needed an allowance to hire bearers for his palankeen, given the great distance of the cemetery from the European quarter of the city. The council allowed Rev Parry 30 rupees for bearers.

To inaugurate a new hospital was more expensive, and it took longer. Kathleen Blychenden informs us that 'in 1768, a house was purchased from a native gentleman for the purpose of a hospital'. This was also far away, 'to the south of the Esplanade, the Maidan, practically in the country'. This house became the Presidency General Hospital.

Following Clive's victory at Plassey, Calcutta began to grow rapidly. While Calcutta grew and spread, elsewhere in the province of Bengal there arose problems, which, though political, nonetheless subsumed medical practitioners much in the same as Boughton and Hamilton were appropriated into the history of the English in Bengal. As the Rev James Long points out, doctors in old Calcutta 'were few, badly paid, and in various cases, badly educated'. 'Great complaints were made', Rev Long notes, 'of the negligence and peculation of the doctors in the hospital'. Hence the council decided that they would visit the hospital by rotation. Certain problems remained unchanged until the turn of the century. Houses in Calcutta remained one-storied and damp, claiming thereby the lives of many of the Writers. Sanitation was poor, and the surrounding swamps made for fever. Pestilence and medical ineptitude generally combined to fill up the burial grounds and enrich undertakers. Despite all this, there were doctors who strove to understand the climate and its endemic diseases alongside local modes of treatment. Howell had practiced medicine for 20 years, and he was by nature observant. History popularly remembers him in relation to his account of the Black Hole but, as the next chapter will show, his medical tract is many times more interesting.

CHAPTER THREE

THREE SURGEONS AND THE PATNA MASSACRE

Clive's victory made Mir Jafar Nawab of Bengal but did not settle matters politically. Clive left Calcutta for England on 25 February 1760, his departure being followed, as J Talboys Wheeler writes, 'by what may be termed the revolutionary period'. Indeed it was a period of great change. At Delhi, uncertainty attended the slow but certain dissolution of the Mughal Empire. Occasional raiders took advantage of this confusion and made successful forays into imperial territories, like Nadir Shah's infamous invasion of 1738-39. The Emperor, Alamgir II, became the subject of contention, his life and reign forfeit to the powers that had placed him on the throne. The most important among these was Ghaziuddin Khan Feroze Jung III, the Imad ul Mulk. The heir apparent, Alamgir's son, Ali Gauhar, fled to Rohilkhand in 1758, and away from the machinations of the Imad ul Mulk. He thereby presented himself thereby as a pole to which drew persons who resented his father's adviser. These persons were mainly opportunists, seeking to carve out their own satrapies. As an initial measure towards establishing his supremacy, they advised the prince to seek the submission of the subahs of Bengal, Bihar, and Orissa. The prince's instigators considered that this submission would easily be achieved since the recent battles between the Nawab and the English, as well as the heavy indemnity that Mir Jafar had been forced to accept, had weakened these provinces. Additionally, these advisers had their own agendas to fulfil. Muhammad Quli Khan of Allahabad, Shuja ud Daulah of Oudh, and Raja Balwant Singh of Varanasi prominently instigated Ali Gauhar to move against Mir Jafar in 1760. Shuja ud Daulah had a deeper interest, for he intended to take Allahabad while Muhammad Quli Khan was away campaigning in Bihar with the prince. At this time Raja Ram Narain was the Naib of Bihar, in residence at Patna. Ram Narain had been implicitly trusted by Nawab Alivardi Khan, Siraj ud Daulah's grandfather. Mir Jafar had no reason to move against Ram Narain but he placed his son, Mir Maran, in nominal charge of Bihar, and demoted the Raja to

Naib. Hence when news began arriving at Mir Jafar's court in Murshidabad, of the gathering of the prince's army, the Nawab panicked. His treasury was empty, and his soldiers disaffected because they had not been paid. None of the local financiers were willing to lend to the Nawab. Mir Jafar found it hard to rely on Ram Narain's fidelity. So the Nawab vainly sought the assistance of the Marathas, and then tried to open negotiations to buy off the prince and his generals, promising them money as soon as it became available. This too had no effect. Desperate to save his newfound realm from depredation, Mir Jafar then applied to the English for help.

In any case, the English were soon drawn into the fight since Ali Gauhar wrote to Clive seeking English aid in forcing Mir Jafar's submission. This was followed by a missive from Delhi in which the Emperor sought English help in subduing 'his misguided and rebellious son'. The Imad ul Mulk too wrote in similar vein to Calcutta. Clive refused Ali Gauhar any help stating that since they acknowledged the nominal authority of Alamgir, the English were bound to follow the orders of the Emperor in putting down rebellions in the empire. Ali Gauhar, unable to bring the English to his side despite his promise to make generous grants, turned to the French for help. This made the English realise that they needed to urgently join the fray.

25 February 1759, English troops marched from Calcutta to Murshidabad. This column, commanded by Clive, included 450 Europeans, 2500 sepoys, and some artillery. The English contingent was joined by a column of the Nawab's army under the command of Mir Maran, and together they marched for Patna on 13 March. In the meantime conflicting information about Raja Ram Narain's activity was received. He had reportedly changed sides and was ready to hand over Patna to the prince. Clive wrote a rebuke to the Raja, and the latter answered that he had been awaiting reinforcements. Like Mir Jafar, Ram Narain too had received exaggerated information about Ali Gauhar's force. Based on these reports, Ram Narain deemed it impossible to hold Patna, and sought advice from the chief of the English factory, Amyatt. In any case, Ram Narain wanted to know if he could count upon the few companies of sepoys under European sergeants, which were there for the protection of the factory and English trade. Amyatt told Ram Narain that he and his council would leave the factory and go downriver to a point accessible to Bengal, and there await orders from Calcutta. Under these circumstances, Ram Narain behaved more courageously than Amyatt because he went to the prince's camp, where he was ceremoniously received. In fact, Ram Narain shrewdly assessed the fact that Ali Gauhar's forces were far less than had been reported. He also realised that Ali Gauhar's generals were not

interested in the imperial cause but personal gain. So Ram Narain returned to Patna, and readied for a siege, corresponding all the while with Clive. The prince's camp soon realised the duplicity and attacked Patna on 23 March 1759. The defenders, including the Company's sepoys, fought off attacks until 5 April, when reinforcements under Ensign John Matthews, rushed by Clive by forced marches, arrived. Ali Gauhar disengaged and retreated, particularly because his allies had broken out amongst themselves, Shuja ud Daulah having seized Allahabad per plan while Muhammad Quli Khan was fighting at Patna. Muhammad Quli Khan was imprisoned en route by Raja Balwant Singh, on the orders of Shuja ud Daulah, and later executed. Ali Gauhar's other officers too dispersed variously and he was reduced to writing abjectly to Clive 'for some pecuniary assistance to enable him to effect his retreat'. Clive sent him 500 gold mohurs, upon which Ali Gauhar went off with his French escort towards Bundelkhand. Clive reached Patna on 8 April 1759 and set about repairing the fort. Then he toured the surrounding districts, where roving bands were pillaging, and restored peace. Clive left a company of European troops, 2 guns, and 5 companies of sepoys in Patna and returned to Calcutta in June 1759, accompanied by Mir Jafar and Mir Maran. The Nawab had been profusely grateful to Clive, and made him a personal gift, making him landowner of a large tract to the south of Calcutta.

These events made Mir Jafar only more acutely aware of his instability and complete dependence on the English. To counter this, he secretly encouraged a Dutch proposition to bring a powerful army into Bengal. Matters came to a crisis in October, when a Dutch force larger than the English, sailed up the river to Chinsurah. It included 750 Dutch soldiers and 800 Malay regulars, as against 500 Europeans in Calcutta including English, Armenian, and Portuguese able-bodied civilians, and 1200 sepoys, plus 3 East Indiamen in port. Moreover, Dutch agents were busily recruiting sepoys in Cossimbazar, Chinsurah, and Patna. Mir Jafar stationed himself halfway between Hooghly and Chinsurah to watch events unfold. Clive decided to prevent the Dutch fleet from landing its troops at Chinsurah but he could not declare war on a country at peace with his in Europe. In November the Dutch opened hostilities, making things easier for the English. Clive's decisive action and the bravery of the English forces made them completely victorious by 25 November 1759. Robert Clive left for England on 25 February 1760, having made over the government of Bengal temporarily to Joseph Zephaniah Holwell, until Henry Vansittart reached Calcutta from Madras.

At the end of 1759, the Emperor Alamgir was assassinated at the orders of the Imad ul Mulk, who placed a younger son on the throne as

Shah Jahan III. Ali Gauhar was at this time once again moving towards Bihar with most of his former allies. As soon as he received news of his father's death, he assumed the imperial privileges, calling himself Shah Alam. He appointed Shuja ud Daulah his vizier, and gained the support of the Rohilla chieftain, Najib ud Daulah. Shah Alam wrote to Ahmad Shah Abdali, the ruler of Afghanistan, who was then moving into India for the second time to fight the Marathas, for support in recognising his authority as Emperor. By the beginning of February 1760, Shah Alam reached Patna. Meanwhile, Clive had dispatched, before his departure, a force of 300 Europeans, 1000 sepoys, 50 gunners, and 6 cannon, under the command of Major Calliaud, to Murshidabad, whence the force, augmented by 15,000 infantry and cavalry and 25 guns commanded by Mir Maran, resumed its march to Patna on 18 January 1760. Raja Ram Narain had presumed to initially rely on his previous skirmish with Ali Gauhar. The prince was now the Emperor, and many more allies rallied to his flag, while his vizier stamped coins in his name. Nonetheless, Ram Narain was unfazed. He summoned his vassals to his army, and amassed an army of 40,000, larger than Shah Alam's. He then marched out of the city and took up a suitable position for battle. Ram Narain had been cautioned by Calliaud not to initiate hostilities but to stay quiet until the reinforcements arrived. There were 2 important aspects to this. Unlike the previous encounter, Ram Narain now had with him an English military detachment commanded by Captain Cochrane. This detachment included 1 European company, 2 guns, 70 gunners, and 8 companies of sepoys. Cochrane's responsibility was to protect the person of Ram Narain, and he urged the Raja to locate with the English detachment, which was placed in reserve. However, Ram Narain refused this offer. The other aspect has to do with the Nawab's troops, who as usual had were in arrears of pay and discontented and, therefore, unreliable.

Raja Ram Narain marched out with his troops on 9 February 1760 to fight the enemy. This was a disastrous decision. Treachery soon reduced the Raja's army substantially, while Ram Narain continued to fight valiantly. Isolated and wounded many times, he sent to Cochrane to be rescued. Cochrane marched with 4 companies of sepoys to his help. These troops faced terrible odds against a much superior and determined enemy. They reached the Raja and covered his retreat but the repeated attacks of the enemy soon took toll. All the English officers, Cochrane, Ensign Winklebeck, and Mr Barwell, a volunteer, were killed. Only 25 sepoys led by 1 European sergeant returned alive to the main body of the English force. This detachment had also been repeatedly and severely attacked. The infantry left in charge by Cochrane and the gunner officer, had both been killed. The only English officer alive was the surgeon, Dr William Fullerton. Fullerton behaved with exceptional courage, and organised the remnants of the English force, fought off enemy sorties, and with the 2 guns, marched steadily towards Patna. The carriage of 1 gun was broken, and it was spiked. The other fell off its tumbrel but Fullerton halted his force and resumed the march only after it had been righted. By his exemplary leadership William Fullerton led his force safely back to Patna. Ram Narain, though wounded, had also reached the city, which he set about preparing for a siege, even as he opened negotiations with Shah Alam. Shah Alam, on the other hand, could have pursued the retreating troops and taken Patna, had he not paused to celebrate his victory and bury the dead. Soon Patna was besieged but only until 19 February 1760, when Calliaud and Mir Maran arrived within 30 miles of Patna with their army. Shah Alam and his force moved out to defeat them. After some delays, the battle was finally joined on 22 February, and Shah Alam's army was routed. Mir Maran was unwilling to follow the enemy and Major Calliaud did not have enough troops to commit to this. Hence matters stood thus until 2 March, when it was discovered that Shah Alam and his remaining troops had marched along the river towards Bengal.

The brief military action with the Dutch had proved that insufficient English troops were available in Bengal, and these were mainly scattered in the districts. On the approach of Shah Alam, many local rulers declared their allegiance to him, which alarmed Mir Jafar, Mir Maran, and the English. Major Calliaud took to the boats and travelling downriver, soon closed upon Shah Alam, whose march was slowed by his guns and baggage. Shah Alam decided to send off his guns and baggage, and took a shorter but hitherto untraveled route across hill and jungle to shake off the English.

Other alarms shook Calcutta at this time. A substantial Maratha force had entered the district of Midnapore, around 100 miles from Calcutta. Again the volunteer civilian force was called up. Mir Jafar had sallied out towards Rajmahal with an army including 200 Europeans commanded by Captain Spear to help his son fight Shah Alam. However, the Maratha incursion placed at peril not only Calcutta but also Hooghly and Burdwan, besides placing them in a position to assist Shah Alam when he appeared before Murshidabad. Mir Jafar returned to his capital and requested English help. They gave him 100 European soldiers, 200 sepoys, and 2 guns with gunners, to help him protect Burdwan. Mir Jafar sent his son-in-law, Mir Kasim, with 1500 cavalry with this force but ordered him to stay put at Katwa, through which any force from the southeast or east would have to proceed, to take Murshidabad. Mir Jafar, now in great panic, dithered over what he should do to save himself and his province. However, the English were reinforced at the right moment by 2 battalions of sepoys under Captain Maclean, who was returning from the Northern Circars. Maclean was ordered to move directly to Burdwan, while the English at Katwa were further reinforced. The Nawab and the English were harrying Shah Alam into where they wanted him. Calliaud and Mir Maran were in pursuit, and the Nawab, with Mir Kasim and Spear awaited his arrival in Burdwan to prevent a juncture between the Marathas and Shah Alam, while Captain Maclean was marching down Midnapore to engage the Marathas. Shah Alam could have taken a more direct route to Murshidabad, which was relatively defenceless but he chose to walk into the trap. Mir Jafar, in keeping with the usual practice of the time, had, unknown to the English, negotiated with Shah Alam, offering his submission. Hence the battle would have been fought between the English and Shah Alam, with Mir Jafar playing a recalcitrant role.

On 1 April 1760 Shah Alam arrived within a few miles of the Nawab's position at Burdwan. On 4 April 1760 Calliaud and Mir Maran joined the Nawab. However, the English had no cavalry with which to force the Marathas and Shah Alam to battle. Repeated pleas by Calliaud to Mir Jafar to send his cavalry to harry the enemy were rejected. Finally, Shah Alam aware that the odds were against him, burned his camp and retreated towards Patna on 10 April. Calliaud sent a force on 16 April under Captain Knox to supplement the English detachment there by the river route up to the closest point from where they could cross the river to the northern bank and reach Patna fast. On 28 April Shah Alam's army, bolstered by a small but determined French detachment, attacked Patna, whose defences since the last assault had not been repaired. The English garrison included Dr William Fullerton, who volunteered his service once more. Fullerton and his small troop of sepoys rushed to dislodge Zainul Abedin, one of Shah Alam's bravest officers, who had successfully breached the eastern wall and ascended the ramparts. Fullerton and his men fought desperately, and Zainul Abedin was killed, as a result of which his men retreated. Soon Captain Knox arrived with his force, and the enemy retreated.

The entire episode had concluded by the end of July 1760, Mir Maran having been killed by a bolt of lightning during a storm earlier in the month. Henry Vansittart reached Calcutta in July, and took over a government whose treasury was empty. The huge sums promised by Mir Jafar had mainly been to individuals, while the Company had neither gained much from these grants nor from the territories newly added and trade had suffered during the attrition that covered the previous 4 years. So straitened was the Bengal council that they had to resort to heavy drafts on the Company in London. The fact remained that Mir Jafar's reign had been full of continuous warfare, into which the English had been drawn, resulting in still greater costs. This provided the basis of the argument that Mir Jafar had to be replaced by a more effective ruler in the interests of trade, for the Company was still only a trading corporation, and not a military power in search of conquests. Hence Calliaud, now promoted to Lieutenant Colonel, added his voice to the need for a change in the Company's dealings with Mir Jafar. The Company would seek a firman from the Emperor, reinforcing the Nawab's feudatory status by making him cede more territory to the Company as indemnity. Many of his ministers, would have to be dismissed, his administration thoroughly overhauled, and his rabble of an army discharged. Seeing this as a means of recouping its losses in the fighting in Bengal and Bihar, a Select Committee of Calcutta council entered into a secret treaty on 27 September 1760 with Mir Kasim, who had been catapulted into primacy in the local government following Mir Maran's death. Mir Kasim was to be Deputy to the Nawab, and run the administration, while Mir Jafar nominally retained his office and all his dignities.

In return for his elevation, Mir Kasim had to make liberal personal payments. Allegedly and most prominently, Henry Vansittart got 500,000 rupees, Holwell 270,000 rupees, and Calliaud 200,000 rupees. The Company's interests were looked after as well. The amount outstanding since 1757 was to be paid, and the jewels and plate pledged by Mir Jafar redeemed through cash payments. The districts of Burdwan, Midnapore, and Chittagong were to be assigned to the Company in return for military aid whenever needed. Mir Kasim also promised to advance 500,000 rupees to the Company to meet war expenses in Madras. The usurpation was planned and almost immediately affected. Henry Vansittart and Colonel Calliaud went to Murshidabad with a substantial force, and on 19 October 1760, Mir Jafar was forced to accept the Company's decision. Mir Jafar refused to remain Nawab and in Mir Kasim's power, and so he abdicated. The former Nawab was escorted to Calcutta under European guard and he and his family settled into some houses in Chitpore. Mir Jafar thus exited Bengal politics for the time being.

Mir Kasim became the Subhadar of Bengal on 20 October 1760. He was acutely aware of the fact that to retain his throne, he would have to immediately meet the terms under which the English had agreed to support him. At the same time, like Siraj ud Daulah and Mir Jafar, he was restive under English dominance and looked for freedom. Mir Kasim found himself in the same financial condition as his predecessor, since the treasury held only 50,000 rupees, and jewels and plate worth 400,000 rupees. By various means, including confiscation of the estates of several ministers and high officials of the former regime, Mir Kasim soon forwarded 250,000 rupees to the Company for Madras, and 700,000 rupees for the maintenance of the English and Nawab's armies in Patna.

Shah Alam was still in the vicinity of Patna and his presence required action. Major Carnac, commanding at Patna, decided to confront Shah Alam's force which, headquartered at Bihar Sharif, dominated the entire region to a few miles close to Patna. The Nawab's army, still cavilling about arrears of pay, initially refused to march with Carnac and his troops to the village of Suan [Sukiyawan?], situated beside the stream called Banowra. Here they found Shah Alam's army on 15 January 1761, camped on the other side of the stream. The battle commenced and Shah Alam's army was dispersed, while its French detachment, under Monsieur Law surrendered. Shah Alam again made a rush for Patna but was headed off by Carnac, and turned southwards.

Unknown to Shah Alam and the English, the Third Battle of Panipat, was fought on 14 January 1761. In this battle, Ahmad Shah Abdali, the ruler of Afghanistan, allied himself with Shuja ud Daulah, Nawab of Oudh, and the Rohilla Afghans under Najib ud Daulah, and defeated and massacred his opponents, the Marathas. In the meantime, harried by the English, Shah Alam and his army moved from place to place, short of money, and unable to find provisions anywhere. Finally, on 6 February 1761 Shah Alam agreed unconditionally to peace with the English. He reached Patna on 14 February 1761 in the company of Major Carnac, the English having agreed to honour him as Emperor. Raja Ram Narain had agreed to pay the Emperor 1000 rupees a day for his expenses. Meanwhile Shah Alam had received news of his recognition as Emperor by Ahmad Shah Abdali, and he wished English support in regaining his throne in Delhi. The Calcutta council was drawn to the idea of helping the Emperor to Delhi, in return for still greater trade and territorial gains. However, the affairs of the Select Committee, particularly the personal fortunes made by its members, had divided the council, even though the Committee's measures were carried because Vansittart had the majority. Further involvement in Indian politics would carry additional expense, which would not be immediately recouped, and which the Company could ill afford, especially since it had been at war in Bengal and Bihar from 1757, and was still engaged in fighting in the Carnatic. There were not enough of the Company's troops in the province to provide military support to the Emperor without endangering their own territories.

Mir Kasim was anxious about the Emperor's presence in Patna, since it gave the English easy access to his nominal feudal lord, who had the power to grant concessions and territories at will. So the Nawab went to Patna, where he was formally received by the Emperor on 12 March, and invested with the authority of the Subhadar of Bengal, Bihar, and Orissa. Shah Alam, finding that the English would not accompany him to Delhi, sought and received the support of his allies, including Shuja ud Daulah of Oudh, and Najib ud Daulah of Rohilkhand. In June 1761, Shah Alam left Patna and journeyed towards Delhi. Mir Kasim, still hard up for money, now looked to Raja Ram Narain's treasury for sustenance. He demanded the payment of longstanding dues, which the Raja denied and offered the accounts for audit by the English. Major Carnac and, later, Colonel Eyre Coote, both sided with the Raja against the Nawab. The relationship between these two officers and the Nawab worsened until Calcutta recalled them at Mir Kasim's behest in July 1761. Coote returned to Calcutta in July itself, and Carnac followed in August, thereby abandoning Raja Ram Narain to the machinations of Mir Kasim. Ram Narain was deposed, and imprisoned, and his property and money confiscated. Almost all his officers and supporters suffered the same fate. This allowed Mir Kasim to meet his financial commitments to the Company, which was the likely reason for the council's recalling Coote and Carnac from Patna.

With the turn of the year, changes occurred in the council at Calcutta. Several members were recalled home, and Francis Ellis, whose animosity to Mir Kasim was well known, became the chief at Patna. In the meanwhile the Nawab had turned his attention to the other regions of his province, whose chiefs suffered as Ram Narain, being forced to pay up. Mir Kasim also began reorganising his army on the European model. The rabble of the former regime had been discharged, and a new army of 16000, composed mainly of Rohillas, Afghans, and Persians, was formed. The artillery was similarly reorganised with newly cast guns of great efficiency and accuracy. This army was many times better disciplined and equipped, being officered by Europeans like Walter Reynaud or Reinhardt, known variously as Sombre, Sumroo, and Somers, and Armenians. The gunners were also Europeans, mainly Germans, Portuguese, French, and Armenian. Through February and March 1762 relations between the Nawab and Ellis worsened to the extent that Warren Hastings was sent to mediate. While the Nawab received Hastings, Ellis refused to see him, and Hastings' mission turned futile. Soon the Nawab took up the issue of the flagrant abuse by the English of their trade concessions for private gain. Soon Englishmen in Bengal were speculating privately on an enormous scale, avoiding paying cess of 10% to 20%, which was applicable to all goods not meant for import or export. Europeans often made very profitable agreements with local merchants, who thereby avoided paying the local government any taxes for the movement of their goods. Any of the Nawab's officials who objected to these arrangements were punished by the English. Complaints by Mir Kasim were mainly disregarded. Henry Vansittart vainly sought to correct them for he was in the minority now. In April 1762 Warren Hastings wrote to Vansittart that he was amazed to see every boat he passed on the river had an English flag, 'I am sure', he wrote, 'their frequency can bode no good to the Nabob's revenues, the quiet of the country, and the honour of the nation'. As nearly all Englishmen in Calcutta had by then invested in this hugely lucrative trade, it soon assumed an enormity that could not be ignored any more. The Nawab's complaints became vociferous, and even the majority in the council, who were deeply engaged in private trade, realised that they needed to address these complaints. So they authorised Henry Vansittart to travel in January 1763 to meet the Nawab and make terms. The Nawab was at Monghyr, where he agreed to allow the English to trade privately by paying 9% cess, less than the local merchants. Mir Kasim added that this reduced tax too would be violated, in which case he would abolish cess for all, which would provide all merchants with equal opportunity to trade. Vansittart signed an agreement with Mir Kasim along these lines and returned to Calcutta in February only to find that his council disapproved of the terms he had signed to. The Nawab was correct in presuming that the English did not want to pay any taxes for local trade. Meanwhile, Mir Kasim, although told that Vansittart's signature meant little without the approval of the majority of the council, informed his officers of the new terms. At once all English commodities then in passage became subject to the new levy. The English, whose goods were held up until the taxes were paid, were furious, as was the council. It was decided that the new tax was illegal, and the English would only pay 2 ½ % duties on salt. The English would settle all disputes relating to cess, which was completely against the principles of justice since the English were an aggrieved party to these disputes. As Hastings had prophetically pointed out in his letter to Vansittart on this subject in April 1762, 'You are sensible, Sir, that it is from such little irregularities, too trivial perhaps for public complaint, and continually repeated, that the country people are habituated to entertain the most unfavourable notions of our government, and by them the English credit suffers much more'.

By March 1763 Mir Kasim was subjected to severe provocation, on the one hand by William Ellis at Patna, who reacted in extreme fashion to every minor occasion that offered scope of humiliating the Nawab and on the other by the barefaced insolence and greed of the English traders. Enraged by reports of English traders and agents being unwilling to pay the reduced tax, Mir Kasim did as he had told Vansittart he would – he removed all taxes, thus levelling the field for all merchants. This immediately deprived the English of all profit in local trade. As a result, the majority in the Calcutta council, readied to commence hostilities against Mir Kasim, despite Vansittart's and Hastings' dissent. William Ellis was permitted by order of council to prepare for aggression but not to attack until a formal mission of 2 councillors, Peter Amyatt and William Hay, had met the Nawab and attempted to convince him to remove all taxes on the English. The council was very unfairly forcing Mir Kasim to opt for war, even as it was readying itself for conflict. At Patna, Ellis repaired and set up his defences openly, and soon boatloads of armaments for Patna were seized by the Nawab's officials at Monghyr, where Amyatt and Hay were negotiating with the Nawab. This was during May – June 1763. The Nawab repeatedly told these councillors that he did not want to fight the English, despite the provocations being offered him. To maintain peace, he suggested that the army detachment at Patna be withdrawn, which the council at once rejected. Meanwhile, some sepoys had deserted the Company's service at Patna, as a result of which Ellis placed all troops on active service with effect from 6 June 1763, which increased their salary since they immediately became entitled to *batta* or special pay. Against the Nawab's reformed army, which had been tested in minor battles, the English had 1500 Europeans and 10,000 sepoys in Bengal. At Patna, Ellis had at his command 4 companies of Europeans, 1 of artillery, and 3 battalions of sepoys, or 800 Europeans and 2500 sepoys.

In mid-June the council concluded that the mission to the Nawab had become redundant, and ordered Amyatt and Hay to make for Calcutta or Patna, as they thought fit, and to inform Ellis of their departure, to prepare him for war. On 18 June the council, through majority decision, resolved that they would have to go to war to protect the Company's lands and trade. This was followed on 20 June by a resolution to restore Mir Jafar. A letter from Amyatt dated 14 June 1763 was received on 23 June at Calcutta, in which the writer said that the Nawab had made the withdrawal of troops from Patna the issue on which the declaration of war depended, and that he had permitted Amyatt to leave Monghyr but not Hay, holding the latter as hostage. The next and final letter from Amyatt, dated 19 June, said that the Nawab was willing to release the boats carrying armaments and to negotiate. On 30 June Cossimbazar reported that communication with Patna had been severed. By the first week of July, Calcutta was rife with rumours that Patna was besieged.

Amyatt, with several others, including Doctor Crooke, had left Monghyr by boat with the Nawab's permission on 23 June 1763, while

Hay and Gulston were kept hostage. When Mir Kasim heard that Ellis had opened hostilities in Patna, presumably after being informed by Amyatt of his departure, he ordered Amyatt's boat stopped, and the English arrested. Challenged and ordered when close to Murshidabad to land and surrender, Amyatt and those aboard his boat, including the sepoy escort, opened fire. The Nawab's boats approached and boarded, and in the fighting all the Englishmen, and most of the sepoys, were killed or taken captive. Amyatt was among the dead. Other versions say that Amyatt and his party were only invited to land and dine with a local general which, having been refused, the refusal attributed to Amyatt's haughtiness, the boat was fired on and boarded.

Meanwhile, in Patna, Ellis prepared to take the city, and having gathered his force in the factory, he attacked early on the morning of 25 June 1763. Using scaling ladders and great stealth, the English soon took the city, with the exception of the Chehel Sitoon, a large building in the city, where the sick had been in the charge of Dr William Fullerton. Fullerton, as was stated in the previous chapter, came out to Calcutta around 1744, and he was appointed to the General Hospital in Holwell's place in 1750. Fullerton experienced the fall of Calcutta in 1756, and its recovery by the English. In 1757 he was Mayor of Calcutta. Fullerton resigned from the Calcutta establishment in 1760, and was appointed to the factory at Patna, where, as we have already seen, he played an important military role in keeping the English troops together in orderly retreat during Shah Alam's attack of 1760. Fullerton, like many of his contemporaries seems to have indulged in private trade, making much profit. In fact, one reason why he had opted to serve in Patna was because he had invested considerably in saltpetre.

The Chehel Sitoon did not fall to Ellis because it was occupied by Muhammad Amin, one of the Nawab's officers, and his troops. Fullerton noted in his diary that he had been called in by Ellis and told to evacuate the sick to boats, to be carried over to the side opposite the city, 'thence tracked up, and crossed over to the Factory'. The evacuation was to take place at 2 am, which was also the time set for the invasion of the city. Since Amin and his men held the English sick hostage, the English did not force their way into the building. Similarly, the city's bastion was held by another of the Nawab's officers, Lal Singh. Rather than taking the citadel, Ellis, his factors, and most of the military officers, returned to the factory for breakfast while the English troops looted the city. Most of the English sick and Dr Fullerton must have been evacuated, since Chehel Sitoon continued to be occupied by Amin and Fullerton spent the day in the factory, looking after the wounded as they streamed in, as Dr Peter Campbell noted.

Dr Peter Campbell was a friend of Captain Carstairs, the officer commanding the European troops at Patna. He visited the factory on 23 June, since they were celebrating the anniversary of Plassey, and noticed the hasty and whispered conferences between Ellis and the military officers. Later, when Campbell asked Carstairs whether he should continue to reside in the city, on which his friend told him to move into the factory the following night. Dr William Anderson too was present at the same party on 23 June, and he knew the details of the impending attack. The following day, after the English had taken Patna, Campbell noted how 'joy reigned in the face of everybody … Biscuits, wine, etc. were sent in to the officers to refresh them'.

In the meantime, the Nawab's troops, commanded by Markar, one of the Armenian officers, reached Patna and scattered the looting English troops. These retreated into the factory, which Markar besieged. He had considerable experience of war, having fought in Holland. He surrounded the factory and kept it under constant musketry and cannonade. The English reply was insufficient. Anderson attended the council that met at 6 the same evening to decide the future course of action. The defence of the factory was the first point to be dismissed, 'the factory being but small and badly provided with provisions' for 1200 sepoys and 200 Europeans, Anderson noted. Both Fullerton and Anderson believed that Markar had been able to surprise the English because at least 1000 sepoys had deserted after the looting. The council was in favour of escaping by boat either towards Bengal or Oudh. The former was no longer possible since the Nawab's forces commanded all territory from Monghyr. The latter was considered feasible, since it was closer, and so farther away from the Nawab's troops. Shuja ud Daulah, the Nawab of Oudh, was friendly towards the Company, and the English expected to be well received by him.

On the morning of 26 June 1763, Ellis sent for Fullerton and gave him a military commissariat task. Fullerton was to take 50 sepoys and commandeer as many boats as he could from the Saran bank opposite the factory. At 12 Fullerton was told to take the boats to the Phaleza Ghat, and wait for the troops there. At 10 pm 700 European troops and 1000 sepoys, with 1 howitzer, showed up at the Ghat. A rear-guard of 1 officer and 30 Europeans had remained behind to cover the retreat of the main body. The bungalows and other buildings had been set afire and they blazed fearfully. Fullerton noted that enemy musketry and cannonade had made the porters cast away the ammunition and bolt. Consequently, there remained only 12 rounds a man. The troops were boated across the river, and they waited until 10 the following morning, when the Company's treasure was brought across. The weary march to the Nawab of Oudh's territory began, with little provisions available, and villagers scared to help the English for fear of reprisals. Campbell's account however states that the boats were not where they had been told to be, that the Europeans marched to the embarkation point at 11 pm, and that the whole party walked up the bank until they found the boats around 3 am, and the embarkation was not completed until 10 am on 27 June 1763. Anderson too states that they crossed the river on boats around at 2 am.

The monsoon had arrived, and they were impeded by heavy rain. Soon Sumroo moved in from Buxar to attack the English column. Dr Anderson had not previously heard of Sumroo. On 30 June he noted some villages on fire nearby, and learnt thus of the presence of 'one Somero', who had with him 3 or 4 companies of sepoys and some guns. Harassed and tired, the English, commanded by Captain Carstairs, deployed to meet the enemy at Manji on 1 July 1763. Campbell recorded the resolution 'to keep our ground on the bank of the river till evening, and if they advanced, to give them a brisk attack, as we had not ammunition to risk two attacks'. Fullerton noted that 'Shimroo' had 3 battalions of sepoys, 8 guns and 10,000 foot and horse, and of his battalions, 2 were armed with 'Europe arms' and 1 with 'country matchlocks'.

The Europeans formed the centre, and the sepoy battalions the flanks of the English position. When they ran out of ammunition, the sepoys charged with great success but were let down by the Europeans, who refused to charge because they had not eaten in a long while and were weary. Carstairs, who was probably attended by Anderson, was shot by a *jingall* ball at 11 am, when he was sitting down. Anderson wrote, 'It entered the inside of his thigh and passed out at his loins/groin'. Anderson felt that 'From the nature of it, it must be mortal'. Carstairs, as Campbell noted, lived until 3 July, when 'his wounds began to mortify' and it became 'very offensive' to those in the boat, which reads strangely as having been written by a surgeon. Several other Europeans were killed, and soon afterwards, the enemy was reinforced.

The boats pushed off with the survivors of the action, and Campbell noted that there were no interruptions that night 'but very dismal thoughts', for it had been decided to 'proceed down the river, and deliver ourselves up'. His boat had 8 Europeans, and 'a number of sepoy women and sepoys'. Anderson was on the same boat, and he noted the presence of 6 women and 6 children. Fullerton had been sent in a dinghy back to Patna, to negotiate an honourable surrender. He reached there the next day, and was well-received by the Nawab, who directed that the English be given safe conduct but before this order could be sent, news came of their capture by Sumroo. In fact, the entire English force, comprising 300 Europeans and 2500 sepoys, had surrendered. The sepoys were disarmed and freed, of whom several joined the Nawab's service, as did many of the Europeans. The remainder were made prisoners and herded, as Fullerton tells us, to Patna on 5 July. Ellis and the others on another boat that had made it to Chapra, were expected at Patna on 6 July, Fullerton wrote. Campbell however wrote in his diary that the governor of Patna 'entertained us in the most obliging, complaisant manner imaginable', having given them a good lunch. In the evening, Campbell noted, he treated them to 'very good arrack and a hookah'. The same day orders had arrived for moving the prisoners to Monghyr but the Governor allowed them to rest that night and depart the following morning. Early the next morning the prisoners set off, with the Governor having given them a 'dressed kid' and bread for their journey. On 8 July, Fullerton received news that Ellis and his companions on the boat, along with 45,000 rupees of the Company's treasure, had been sent to Monghyr as well. This was untrue.

Having reached Monghyr on 8 July 1763, Campbell was surprised to see no one to receive them. They provisioned themselves from the bazaar, and the next day Campbell's servant, Nimmo, ran away with 30 rupees and some combs. The prisoners continued to live on their boat until 10 July, when very strangely they were returned to Patna. Campbell awoke on the morning of 12 July with 'a violent pain' in his instep. This he at once attributed to the weight of 'Dr Anderson's head … as it is pretty heavy, it was generally believed to be the cause by lying on it'. The pain so 'increased to a violent degree', and Campbell concluded that the reason wasn't Anderson's heavy head 'but rather a touch of gout'. Clearly, confinement was not helping professional relations between the two surgeons. The pain continued the next day, 'which puts it past all doubt that it is the gout'. The prisoners now learned that Ellis and his companions were on the way to Monghyr, which amazed them since they were returning to Patna. At this point Fullerton's account veers off, since he was sent to Monghyr on 16 July, 'and there confined separately from the rest of the gentlemen'. Anderson and Campbell and their group reached Patna at 10 am on 18 July 1763, and were received by the Dewan. Then they were 'kept in a sort of Durbar place, immensely close and hot' (Campbell), and 'pestered with flies' (Anderson), until evening when the Governor sent for them and again politely assured them of kind treatment. They spent that night in the Dewan's bungalow where, as Anderson noted, they had little rest 'as it was swarming with bugs and mosquitoes', but were taken the next morning back to their old prison. This was unbearably hot during the day. While the conflict between the Nawab and the English was ensuing, the Dutch had been in their factory all the while, and Campbell noted that they sent a few bottles of wine to their fellow Europeans the next day, which were intercepted by the guards. Mortified, they 'resolved to bear everything patiently'. The following night was spent most disagreeably in the hall, due to the heat, 'bugs, and a noisy guard' (Anderson). That night the guard moved out, so that the English slept on the verandah, which was cooler, and they had 'a little air, and less noise' (Anderson).

They thought that this was to be their home until the war ended, and so reconciled themselves to the place. They got a pack of cards and played whist but as Campbell noted, with despair, 'much troubled with flies, and the time hangs very heavy'. The next day, 22 July 1763, they were taken to a storehouse, which had been cleared for them, and which seconded as dungeons, for Campbell recorded that the first sight that met them there were 'two or three in irons'. The room allotted to the English was full of rats, the floor covered with their holes. Campbell was depressed. 'I retired into it [the room]', he wrote, 'and laid myself down in one of the corners to be free from the gazing of our new companions in irons, and found a small window where I could peep through, and contemplated upon our sad situation'. Anderson, more in control of his feelings, recorded meeting 2 Europeans on the way, who told them that 15 Europeans had been sent down from Monghyr. Anderson noted that the 'compound' where they were confined, was damp and hung with cobwebs, but better for all that since all their belongings had been carefully sent there, and they were more comfortable. Moreover, Anderson wrote, 'We found this a place for state prisoners, and several people of some consequence had been there since Ram Narain's misfortunes'. The guards allowed them to walk along the square, which Anderson preferred to being confined.

By the following day Campbell had recovered his composure, recording that they had spent 'a very agreeable night', and that they were to send to the bazaar for victuals. Their fellow prisoners visited them and condoled with their condition, which made Campbell think that they were 'very sensible men'. The following day was still better, with a 'leg of roast mutton and curry, steaks, etc.' for dinner, and drink or two from bottles sneaked in from the Dutch by their servant, Niccolo.

On 26 July Anderson noted that it was 'close and sultry, which makes the flies very troublesome'. He also recorded their new routine, 'to drink twice a day, dinner at one, talk a while in the evening, and sleep at ten'.

On 30 July 1763 they sent Niccolo to the Governor with a petition for a daily allowance for food, and permission for a bottle or two of liquor, which was granted. Niccolo now became their contact with the outer world, bringing in formation, typically a mixture of truth and rumour, about the progress of the English army from Calcutta. The English prisoners had also begun drinking more liquor, with Campbell justifying bulk purchases from the Dutch through Niccolo, as economical compared to 2 bottles a day. Drinking too much probably led to quarrels, for Campbell noted on 3 August 1763 that 'Dr Anderson was a little out of humour today, and did not eat his dinner as usual, owing to a mistake made in describing a house that he and some gentlemen built at Neg's (that they had built a house without any dimensions)'. Campbell wryly added, 'he [Anderson] is nearly related to my countrymen, I believe, for he seems to have established a maxim that it is not right to give up a point'. Maybe Campbell said some such thing to Anderson, for he recorded the next day that Anderson was 'highly offended' with him at dinner 'for having wanted to drink out of the cup before he had finished what he calls his daily allowance of gin'.

Fullerton wrote on 10 August that the Nawab had left Monghyr, and Fullerton, who had continued to be housed separately, was allowed to treat Captain Turner, who died soon 'of a flux'.

In the meanwhile, Mir Kasim wrote on 28 June to Calcutta, stating that the Company would have to take the responsibility of the pillaging of Patna, in the same way in which they had sought indemnity for Calcutta in 1757. For this, the Nawab demanded, 'in the same manner in which you took Burdwan and the other lands, you must favour me in resigning them'. This missive reached Calcutta on 7 July 1763, and on the same day the council issued the proclamation of war by the Company on behalf of Mir Jafar, against Mir Kasim. The factories in Murshidabad and Cossimbazar were soon besieged, and war commenced. Cossimbazar soon fell, and its English population sent to Monghyr. However, there was hardly enough money in the Company's account in Calcutta to fund a prolonged conflict. Mir Jafar promised 3,000,000 rupees as war expenses and donations of 2,500,000 rupees and 1,25,0000 rupees to the Company's army and navy, besides directly funding a corps of 12,000 cavalry and 12,000 infantry.

On 19 July 1763 a decisive battle was fought near Plassey, at which the English defeated a force commanded by Muhammad Taki Khan. Murshidabad fell on 23 July 1763, and Mir Jafar was proclaimed the Subhadar of Bengal, Bihar, and Orissa 2 days later. By 27 July the English force comprised 1000 Europeans and 4000 sepoys, and it crossed the Bhagirathi River to begin its march towards Monghyr and Patna. They next crossed the Bansli Nullah on 1August and found the enemy drawn up to meet them at Gheria, at the junction of the Bhagirathi and the Bansli. Mir Kasim's army was 40,000 strong, including 12,000 cavalry and a detachment of rocket-men. The English position was very strong, since they had the rivers to the right and left, which protected their flanks and allowed them to concentrate their troops and artillery. Mir Kasim's army advanced to the battle the next day, having made the mistake of allowing the English to cross.

Mir Kasim's was defeated after another hard-fought battle, and the English advanced to Rajmahal, reaching there on 6 September 1763. In the meantime, Mir Kasim, at Monghyr, was growing restive. He wrote to Major Adams, commanding the Company's forces, on 9 September to restrain from further incursions, with the dire warning, 'if you are resolved on your own authority to proceed in this business, know for a certainty that I will cut off the heads of Mr Ellis and the rest of your chiefs and send them to you'. To this Major Adams replied as threateningly, 'It is true you have Mr Ellis, and many other gentlemen in your power; if a hair if their heads is hurt, you can have no title to mercy from the English, and you may depend upon the utmost fury of their resentment'. Fullerton noted that Ellis and his group were sent down from Monghyr on 13 September 1763 to Patna, and confined in Haji Ahmed's house. On 19 September Fullerton was ordered to Patna, and imprisoned alone in the bastion.

It had rained heavily through August at Patna, and many of the English were sick, including Campbell. Hence, between 16 August 1763 and 11 October, we hear no more from Campbell. Major Adams' letter to the council from Patna dated 18 October informs us that Dr Campbell had been sent to Chehel Sitoon, where the English sick were. There he was killed with the others by Sumroo's men on 11 October. Anderson probably also died at the same place, since the last entry in his diary records, 'Heard this morning that Mr Ellis and 47 gentlemen were cut off last night, so that doubtless our fate must be in 24 hours, for which God prepare us all!' The same day Anderson wrote a letter to his friend, Dr Davidson. He wrote, 'Sumero and his Sepoys arrived here last night, and I suppose to effect his wicked designs, for last night Mr Ellis and 48 gentlemen were murdered, and as almost an equal number remains, of soldiers and us, I expect my fate this night'. He was not afraid of dying, for he had long expected such an end, 'I must therefore, as a dying man, request you to collect and remit home my fortune as soon as possible, and write home a comforting letter to my father and mother'. Yet, sorrow at an untimely death broke through, and Anderson wrote, 'Oh, Davidson, be not over anxious for a fortune; let mediocrity satisfy you, and go home, and comfort your friends and mine'.

In his last hours Anderson was perhaps regretting his decision to serve in Bengal.

At this point, successive defeats made Mir Kasim suspicious of his Armenian commanders, particularly Khoja Gregory, who had relations living in Calcutta. Khoja Gregory was popular with his troops, which Mir Kasim also resented. Hence Gregory was assassinated in his camp on the night of 2 October 1763. Another event that might have precipitated this action was the surrender of Monghyr by its commander the same evening. Mir Kasim had moved to Patna, and the fall of Monghyr infuriated him such that he ordered the immediate execution of all the English prisoners, which was carried out on 5 October 1763 by Sumroo. Among the dead were Ellis, his wife, and their child. The English sick and wounded in the Chehel Sitoon were killed on 11 October. Dr William Fullerton, who was much respected by Mir Kasim for his professional skill, had been permitted to live in the Dutch factory, which ensured his survival. Soon Fullerton escaped and joined Major Adams's force, as did 4 sergeants, who had similarly run away. The author of the *Siyar ul Mutaqherin* noted that 'Of all the prisoners, not a man remained alive, save Dr Fullerton, who, by assisting most of the grandees of the court, had endeared himself to them: he even had Mir Kasim himself for an acquaintance and friend'.

Patna fell by assault in November 1763, and Mir Kasim fled into Oudh, vainly pursued to the border by an English detachment. Major Adams, ill and fatigued, left the command to Major Knox in December 1763 and returned to Calcutta, where he died on 16 January, just before he was to leave for England. Knox too was unwell, and he gave the command to Major Sherlock, and similarly proceeded to Calcutta, to die there like his predecessor. In the meantime, the English army was rocked by a series of mutinies in which Europeans and sepoys participated, dissatisfied due to their feeling that they had not been adequately compensated despite Mir Jafar's promises of a bounty. Eventually Major Hector Munro's arrival precipitated matters, bringing Shuja ud Daulah, who had already fought the English earlier in 1764 to a conclusive battle on 23 October 1764, the Battle of Buxar, which permanently established English dominance in the region. Mir Kasim eventually escaped, and lived the life of a vagrant, moving from place to place as a supplicant, until he died on 6 June 1777 in extreme poverty near Delhi. Mir Jafar died on 5 February 1765, aged 74, and was succeeded by his second son, Nawab Nazam ud Daulah, who ruled for only a year, and on his death was succeeded by his younger brother, Saif ud Daulah, who perished at the age of 17 in the smallpox epidemic that assailed Murshidabad in 1770. The title of the Nawab of Bengal was abolished in 1880, the last Nawab being Mansur Ali Khan

(1830-1884). The title had been made redundant in 1773 by the appointment of Warren Hastings as the first Governor General.

Sumroo deserted Mir Kasim's service as soon as he saw his former employer defeated, with no hopes of regaining his realm. With his troops, whose ferocity matched his, he reportedly robbed Mir Kasim's treasury, and went first into the service of a Rohilla chieftain, then the Raja of Bhartpur, the Maharaja of Jaipur and, finally, the Emperor, Shah Alam through his vizier, Najaf Khan. Najaf Khan hired him and his men for a monthly salary of 65,000 rupees. He was granted the *jagir* of Sardhana, 40 miles north of Delhi, where he settled down and fortified the place. After 1763 he seems to have been in constant fear of being apprehended by the English through betrayal, for they wanted him for the massacre he had perpetrated. Sumroo also married, at Sardhana, a beautiful young lady, who thereafter became famous as Begum Sumroo. Sumroo died on 4 May 1778, aged 58, and was first buried in the garden of his home, his remains being later disinterred and buried again in the churchyard of the Roman Catholic Church there. Begum Sumroo died in 1838, at a highly advanced age.

While Fullerton's account following the incident lists Campbell as a merchant, those who find no mention in any contemporary account are the 8 'Black Doctors' attached to the sepoy battalions in Patna. The 2nd and 3rd battalions both had 3 'Black Doctors' each, while the 5th had 2. No one knows what their fate was. The interesting thing is that they were rated after the lascars and washer men. Were these 'Black Doctors' trained surgeons' mates, or were they only medical assistants? Of Fullerton, little remains of direct interest to the subject of this book. He was accused of treason by General Carnac in November 1765, on the ground that he had deliberately concealed knowledge of traitorous correspondence between Raja Nandakumar and Raja Balwant Singh in 1764. In a letter dated 24 March 1766 addressed by the Calcutta council to the Company, we find that Fullerton was called down from Patna to 'vindicate himself', which he did on 25 February 1765. Subsequently Fullerton was acquitted of 'any ill-design in concealing his knowledge of the letter from General Carnac' but was censured for not having given him 'intelligence of the discovery'. In any case, Dr William Fullerton, after a long and full career in Bengal, seems to have sailed for England in April 1766, with the feeling that he had been wronged and, possibly, enough money for a comfortable life at home.

CHAPTER FOUR

JOHN ZEPHANIAH HOLWELL: SURGEON, COUNCILLOR, GOVERNOR

One of the earliest medical tracts on disease in Bengal is by John Zephaniah Holwell (1711 – 1798), he of the 'Holwell Monument' fame, whose recounting of the Black Hole of Calcutta created an everlasting and contentious myth. Holwell was born in Dublin to Zephaniah Holwell, a timber merchant. He was educated at Richmond Green and Rotterdam, to be an accountant. He fell ill there and returned to England, where his father, finding him uninterested in business, apprenticed him to a surgeon, Mr Forbes, in Southwark. In 1729 Zephaniah Howell died, leaving his widow and son a small inheritance. Zephaniah's death was followed by that of Mr Forbes, which allowed Joseph to become apprentice to Mr Andrew Cooper, senior surgeon of Guy's Hospital, London. Following Cooper's death in 1732, Holwell found a job as surgeon's mate aboard the East Indiaman *The Duke of Cumberland*. He sailed to Calcutta, and was appointed there to a frigate belonging to the Company. He next sailed from Calcutta to Persia and back. He spent much of his leisure time learning Arabic and some local languages. In 1734 he voyaged to Surat aboard another East Indiaman. On returning to Calcutta, Holwell was appointed 'surgeon-major' to the 'Patna Party', an annual exercise during which 400 European infantry travelled from Calcutta to the factory at Patna at the end of September every year. Next Holwell sailed again to Arabia, which helped him perfect his knowledge of the language. Then he once more became doctor to the Patna Party, after which he became tired of wandering, and was appointed surgeon to the factory in Dacca. During this time he learnt Urdu and Hindi. He returned to Calcutta at the end of 1736, and in 1740 became assistant surgeon at the Company's hospital. He had spent the intervening years as an alderman at the Mayor's court. In 1746 he became senior surgeon of the hospital and, successively, Mayor of Calcutta in 1747 and 1748. In 1749 he returned to England, and presented a detailed paper on the finances of Bengal to the Court of Directors, as a result of which he was appointed to the Company's covenanted service as

Collector of Calcutta, and placed twelfth in council though under condition that he would receive no further promotion. Holwell returned to Calcutta in 1751 and assumed his responsibilities in this capacity.

His financial measures soon proved so effective in eradicating malfeasance that the Directors removed the bar to his promotion and granted him an increase in salary of 4000 rupees a year. In 1756, when Siraj ud Daulah invaded Calcutta, Holwell was seventh in council. Released from captivity on 31 July 1756 by Siraj ud Daulah, Holwell was permitted to return to England to report to the Court. He famously reached England in February 1757, and was back in India towards the close of the following year. Although he had not been allowed to rise higher than seventh in council, he found that circumstances had promoted him to fourth, and in 1759 Holwell became second in council, under the governorship of Clive. With Clive's departure to England, Holwell became the temporary governor of Bengal on 28 January 1760, achieving thereby his coveted promotion. However, he had served the Company as a covenanted servant for only 9 years, and despite his bravery in action in 1756, there were other, more eligible Company's employees in India, looking to the same post. Holwell was superseded on 27 July 1760 by Henry Vansittart, and he resigned the Company's service in September 1760 and returned home. It was well that he had resigned, since he and several others were dismissed by the Company in 1761 for sending a despatch to London the previous year, opposing Vansittart's appointment. He lived another 38 years there, publishing several works but earning little money, due to which he died nearly penniless on 5 November 1798, having lived a long life, full of adventure. None of his contemporaries survived as long as he did. He was rightly disappointed with the Company for having given him little in return for his service.

Holwell's book is titled, *An Account of the Manner of Inoculating for the Smallpox in the East Indies with Some Observations on the Practice and Mode of Treating that Disease in those Parts*. Published in September 1767, ten years after the Battle of Plassey, this tract is remarkable in that Holwell declares that his intention in publishing this book is fuelled by 'the great benefit' that mankind would gain, in comparing the method of inoculation practiced 'time out of mind,' by the Brahmins of 'Indostan,' with the then current method in Europe, which has given 'such marvellous success'. In 1767, Holwell had been back home 6 years, and he presumably wished to begin practicing surgery again. It is interesting to note that Holwell, still sailing on his reputation as the semi-official historian of the Black Hole incident, was also made a Fellow of the Royal

Society the same year, but for his original research as published in this book.

Holwell is aware that in taking up the pen to write on a medical subject, he is about to begin discussing matters, which had not been in his 'thoughts and attention' for 26 years. Equally remarkable is Holwell's willingness to advocate the ancientness of Indian medical practice: 'the same salutary method' of inoculation, 'so happily pursued' in England, the fact notwithstanding that it 'has been seemingly blundered upon', actually having 'the sanction of remotest antiquity', as understood through its established use by Indian medical practitioners. Further, 'inoculation in the East, has natural fears and superstitious fears, to encounter, as well as in the West'. Considering that Holwell had survived the Black Hole, his advocacy is unique, when compared to the generally violent, revengeful, and denigrating, attitude adopted by Europeans towards natives during and after the Mutiny. Holwell's contribution in tracing the roots of the ancient Indian practice of inoculation is singularly praiseworthy.

Holwell traces small-pox back to 'the period in which the *Aughtorrah Bhade* scriptures of the Gentoos were promulgated (according to the Brahmins three thousand three hundred and sixty six years ago; this disease must have been of some standing, as those scriptures institute a form of divine worship, with *Poojahs*, or offerings, to a female Divinity, styled by the common people *Gootee ka Tagooran* (the Goddess of Spots) whose aid and patronage are invoked during the continuance of the Small Pox season, also in the Measles, and every cutaneous Eruption that is in the smallest degree epidemical'. Holwell was referring to the *Atharva Veda*, which contains, among other matters, incantations and spells to protect against, and heal, diseases. When writing this treatise sitting at his desk in England, Holwell must have been recalling Bengal rather wistfully. It probably wasn't just the climate, even though he states that 'from the middle of October to the middle of February is the cold season, which never rises to a degree of freezing; the whole globe does not yield a more desirable or delightful climate than Bengal during these four months'. The style of life he had been leading in Bengal would have been prohibitively expensive back home. In Bengal he had the authority to deal with Rajas and Nawabs, to sit in council and decide upon the fate of a realm larger England, and many times wealthier. It was only possible in India to arrive an assistant surgeon, and rise to become a Governor.

Inoculation against smallpox in India, Holwell writes, is the task of a special class of Brahmins, who have been trained in this task, at 'different Colleges of Bindoobund [Vrindavan], Eleabas [Allahabad], and Banaras.' Their method is to divide themselves into small groups of three or four each, and 'plan their travelling circuits in such wise as to arrive at the places of their respective destination some weeks before the usual return of the disease'. They reach Bengal in February, when the weather is best. Holwell, still recalling his years there, says that it is 'the freedom of living, which the Europeans fall into at this season, sow the seeds of those diseases which spring up in all the succeeding months of the year'. The hot season, which covers the period from March through July, is not too bad either, in Holwell's opinion, so long as the air is often 'agitated and refreshed' with North Westers, and people do not expose themselves to the hot winds. Otherwise, he says, this season produces 'high inflammatory disorders of the liver, breast, pleura, and intestines, with dysenteries, and a deplorable species of the small-pox'. Holwell's constant reminiscing about his time in Bengal adds to the historicity of his treatise. He recalls, for instance, that in 1744 – 45, there was no rain from the 20 October to the 20 June. These personal touches make his patently scientific work unique. The worst weather, from the medical perspective, covers the period July – September, when 'the atmosphere is loaded with suffocating heat and moisture, the parents of putrefaction … and nervous putrid fevers (approaching sometimes to pestilential) take the lead, and mark the dangerous season'. While locals recover from these distempers, Europeans usually do not, 'especially if they in the preceding May and June indulged too freely in those two *bewitching delicacies, Mangos* and *Mango Fish*, indiscriminately with the free use of *flesh* and *wine*' [Holwell's emphasis]. All these burden the European physic that death never fails to reap a harvest in this season. Holwell names the pestilential, putrid fever endemic to this season the '*Bengal Fever*,' and proceeds to deliberate its peculiarities.

The preliminary symptoms, which are insidious, occupy the first 2 days, and are not taken seriously, include an 'unaccountable lassitude,' aided by the lack of adequate sleep, the 'failure of natural moisture in the mouth,' and an overall depression, but with 'no acute complaint whatsoever, nor preternatural heat, that should indicate a fever'. The European patient addresses these symptoms by attributing them to the season, and staying at home, or going out oftener, in order to suppress the depression and lassitude. The increase in these symptoms on the third day alarms the patient, who sends only too late for the doctor to be of any help. Holwell writes that 'in the course of eighteen years' practice I never knew an instance of recovery from this genuine fever, where the first three days had elapsed without assistance, and the patient in this case died on the fifth or seventh day'. The physician's findings would include either a 'full, equal, undisturbed pulse, but obviously greatly *oppressed*,' or 'a low and *depressed* one, but equal, and undisturbed also' [Holwell's emphases].

Doctors new to the diseases of Bengal would make the error of misreading the 'full' pulse, 'which they thought indicated the loss of blood', that is, indicated the need for blood-letting. Once mistaken, 'they followed the suggestion, the pulse suddenly fell, and when that happens from this cause, the art of man can never raise it again, the patient dies on the fifth or seventh day', the consequence being exactly the same, 'if Nature, being overloaded, attempted to free herself of part of the burden' by a haemorrhage or through the intestines, on the second or third day. Holwell recommended a critical examination of the urine on the sixth day. If the fever remained even, and the urine 'natural,' there was hope; if the fever rose suddenly and the urine appeared 'crude and limpid,' 'it was a sure presage of death on the seventh'. If treated 'judiciously' by the physician from the very beginning, the urine on the tenth day showed 'a copious sediment and separation', and there followed a crisis on the eleventh day, which appeared 'in a multitude of small boils, chiefly upon the head, or in small watery bladders thrown out upon the surface of the skin, but in the greatest abundance on the breast, neck, throat, and forehead'. It was vital to now keep the patient well-guarded from the cold, for if by 'any inadvertent exposure to the cold air, these eruptions were struck in, the repelled matter fell instantly upon the brain, and convulsions and death followed in a few hours, and small purple spots remained in the places of the eruptions'. This, Holwell asserts, is the course of 'the *genuine putrid nervous fever of Bengal*' which responds to only treatment employing the application of blisters, 'supported by the strongest alexipharmics' [Holwell's emphasis]. Sometimes a patient may linger on for months, or may, at other times, linger on, 'in a dying way,' until February, when the season changes. The patient's health however, remains impaired until the return of 'the salutary *mango season*, which fruit, eaten with milk, proves an effectual and never-failing restorative'.

The 'Inoculating Brahmins,' prescribe a preparatory diet for those wishing to undergo inoculation, to be followed for a month preceding the operation. This diet involves abstention from fish, milk, and ghee. Only if a patient has undertaken with absolute commitment the necessary diet, will they proceed. These Brahmins would move from house to house, operating at the door, and asking, so Holwell tells us, 'the Parents how many Pocks they choose their Children should have … [and] true it is, that they hardly ever exceed, or are deficient, in the number required'. 'Vanity, we should think', Holwell wrote, 'urged a question on a matter seemingly so uncertain in the issue'. The fact was, as he admiringly found, that 'they hardly ever exceed or are deficient of in the number required'. Holwell admiringly wrote, 'of the multitudes I have seen inoculated in that country, the number of pustules have been seldom less than fifty, and hardly ever exceeded two hundred'.

They inoculated males midway between the wrist and elbow, and females between elbow and shoulder. The method of inoculation was simple. It began with 'a dry friction' of the intended part for around 10 minutes with a cloth. By this means 'the circulation in the small sanguinary vessels is accelerated'. Then, using a small instrument, 'four and a half inches long', the size of 'a large crow quill', of which the middle is twisted, and 1 inch of one end is steeled and flattened, the extremity having a 'very keen edge' and two sharp corners. The other end of the instrument was 'an ear picker' of the sort used by Indian barbers 'to cut the nails and depurate the ears of their customers'. Next the 'Operator of Inoculation holds the instrument as we hold a pen, and with dextrous expedition gives about fifteen or sixteen minute scarifications with one of the sharp corners of the instrument' of circumference of a 'silver groat'. Their precision is such there only is 'the smallest appearance of blood'. Taking a cotton wound inside a 'linen double rag (which he always keeps in a cloth round his waist) a small pledgit of cotton charged with the variolous matter, which he moistens with two or three drops of the Ganges water, and applies it on the wound'. The Ganges water causes the variolous to be 'readily and eagerly received', while sanctifying the process at the same time. In Holwell's view, Ganges water 'may have as much efficacy as any other holy water'. This bit of cotton is fixed on the wound with a loose bandage, and ordered to be kept unmoved for 6 hours, after which the bandage is removed while the cotton allowed is to stay in place until it falls of its own. Rarely the inoculators squeezed a drop of water from the cotton on to the wound before placing it. Holwell testily dismisses arguments over the best method of scarification, presumably contentions over the supremacy of European methods, saying 'I cannot help thinking that too much has been said (pro and con) about nothing … provided the matter is thrown into the blood, it is certainly a consideration of most trivial import by what means it is effected'. The inoculation is a most solemn occasion, as represented by the serious demeanour of the inoculators, who chanted appropriate sacred verses while inoculating.

Howell particularly noted that the cotton employed by the inoculators was 'saturated with matter from the inoculated pustules of the preceding year, for they never inoculate with fresh matter, nor with matter from the disease caught in the natural way, however distinct and mild the species'.

The patient was required to follow a strict regimen. Fish, milk, and ghee, were prohibited from the diet, and following the onset of fever, the patient is allowed 'all the refrigerating things the climate and season produces, such as plantains, sugarcanes, watermelon, rice, gruel made of white poppy-seeds, and cold water, or thin rice gruel for their ordinary drink'. Analysing this from the standpoint of contemporary European medical theory, Holwell opined that fish constituted a 'viscid and inflammatory diet, tending to foul and tending to obstruct the cutaneous glands and excretory ducts, and to create in the stomach and first passages a tough, slimy phlegm, highly injurious to the human constitution'. The forbiddance of milk, however, surprised him, since the local diet included the consumption of milk and milk products, until he learned from local practitioners that 'milk becomes highly nutritious, not only from its natural qualities, but also from its ready admission into the blood, and quick assimilation with it'. Therefore, milk was a 'warm, heating diet', which 'must have a remote tendency to inflammation, whenever the blood is thrown into any preternatural ferment', particularly during sickness. Holwell extrapolates this further by saying that local women do not partake of milk 'during the course of their periodical visitations', since this could, 'upon any accidental cold, dispose the uterus to inflammation and ulceration'. He proceeds to state that 'our European women, resident in India', drawing directly from this experience, 'have adopted the same precaution … and will not, from any consideration, at those times, mix the smallest quantity with their tea'. European women in India, he says, learnt this from the midwives attending them, who were locals, and 'instructed in their calling by the Brahmins and other Practitioners in the Physic'. The prohibition of ghee involved a prohibition of 'all fat and oily substances'.

From the morning of the day following the inoculation, the patient was to be doused in 8 gallons of cold water from the head downwards, every morning and evening, until fever set in. The water was collected in vessels the evening before, and left overnight to collect the dew and become intensely cold. 2 servants would pour the water on the patient's head from 'a distance of six or twelve inches above the head'. Taking up the argument whether immersion in cold water was more effective than cold bathing, in relation to whether 'the weight and pressure of the circumambient body of water' was more important than the shock of being doused in cold water, Holwell concluded that the latter was more effective. It had a 'longer continuance … the severity of one being nothing comparable to the other'. 'I never had a patient', Holwell asserted, 'that did not aver the same, who had undergone both trials'. In fact, the shock of cold bathing was so intense that for his European patients, 'in many cases, when the subject was deeply exhausted and relaxed, I have found it absolutely necessary to begin the course only with a *quart* of water'. The 'Eastern' explanation for the usefulness of cold bathing was that 'by the sudden shock of the cold water, and increased motion of the blood, all offensive principles are forcibly driven from the heart, brain, and other interior parts of the body, towards the extremities and surface, and at the same time the intended fermentation is thereby more speedily and certainly promoted'. Cold bathing was useful for the same reasons in 'Palsies, Rheumatisms, general relaxation of the solids, and particular relaxation of the stomach and intestines'. The twice-daily regimen of cold bathing provided fresh impetus to the blood to drive the '*immediate*' cause of smallpox to the pustules. Holwell wrote, 'I have myself been an eye witness to many instances of its marvellous effect, where the pustules have sunk, when the patient appeared in imminent danger, but almost instantly restored by the application of three or four collans of cold water'.

Fever usually struck from the evening of the 6th day after inoculation. The patient was then 'to desist until the appearance of the eruptions', which took place at the close of the 'third complete day' from the onset of fever. Bathing in cold water resumed until the scabs of the pustules fell off. In fact, the pustules were ordered to be opened with a thorn as soon as they changed colour and 'whilst the matter continued in a fluid state'. To Holwell this practice was 'so important, so self-evidently rational and essential', that 'it effectually prevents inflammation and weakness of the eyes, biles, and other eruptions and disorders, which commonly succeed the disease'. In very severe cases, Holwell has seen these inoculators at work for hours, with 'amazing patience and solicitude', opening the pustules themselves. 'I hardly knew it fail', he recorded, 'of either entirely preventing the *second fever*, or mitigating it in such sort, as to render it of no consequence'. It was important to use 'a very fine sharpened thorn' in preference to European instruments like lancets, scissors, or needles. The method use by the locals is unique, since they apply the thorn to 'the most prominent part of the Pustule, and with the sides of the thorn, press out the pus'. They wash the area thus covered with 'a calico rag, dipped in warm water and milk'. The orifice made by the thorn is so small that it closes immediately after the pus is squeezed out, 'so that there is no admission of the external air into the Pustule, which would suddenly contract the mouths of the excretory vessels, and consequently further secretion of the variolous matter from the blood would be thereby obstructed'. Those European practitioners in favour of opening the pustules advised the use of scissors, which Holwell objected to, 'as the aperture would be too large'.

Contrary to the usual European practice of confining the patient indoors with the onset of fever here 'Confinement to the house is absolutely forbid, and the inoculated are ordered to be exposed to every air that blows'. Even at the height of fever, the patient is allowed to lie on a mat at the door. Once the fever abates and the pustules fall off, the Goddess is worshipped, and the inoculator receives his money, a pound of 'cowries', equivalent, in Holwell's time, to 'a penny sterling'.

In the final analysis, since this system of inoculation provided safety from the disease, Holwell concluded in a manner that would become both unfashionable and illogical less than a century later, that since 'this practice of the East has been followed without variation, and with uniform success from the remotest known times, it is but justice to conclude it must have been originally founded on the basis of rational principles and experiment'. As a European surgeon, Holwell admitted that he was 'very early prejudiced in preference of the cool regimen and the free admission of air, in the treatment of this disease', he nonetheless felt that 'the Brahmins carried both to a bold, rash, and dangerous extreme'. Soon practical experience convinced him of 'the propriety of their method', and he successfully pursued the same treatment. 'I will venture to say', Holwell added, 'that every gentleman in the Profession who did not adopt the same mode (making a necessary distinction and allowance between the constitutions of the Natives and Europeans) have lost many a patient which might otherwise have been saved'.

Holwell propounded local medical belief that all epidemics, especially smallpox, arose from 'an *immediate* (or instant) cause' that 'exists in the mortal part of every human and *animal* form', which was stirred up and thrown into 'a state of fermentation' by a '*mediate* (or second) *acting* cause'. This second cause consisted of 'multitudes of *imperceptible animalculae* floating in the atmosphere'. These pass in and out of the body with the breath, causing harm only when the food they cover is eaten. Only then do 'their malignant juices excite a peculiar fermentation'. Stating that this theory is not unique to Indians, Holwell presents it as a tenable explanation to why particular parts of the globe are prone at certain times of year to epidemics. 'I hope I shall not be thought to refine too much on the argument', he wrote, 'if I give it as my opinion that epidemical blights, and epidemical diseases of one kind or other may be observed to go often hand in hand with each other, but from the same identical cause'.

The 'Eastern practitioners' disagree with the European practice phlebotomy and the use of cathartics. Venesection 'weakens the natural powers', while cathartics counteract 'the regular course of nature'. Holwell concluded his treatise by hoping that the Indian practice of smallpox inoculation would throw 'new and beneficial lights on this cruel and destructive disease'. His particular hope was that European doctors would bring into '*regular and universal practice the cool regimen and free admission of Air*'.

Holwell was willing to learn from his medical experience in Bengal, and apply the knowledge thus attained to the betterment of his people. As we shall see in the next chapter, this was not an unusual attitude. Racial superiority was yet to colour common sense. In a sense, the sequel to Holwell's tract is Major S P James' *Smallpox and Vaccination in British India* (1909). James quotes Holwell extensively, and notes that the successful inoculation recorded by Holwell derived from the fact that the inoculators or '*ticcadars*' followed the 'rules' of hygiene as prescribed in European medical theory. James entirely misses the fact that the Indian inoculators were vaccinating people long before it had become popular in Europe, and this was the reason why Holwell observed the process so closely and recorded it. James is also supercilious in saying that another reason for successful inoculations in Bengal, Assam, and Burma, where the process described by Holwell was practised, was that people there 'lived in small villages or hamlets, each house being some distance from the next, and each village or hamlet a mile or more from neighbouring ones'. Hence 'with the strict rules of segregation in force, the danger of spreading the disease set up by inoculation was not great'. The increasing obtuseness of English doctors in accepting the possible superiority of local medical practice is exemplified by James' further statement that by the 1830s, an established cause of the spread of smallpox in Calcutta was the arrival of inoculators. These persons no longer followed the 'rules' formerly enforced. Additionally, they charged exorbitant fees. Inoculating a male child in 1850 was 4 annas and some rice, and for a girl, 2 annas. Other writers, James tells us, recorded that the lowest fee charged was 2 or 3 rupees, while the highest was 16 rupees and a shawl. In the same year, 1850, James quotes the report of the Civil Surgeon of Serampore, whose questioning of an inoculator revealed that he had vaccinated 400 persons, of whom 200 had died. James also referred to the finding of the Smallpox Committee, on the authority of the editor of a 'respectable Bengali newspaper – the *Bhaskar*' that of 1000 children who were inoculated by local methods, 300 had died. Further, since the inoculator was paid only if fever and eruption followed inoculation, James noted that in order to achieve this quickly, they often gave a 'small quantity of smallpox matter internally' when the cutaneous procedure seemed slow. James noted that in France smallpox inoculation had become illegal in 1763, while in England it required Jenner's demonstration of vaccination to make inoculation unlawful. Lord Wellesley had vainly striven to pass a law in 1804 against inoculation in Calcutta and it was only in 1865 that inoculation was banned by law in Calcutta and its suburbs, before being finally declared illegal in British India on 13 November 1870.

James records the excitement caused in medical circles in Calcutta in 1804, when news of Jenner's successes was received. He refers to Dr John Shoolbred, who reported the arrival of this news in his paper, 'Report on the Introduction and Progress of Vaccine Inoculation in Bengal'. Shoolbred wrote that doctors 'anticipated with anxiety and pleasure the acquisition of a discovery which promised an exemption from pain, misery, and premature death, to so large a portion of mankind'. Edward Jenner seems to have put a book on vaccination and a container of lymph aboard an East Indiaman, the *Queen* in 1799, which, having been wrecked, never reached Bengal. James writes, 'Jenner … then engaged that if twenty recruits who had not had smallpox were selected and he were allowed to select a surgeon to attend them, vaccine should be conveyed in the most perfect state to any of our settlements'. This was not a feasible means of transmitting the vaccine, until some years later, when it was carried most precariously overland from London via Vienna and Constantinople to Dr James Short in Baghdad, where a child was vaccinated, and sent down to Mr Milne, surgeon at the port of Basra, from where the collected lymph was despatched to Bombay, where Dr Scott made a successful inoculation on the arm of 3-year-old Anna Dusthall on 14 June 1802. The vaccine was sent on to Ceylon and most parts of India, except Bengal, to which all attempts at despatch failed until a means that appears terrible to us today, was adopted. A boy, John Creswell, aged 13, was vaccinated in Madras by Dr James Anderson, and accompanied aboard a ship to Calcutta with a number of other children, which sailed on 10 October 1802. On the ship, Anderson next vaccinated a girl on 22 October and from her a Malay boy on 2 November, and from him Charles Norton, 15, 'who arrived at Calcutta on the 17th November 1802, with a genuine pustule of the sixth day on each arm'. Almost immediately on landing, several English children were vaccinated, and in this way the vaccine was kept alive. Dr William Russell was appointed Superintendent-General of Vaccination, and in 1804 Dr Shoolbred took over this post from Russell. Shoolbred's opposition to local inoculators led to disaffection and resistance, to overcome which pensions for life were granted in February 1805 to the ticcadars. This was followed by a signed declaration by 26 ticcadars on 23 April 1805 that they believed in the efficacy of vaccination as an improvement on inoculation. Vaccination was encouraged by doles of rice and payment in lieu of vaccine crusts collected by locals. In May 1806, the inhabitants of Calcutta gifted Dr Edward Jenner £4000, Bombay £2000, and Madras £1383.

The further history of smallpox vaccination in India need not detain us. James tells us that between 1802 and 1836, the Company spent over 3,500,000 rupees on 'vaccine establishments'. By 1838, the 'dispensary system of vaccination' had been established throughout the Presidency of Bengal, which involved the setting up of dispensaries supervised by civil surgeons in 12 towns in the Presidency. 'An educated native sub-assistant surgeon' was in charge of the dispensary, and he was helped by some trained assistants. This system in more or less the same form remained in place until the twentieth century.

CHAPTER FIVE

FRANCIS BALFOUR AND THE SOL-LUNAR INFLUENCE IN FEVERS

Little is known about the early life of Francis Balfour. After obtaining an MD from the University of Edinburgh, he joined service in the Bengal Army on 3 July 1769 as assistant surgeon. On 10 August 1777 he was appointed surgeon. Between 1784 and 1789 he was in charge of the general hospitals at Varanasi, Chunar, and Calcutta. During this period he studied the fevers of India and wrote treatises on their treatises. He left for England in May 1789, and spent his time on the voyage reworking his theories. Balfour was in Britain during 1790-92. He was in Bengal in 1793, and remained there until 1798. Balfour returned to Bengal for the second time in 1800. By 1805 he had compiled his tracts on the fevers in Bengal into one volume, which he dedicated to the Governor-General, Lord Wellesley. Unlike most of his contemporaries, who either died or resigned the service, Francis Balfour retired on 16 September 1807, at the end of 37 years of service in India. He returned to his native city of Edinburgh, and we know nothing about his subsequent life, other than that he was alive in 1815, since the third edition of his book, *A Collection of Treatises on the Effects of Sol-Lunar Influence in Fevers with an Improved Method of curing them*, appeared in London that year with a memorial prefaced to it by Balfour. In fact, this book was his swansong, for in the preface he writes that he is 'On the eve of bidding adieu to every controversy on the subject of medicine'. In Balfour's view, the diseases of Bengal 'belong chiefly, and almost wholly, to the class of fevers, in which are included dysenteries, etc'.

Balfour's first treatise is titled *On the Influence of the Moon in Fevers* (1784). He begins by declaring that his stay of 14 years in India has convinced him of the influence of the moon on fevers, and this conviction has 'directed my practice on every occasion'. This led him to 4 axioms: first, that 'in Bengal, fevers of every denomination are, in a remarkable manner, connected with, and affected by, the revolutions of the moon'; second, that 'in Bengal, a constant and particular attention to the revolutions of the moon, is of the greatest importance in the cure and prevention of fevers'; third, that 'the influence of the moon in fevers prevails, in a similar manner, in every part of the globe'; and finally, that 'the whole doctrine of the crisis of fevers may be readily explained, from the premises established … in these disorders, at the full and change'.

We learn from Balfour that in Bengal, 'the bilious intermittent fever, which appears for the most part in the form of a tertian, or of a quotidian, and seldom in that of a quartan, is by far the most common fever in this country'. 'I have almost invariably observed', he wrote 'that its first attack is on one of the three days that immediately precede the full of the moon'. The full and change of the moon also causes relapses, which 'few Europeans, who have resided for any time in this country' have not seen either in their own cases or of their friends'. Addressing those who would doubt this conclusion, Balfour asserts that 'whenever a number of the sick are collected in one place, and a multiplicity of corresponding proofs are repeatedly presented at the same instant, persuasion follows insensibly, and every doubt is removed'. During 1773-74 he was surgeon to a regiment of sepoys in Cooch Behar, in the Himalayan foothills. The sepoys were ill with 'chiefly fevers or fluxes attended with fever'. At first 400 sepoys fell ill, a number which was reduced to 70 or 80 through treatment. However, those who recovered did so in the 8 days between the full and change of the moon, and increased to double this number at every full and change. This did not mean that fevers and relapses were absent during the interval between full and change, 'But these happen much less frequently at this time, and when they occur, furnish arguments to support the proposition we are trying to prove: for the fits are now less severe, of shorter duration, and yield much more easily to medicine'.

The other type of fever common in Bengal is the 'remittent fever'. These are either 'purely bilious or of a putrid tendency', like the infamous 'pucca fever of Bengal', or 'rheumatic and nervous fevers' or yet that which accompanies smallpox. In all these fevers too 'the influence of the full and change never failed to show itself in a remarkable manner'. In cases of headache, toothache, 'inflammations of the eyes, asthmas, pains and swelling of the liver and spleen, fluxes, spasms and obstructions in the bowels, complaints in the urinary passages, eruptions of different kinds, and a great many more', full and change intensify the disorder, which 'diminish and disappear' during the interval. 'I am fully convinced myself', Balfour asserted, 'of the truth of this conclusion from my own experience, and … in almost every case where I have had an opportunity of attending to fevers at the period when the full or change expired, I have observed almost invariably, either some symptom of the abatement of the fever, or a perfect solution'. He concluded that the interval represented a '*favourable critical period*' in fevers, while the full and change stood for the opposite, an '*unfavourable critical period*' [Balfour's emphases]. He called for detailed experiments along these lines, to establish his theory that certain changes took place in the '*state or quality in the air*' during these periods which, during full and change, increased fever and took it to an unhappy termination, and during the intervals, diminished the fever, allowing the physician to act quickly to help nature. In other words, the febriferous influence decreased during the intervals, and increased during full and change. In some cases, 'the symptoms run extremely high', and the influence of the moon, operating through the favourable and unfavourable critical periods, might not be discernable to the physician, although Balfour would hasten to reassure him that such influence 'still continues to be exerted', and must therefore be taken into account for treatment.

Balfour's experience was that 'the attack of intermittents' during the evil influence of full and change was particularly noticeable between 8 am and 6 pm. The remittents also exert their worst during this period, while the remissions are mostly seen between 3 am and 8 am. Balfour particularly affirmed his experience of treating the remittent pucca fever of Bengal during the 'season' of 1769-70 by proactively using 'the bark in powder'. The 'bark in powder' is of course cinchona. Balfour proclaimed the use of the 'bark in powder' as a 'certain cure' for the pucca fever of Bengal, stating that 'it may be given in safety at all periods of the disease; whether in the remission or exacerbation', and should the patient's body reject the medicine by vomiting or diarrhoea, 'opium will in all cases make it sit quietly'. In fact, 'opium may be given in any moderate does, during any symptom, and at any stage of the disease'. Further, 'a speedy termination' of the fever could be achieved 'by an early and vigorous exhibition of the bark'. This checks the fever, and 'prevents the putrefaction from making any advances' while other drugs continued to 'evacuate the corrupted contents of the bowels, and to supply the system with fresh stores of ascescent nourishment'.

Nervous fevers were, Balfour believed, 'nothing more than putrid fevers, in a lower degree', which were also effectively treated with the bark. Similarly, the rheumatic fever, characterised by a 'large secretion of bile', was treated in the same way.

Unlike many doctors then and now, Balfour admitted to his mistakes as well. On being posted to 'the upper and more healthy parts of the country', where 'the pucca fever very seldom makes its appearance', Balfour was 'often misled into a premature exhibition of the bark', while the fevers he encountered there needed nothing more ... than early and plentiful evacuations'. In these cases where the bark had been needlessly administered, it was merely vomited out, or 'if it remained in the stomach, not having the power to prevent the succeeding paroxysm, it seemed to render that more uneasy'.

Patients, in whom the liver was palpable and painful, Balfour said, 'even a slight pain of the liver does not prevent me' from administering the bark, 'unless I find it increase to any considerable degree'. In a footnote, Balfour wrote, 'The large size of the liver, its warm situation in the body, and the languid circulation and peculiar nature of the blood that passes through it, suggest the probability of relaxation, accumulation, obstruction, stagnation, corruption, and irregular secretion in this organ, in warm climates'. Consequently, 'the livers of Europeans who residing in this country are rarely to be found in a sound state'. The physician was thus advised to disregard complaints of painful livers and proceed with the administration of the bark. The aim was to stop the fever, especially 'in a country, where weakness always disposes to a relapse'. It was also the physician's responsibility to see to it that 'the want of proper sick-bed attendants' was not a hindrance. Often it happened that the 'evacuations, absolutely necessary, after every fit, whether the bark is given or not', did not take place because the drugs were not given to the patient at the proper time, which often happened at night, or because the patient vomited it, and no substitute was given, or the patient refused to take the drug, and 'a false report is made to the surgeon in the morning'. Due to this, 'bowels and circulation get loaded with bile', and 'the stomach becomes so weak and irritable, as to receive neither medicine nor nourishment'.

'I attribute my success', Balfour said, 'to the despatch and freedom with which I go through the first evacuations; to the particular care I always take to be certain that these have been properly effected'. In some cases of remittent fevers, in which it was not possible to bring about 'evacuations downwards', Balfour 'saved the patient's life by preparing the stomach with a large dose of opium, and throwing in, during its operation, a quantity of bark, sufficient to stop the fever'. In cases of fever accompanied by inflammations of the liver, 'venesection must be instituted freely ... and in many cases blisters are necessary'. Should none of these show any effect in abating the inflammation, Balfour advised the physician, 'the bark is to be given without hesitation'.

This theory of the vigorous use of the bark, combined with the influences of the moon, gave the physician ample time during the interval of full and change, 'both for plentiful evacuations, and for the bark'. However, the physician also had to beware of relapses, which occurred on the full and change, by making the patient avoid 'the common occasional causes of fever', like 'exposure to the sun, full meals of animal food, or whatever heats or irritates, and, in short, excesses of any kind'. Should his precautions for a relapse fail, 'we are then taught to remove him from with all expedition to a climate where the influence of the moon is less perceivable, and less prejudicial than it is in Bengal'. Madras was such a place, 'and a removal to that settlement from Bengal is, in many cases, almost a certain cure'.

In the case of remittents, the moment of remission was to be carefully noticed, 'and purgatives must in all cases be administered on the first signs of a remission'. 'This period', Balfour said, 'is also the proper season for throwing in the bark, and it is often of the greatest consequence not to allow a moment of it to escape'.

Though he had not much experience with smallpox inoculation, Balfour wrote, 'I am perfectly satisfied, that the full and change of the moon, interfered with the eruption, and increased the fever to a dangerous degree'. In particular, Balfour felt that his conceptualisation of the favourable and unfavourable critical periods would not only assist physicians in preventing and curing fevers in Bengal, but also 'PREDICT and EXPLAIN their various CRISIS, on grounds that are consistent and satisfactory' [his emphases].

Balfour's second treatise is titled *On Putrid Intestinal Remitting Fevers* and it was written aboard the East Indiaman *Kent*, by which he was returning to England, on 20 May 1789. His previous tract on the influences of the moon seems to have been received derisively by the medical fraternity, since Balfour writes in the preface to the second tract that 'Perceiving … upon the eve of my departure from India, that five years had elapsed without contributing anything new to establish this discovery … I instantly determined to employ the leisure of my voyage, in arranging the observations and remarks I had made myself since my first publication'. 'In the beginning of June 1788' he had explained the system of employing the favourable and unfavourable critical periods to 'the medical gentlemen who acted under me in the general hospital at Calcutta', to great success in curing fevers. To this end he begins the new treatise by stating that all remitting and putrid fevers, whether low or violent, 'all resemble one another in the *peculiar fetor* which distinguishes their stool, and marks the seat and nature of the disease'. Further, 'They are all infectious; they prevail under the same circumstances of heat, moisture, confinement, etc', and so Balfour categorised them all as 'putrid intestinal remitting fevers'. For Balfour dysentery is also a form of the same fever. His experience had in fact led him to conclude that in these fevers, 'the mucus which lines the intestines, especially the smaller, is infected, and in a putrefying state; and that this not only produces the peculiar fetor which distinguishes the seat and nature of this disease, but being absorbed and mixed with the blood, becomes the cause of that remarkable change in the system which constitutes the *febrile state*'.

The contagion, 'in all cases, found to proceed from some putrefying or putrid body' is, in this ailment 'first conveyed into the stomach and bowels along with the saliva'. With the progress of the disease, during which the 'corrupted matter' in the intestines is invariably absorbed into the blood, 'the degree of the febrile state is constantly increased when the contents of the bowel are long retained, and are become highly offensive; and as constantly prevented from increasing, when they are maturely and completely evacuated'.

Besides the peculiar fetor, the stools of the patient bore mucus 'in a loose, frothy, putrefying state'. Other symptoms included restlessness, rapid pulse, disturbed sleep, flushing of the face, redness of the eyes, and tendency to delirium and headache. In fact, Balfour wrote, 'From the observations I have made in India, not only upon men, but upon dogs and horses, I am much inclined to believe that in all animals, even when in health, there prevails in the bowels, during the lunar periods, *a stronger tendency to contract, and to retain their faeces, than during the interlunar periods*' [his emphasis]. On viewing these symptoms, the physician was to conclude that the fever was due to 'a *spasmodic affection of the vascular system*, excited and supported by the *morbific matter* absorbed from the intestines into the blood'.

From this Balfour proceeds to propound the axiom that 'the critical disposition of the febrile state' seldom resolves before 4 days have passed, with a maximum period of 21 days. Balfour encouraged the physician to observe the remissions and paroxysms as they occurred within this period by following the stages of the moon. Further, Balfour's theorem posited that 'the superior force of sol-lunar influence at the autumno-equinoctial period, first, by exciting the attacks of fevers during these periods in such as are already infected, then by propagating and spreading the infection from these to others, and again by exciting these to attack, and so forth, MORE powerfully and frequently than in the inter-equinoctial intervals, operates in a circle, and thus becomes the cause of the superior frequency, violence, and obstinacy of fevers in the autumno-equinoctial period'. The physician was advised that fevers achieving their crises in the autumn-equinoctial period were likely to be far more severe than in the inter-equinoctial period. Further, fevers passing from the autumno-equinoctial period to the winter inter-equinoctial interval, held good prognosis, tending 'to subside and terminate'.

The aim of the physician thus was to ensure evacuation of the system before the contagion severely affected it. Balfour recommended for this purpose calomel, which 'possesses the property of loosening and detaching the mucus in the intestines'. The dose for an adult was 6 to 12 grains, and it required 6 to 10 hours to work properly, 'and operates best when the patient lies quietly abed, without tossing or moving about'. Determined by the stools, calomel was to be administered 3 to 6 times at the beginning of the fever. Along with calomel, small doses of tartar emetic were to be given, in an infusion of tamarind, in small wine-glassfuls. Additionally, 'every possible means must be employed to prevent the readmission of contagious effluvia into the body, by renewing and correcting the air in which the patient breathes … and by a proper change in his linen and bedclothes'. Nourishment for the patient was a *panada*, 'A mixture of farinaceous substance, with the juice of fresh fruit, seasoned with wine, sugar, and nutmeg, or cinnamon'. This would 'counteract the putrid tendency of the disease' and be readily acceptable to the patient. However, the *panada* would have to be given after the operation of the morning laxative and 'before the approach of nocturnal exacerbation'.

The physician was to avoid 'every irregularity that may increase the violence of the fever and concur with the natural tendency of this period' by closely observing the lunar and equinoctial cyclicity. The 'final interlunar crisis' of the fever shall be understood through 'a sediment or a turbid appearance in the urine; spontaneous stools; a clearer, moister, and softer tongue, with a more free and natural discharge of saliva; a more loose and copious expectoration; a free discharge of bile'. During this period Balfour would keep his patient 'exceedingly quiet', evacuate the bowels, and use an antimonial to 'encourage a gentle perspiration'. A false remission could be identified by a quick pulse, foul tongue, 'sleep disturbed by dreams in the night', and 'instead of a proper sediment at the bottom of the glass, the urine should exhibit a suspended mucus-like cloud', even though the patient might seem fully recovered, with a completely restored appetite. In such cases the physician should beware of 'the seeds of the fever … still lurking within', and waiting for the next lunar change to strike again. Every 'young practitioner' was enjoined to learn from Balfour's own several deceptions, and give the patient the bark and opium, which provide 'great security' against the '*more dangerous forms* of these disorders'. Balfour had seen few fatalities from this disease, and of them, most seemed to occur due to an injury to the brain from the violence of the paroxysms. The most effective remedy was the bark, which could be given in wine or wine and water, though Balfour preferred 'to give it in claret without limitation; and with the best effect'.

Bloodletting was needless in India 'when there was no local affection', but became essential in case of inflammation. Aware of the pain accompanying venesection and blistering, Balfour wrote, 'since I began to regulate my practice by the rules which I have so fully explained, I have seldom had occasion to employ them; and I have considered it an improvement of some consequence, independent of its success, to be able to avoid so painful a remedy'.

There was advice for the patient too, on whom these powerful drugs would work. Laudanum would keep the patient in a restful state since one of the aims was 'to compose', but 'let it be recommended to every patient labouring under a dysentery to force himself away from the chair the moment the faeces which occasioned the call are evacuated'. 'The straining is fruitless', Balfour said, 'the best of all is to receive the faeces upon clothes introduced below the patient, for that purpose'. And in addition to the *panada*, 'Gruels, made of rice or oatmeal, are the most proper drink'.

Taking his theory of the sol-lunar influence to new heights in the study and cure of fevers, Balfour addressed the effect of the moon on urinalysis in his third tract, *On the Action of Sol-Lunar Influence* (1791), stating that 'there is to be observed in the state of the urine a *fluctuation* coincident with that of the ocean, respecting the times of the alternate changes which both undergo daily'. Further, 'Taking a comprehensive view of the subject, I think there is much reason to believe that all the different kingdoms of nature, at least the animal, vegetable, atmospheric and aqueous departments, are under the dominion of sol-lunar influence; and that, like the animal constitution, they are subject to daily and monthly revolutions'. Balfour's experience in India is obvious from the notes he appended to this treatise. 'At Calcutta, Benaras, and Lucknow, I have met with a species of ophthalmia attacking about the coming on of the rains in June, the proper method of treating which is probably not generally known'. This disease begins with a grittiness in the eyes, a slight swelling of the eyelids, and 'In the space of 4 or 5 days, the inflammation of the eye has increased, in spite of all common remedies, to so great a pitch, that it is unable to endure the smallest degree of light; the pain now begins to shoot through the head, and to produce a terrible headache, and the sclerotic coat swells and rises above the surface of the cornea'. The ailment is exacerbated during the full and change of the moon, and Balfour recommends the usual treatment of calomel, cathartic salts, and the bark. However, he adds, for the eyes, a topical ointment, whose composition he first learnt from a local: 'Take one tablespoon and a half of fresh butter, keep it boiling in a glazed pot for half an hour, free it of all impurities, and then carefully mix with it in a mortar one scruple of opium and one dram of alum, previously rubbed together in an impalpable powder'. Balfour noted that the original recipe contained 'a small portion of turmeric and neem-leaf, but not being acquainted with the effects of these articles, I was afraid, and left them out'. This ointment, when applied along the inside of the eyelids, caused 'a thin watery discharge … copiously down the cheeks', which greatly relieved the sufferer.

Two or three applications of this ointment, followed by a lotion of lead, and another ointment during the night completed the cure along with calomel and cinchona.

Another note addressed the boil which afflicted Europeans 'most frequently in the months of May and June', being 'exceedingly painful and troublesome'. Here too Balfour recorded the effectiveness of local treatment: 'About eight years ago, when afflicted with this complaint, I was advised by my servants to try an application of the leaves of the neem-tree'. The effect of this was 'sudden and conspicuous' and Balfour subsequently tried it on several occasions with equal success, 'It will produce in one or two days what cannot be effected by common means in eight or ten'. The application was made by taking a handful of neem leaves, and heating them quickly without drying them on an earthen plate or a fragment of an earthen pot. These were immediately applied to the boil, the operation, 'generally performed by the bearers who carry the palankeen', being repeated until suppuration occurred. After suppuration, emplaster diachylon was applied. This, John Ayrton Paris, in his book, *Pharmacologia* (1824) tells us, was used 'as a common application to excoriations, and for retaining the edges of fresh cut wounds in a state of apposition, and at the same time defending them from the action of the air'.

Balfour's fourth tract was *A Treatise on the Sol-Lunar Influence on Fevers* (1794), whose publication costs were defrayed by the Bengal council, under condition that copies of the book were sent to different stations in the Presidency, and 20 copies deposited with the council for despatch to the Court of Directors.

This was good news for Balfour, since his previous tracts had received with incredulity in England. Balfour's disappointment shows in the preface to this fourth tract on the same subject. 'It was natural to suppose that men of science in England', he wrote, 'would be curious to be more fully informed respecting the foundation of a theory which pretended to the discovery of a new and active principle in medicine and philosophy'.

However, 'a general silence and reserve prevailed everywhere on this subject, and left me no room to hesitate respecting the degree of credit it had obtained in my native country'. In particular, Balfour was greatly disappointed when Dr James Lind (1716-94), the naval surgeon who famously discovered in citrus fruits the cure for scurvy, trashed Balfour's theory, having previously lauded it.

Lind finally dismissed the sol-lunar theory in a letter, titled 'Some Remarks on the Supposed Influence of the Moon in Fevers' addressed to Dr Simmons and published in the *London Medical Journal* in 1787. Lind seems to have rather unkindly commented, per Balfour, that 'lunar influence will nowhere be found, but where remitting and intermitting fevers are caused by muddy shores left by the ebbing of the tide'. Lind's letter, however, is forthright. In it, Dr Lind says that he had himself been of the same opinion as Dr Balfour, as evidenced by his 'Inaugural Dissertation on the Marsh Fever, which raged in Bengal in 1762'. 'Upon mature consideration', Lind had since doubted the influence of the moon, and felt 'it ought rather … be imputed to the noxious vapours arising from the swamps, produced by the high tides which happen at the time of the full and change of the moon, and overflowing a great part of the country, leave it at a marshy state at low water, thereby occasioning the frequent attacks and relapses that occur at those periods'. Lind was convinced that the remissions claimed by Balfour on removal from the influence of the moon were due to other reasons. The first reason is, 'this lunar influence entirely ceases when the patient is removed a few miles from the swamps that are left uncovered by the tide at low water', and 'intermittent fevers are not observed to follow lunar periods at many places within the tropics'. Lind gave the example of Canton, where 'by reason of the industrious Chinese keeping the river within its bounds', the intermittent fever does not follow the typical pattern of ebb and flow but rather 'the state of the weather'. Dr Lind consigns Balfour's theory to the bin by concluding that 'what is called a lunar influence will, I imagine, be nowhere found, but where the remitting and intermitting fevers are occasioned by muddy shores left by the ebbing of the tide'.

This dismissal smarted, and was not soothed for Balfour by the Calcutta council's willingness to believe in his theory. His medical colleagues in Bengal were as unimpressed by his theory, for Balfour noted 'the profound silence with which it has been treated, for no less than nine years, by my brethren in Bengal'. This made him fear that his theory would soon be forgotten and buried in oblivion. Considering that we are currently engaged in studying its implications and place in the history of

European medicine in Bengal, Balfour need not have worried about being forgotten by time.

In any case, Balfour decided to bolster his arguments in favour of a definite connection between the phases of the moon and phases of fevers by sending a general letter dated 22 June 1793 to all stations in the Presidency of Bengal, seeking officers' and others' opinions on this. By the time the book went into publication, Balfour had received letters on the subject from 65 officers and servants of the Company, of whom 25 were surgeons and physicians.

Several of his correspondents had lived for 25 years in India. This was a signal rebuttal to Dr Lind, whose theory of the noxious vapours was woven in England, and not based on either actual experience, or discussions with former Company's servants and military and naval officers with long service in India. Balfour included the letters, which are interesting narratives on sickness and medicine in colonial Bengal, in his book. English officers and surgeons wrote in from places as far away from Calcutta as Sylhet and Hazaribagh, recounting their experiences of relapses of fever during the full and change of the moon. One officer, Captain Robert Ogle, wrote from Cooch Behar on 16 July 1793, 'I am sorry to say that my debilitated state from my long indisposition, renders me totally unable, as also my mind too uncollected, to respond fully to your letter, having been confined to my bed, where I still am, these two months past', had nonetheless led him to rise from the sickbed and state that 'I never heard the reality of the moon's influence in fevers in this country yet doubted, as it occurs almost daily at a certain season of the year, when fevers frequently prevail'.

Another interesting letter came from Captain Samuel Knowles, of the same date, written from Midnapore. Describing himself as 'a valetudinarian', Knowles said, 'I shall not hesitate to declare that I have, for the greatest part of my life, been a pretty rigid observer of the precept enjoined Adam by the seraph Raphael, viz. to confine his attention to terrestrial objects, as better adapted to his intellectual strength'. Knowles had spent 24 years in India. Nonetheless, personal experience led him to further declare that 'the moon has, at the periods you mention, a more than ordinary effect on the patient, under almost every complaint I have experienced, and I believe the contents of Pandora's box have been nearly exhausted upon me'. William Chambers, the famous linguist, wrote on 27 July 1793 to Balfour in respect of the sol-lunar influence, 'if only one life should be lost, or one man's health materially injured, in the course of a physician's practice, by an inattention to a point of so obvious a nature, and so easy to be ascertained, I think he ought not to forgive himself'.

Lieutenant J W Hutchinson wrote from Kanpur on 19 July 1793 that, 'Having had for many years successively what in India is termed a jungle fever, I frequently experienced the effect to the sun and moon to that disorder'. Dr Adam Burt, surgeon at Gaya, and Dr James Ross, at Gaya, wrote on 6 August 1793, supporting Balfour's theory with their practical experience. Captain John Rattray, who had also been resident in India for 24 years, wrote from Midnapore on 28 August 1793 that locals, especially weavers, were commonly afflicted with 'a swelling in their legs, a disorder commonly known by the name of Cochin leg'. Rattray had observed that those suffering from this ailment 'complain of its recurring with great violence at the full and change of the moon, at these periods being seized with the most acute pain in the affected limb, attended with a smart fever'.

Dr W Baillie, wrote on 11 September 1793 from Midnapore that he knew a gentleman, 'who had suffered much from fever in this country, and, in consequence, had acquired a feverish tendency, assured me that he was obliged to guard himself against a moonlit night with as much caution as against the midday sun, though the moon might not be at the full; and that from the time he had used the precaution of avoiding moonlight, and, particularly, excluding it from his bedchamber, he had got the better of his feverish habit'. In his letter of 25 July 1793, Lieutenant John Towers listed the places 'where I have known the moon at the full and change to possess influence in cases of intermittent fever: Chitterpore, Chittra, Gayah, Patna, Danapore, Chunargur, Juanpore, Allahabad, and Cawnpore'.

John Miller, a merchant who had spent 30 years in India, wrote a remarkable letter on 10 October 1793. He had been in Bengal in 1758, when the 'reestablishment of British power, and an overflow of riches', led to a conviviality which resulted in his getting 'a severe fit of the piles'. He travelled to Madras but suffered even more, until fear of a surgical procedure led him to 'a rigid diet and abstinence from spirituous and fermented liquors'. He noticed that he suffered most with the new and full moons. Later, in 1772-3 Miller suffered from severe dysentery. As a result, 'I have found it necessary, as have several of my acquaintances', he wrote, 'to be more regular and exact in taking the bark, at the new and full moon, than at other times'.

Alexander Campbell wrote on 2 February 1794 that 'About fourteen years ago, I lived with my friend, Doctor Daniel Campbell, then surgeon general, resident in India for many years, and employed in a very extensive and successful practice: and I can assure you he was a firm believer in sol-lunar influence, and attended to it in his practice'. On the other hand, Dr William Allison had written on 26 October 1793 from Natore, in Bengal, that in his opinion 'the moon has no immediate or direct influence in aggravating or producing disease'. He admitted that fevers reached their crises during the full and change of the moon but 'this has not appeared to me to arise from any direct effect of the moon on our bodies, but from a change which at those periods is almost instantly produced in the temperature of the air'.

Another disbeliever was Dr John Wade, whose tract on medical discipline for sailors on board East Indiamen we shall soon discuss in a separate chapter. Like Balfour, John Wade was deeply interested in Indology, and eventually became famous for publishing a history of Assam. Wade wrote to Balfour on 15 August 1794, stating that 'in all febrile cases of *neglect or maltreatment*, those symptoms are liable to recur at the lunar periods' [my emphasis]. 'In cases where the patients have not been neglected or maltreated', Wade wrote, 'I have seldom perceived any decisive proofs of the existence of this influence'. He was in charge of a hospital in Assam, and except in the case of one European officer, he had seen nothing 'sufficiently obvious to produce conviction'. Wade went on to provide admission and discharge statistics for his hospital. Of 665 admissions, 595 were discharged, while 33 died. Of those admitted, 303 were ill with fever, and of those who died, 23 'Refused or took no medicine'; 5 were brought in from the jungle, having been ill for 10-15 days previously with fever; 2 were patients who had neglected venereal disease; and 3 of fever and fluxes.

The argument for and against the sol-lunar influence continued through the next decade. Francis Balfour read his paper, 'Of Sol-Lunar Influence in the Fevers of India' at the meeting of the Asiatic Society on 7 July 1802. Nonetheless, Balfour continued to be misunderstood. In March 1812, he wrote to the editor of the *Edinburgh Quarterly Review*, refuting misstatements relating to the review of his tract on the sol-lunar influence published in that journal. The first misstatement was about the 'local extent' of his 'personal observations'. The reviewer had written, 'We will do Dr Balfour the credit, to believe that were sufficiently accurate … but these personal observations prove little more than that at Calcutta (a single town) and its neighbourhood, Sol-Lunar Influence has an evident effect on the Paroxysms of Febrile Diseases'.

The second reason for Balfour's ire was that the reviewer had doubted the number of individuals who had recorded their statements and their competence, saying 'With respect to the Testimonies brought before us we cannot allow the majority of them much weight: because the observations were made, not by Medical men, or by Gentlemen whose previous education fitted them for making observations in an accurate manner; they were chiefly made by Officers in the army'. Balfour defended himself, saying that of his 81 correspondents, 5 were Civilians, 26 army officers, and 50 were medical men. Likewise, added Balfour sarcastically, 'most of them were educated at the University of Edinburgh; where they did not, probably, receive any preponderating bias in favour of the Sol-lunar system'.

Worse, the reviewer had questioned Balfour's 'means' of obtaining information from these persons. The reviewer, basing himself on the alleged fact that most of Balfour's informants were army officers, further aspersed that 'Dr Balfour gives some curious reasons why he applied to those Gentlemen rather than the Brethren of his Faculty'. Balfour defended himself by positing that if his means of extracting information had been inexact, the council would not have funded its publication at the Company's expense, nor would have he been permitted to present a paper before the Asiatic Society.

The interesting thing about Balfour's theory was that it divided the medical practitioners into 2 camps: those who believed in medical theory deriving from professional and practical medical circles in Europe, particularly England, and those who had lived and served for long in India, and believed in phenomena, easily discredited in Europe, but which they had seen through experience. In dismissing Balfour's sol-lunar influence, James Lind presented a school whose credence, in turn, was placed in doubt by the Governor General's ordering the funding and official circulation of Balfour's treatise. This divide finds voice in John Elliotson's *Principles and Practice of Medicine* (1839). 'Before I conclude the subject of these fevers in hot countries', he writes, 'I must mention that, in the East Indies, the sun and moon appear to have great influence upon them'. Elliotson refers to Balfour's book and theory and then adds, 'This may appear incredible or whimsical; but I have no doubt of the fact'. 'I have seen medical men who have practiced in the East Indies', Elliotson wrote, 'and they say it is well enough for *us* not to believe it; but they have suffered enough to know that it is perfectly true' [his emphasis]. The pronoun 'us' implies a difference from 'them', and Elliotson, as a writer, did not want his textbook to become controversial and unacceptable to doctors in India. At the same time he knew enough of medical politics in England to not discard James Lind's explanation, so he added the explanation that the sol-lunar influence could not 'be ascribed to the direct influence of the sun and moon on the human body'. Rather, the full and change of the moon affected the tides, 'causing more or less malaria to be disengaged; so that the atmosphere is more impregnated with it at those periods, than at others'.

Modern medicine does not fever as a disease but as a symptom. Hence it is easy today to be sceptical of the sol-lunar theory. Unlike most of his medical contemporaries in Bengal at the time, Balfour at least strove to achieve an effective cure to local ailments. In referring to the contagiousness of the 'putrid intestinal fever' and establishing the proper handling of the patient's clothes as a rule to treatment, he considerably advanced medical practice. Similarly, in advocating the use of the bark, he pre-empted death from malaria, not effluvium but the mosquito-borne parasitic disease. However, Balfour remained misunderstood in Europe and, at best, a historical curiosity. The reason for this was that his obsession with the sol-lunar theory diverted him from other lines of inquiry, which might have led him to great discoveries, like the curing of boils using neem-leaves. In any case, medicine was evolving in Europe even as it was trying to deal with new illnesses in India using a pharmacopeia not much different from the contents of Woodall's surgeons' chests, even though 170 years had passed in the meanwhile.

CHAPTER SIX

THE BRUNONIAN DOCTRINE IN CALCUTTA

Wandering through the tombs in the South Park Street cemetery, I am struck by the comparative youth of the dead: most died in their 20s or 30s, some lived to their mid-40s, and a few were lucky enough to live long lives. In rare cases accident or battle caused premature death, while the majority died of disease. A rare and interesting book explains how patients were treated in the General Hospital in Calcutta, with whose establishment we concluded the previous chapter on this city. Charles Maclean and William Yates collaborated on *A View of the Science of Life* (1801), which not only corrects errors in *The Elements of Medicine by the celebrated John Brown, MD*, but also includes *Cases in Illustration chiefly selected from the Records of their Practice at the General Hospital, Calcutta.* To these are subjoined *A Treatise on the Action of Mercury upon Living Bodies and its Application for the Cure of Diseases of Indirect Debility* and *A Dissertation on the Source of Epidemic and Pestilential Diseases in which it is attempted to prove, by a numerous induction of facts, that they never arise from contagion but are always produced by certain states, or certain vicissitudes of the atmosphere.*

Despite the off-putting title, the preface makes the aim of the book clear. 'Having carried on our practice together, in the General Hospital at Calcutta', write Yates and Maclean, 'and having by chance discovered, that each of us entertained the design to promulgate the doctrine of Brown, with some modifications, in India, we thought it might be more conducive in the end to view, to consider the subject conjointly'. The aim was to draw the attention of medical men in India to their application of that medical principle, 'vulgarly known by the name of Brunonian Doctrine', at the General Hospital in Calcutta, illustrated through case studies.

The Brunonian Doctrine was propagated by Dr John Brown (1735?-88), and for a while it became a popular medical theory, with several doctors implementing it in their practice. He published his only work, *The Elements of Medicine* in 1780, in Latin. It was later translated with substantial prefatory material, including a life and a discussion of 'Dr Brown's Fundamental Propositions', by Dr Thomas Beddoes (1760-1808), in 1795 for the benefit of Brown's family, who were left without financial support following his untimely death. The most elementary principle in Brown's theory is the quality of 'excitability', of which 'a certain portion' exists in all living beings. The more the excitability in an animal, the more susceptible it is to the 'exciting powers'. Brunonian theory posits 2 classes of 'exciting powers', viz. 'External, as heat, food, wine, poisons, contagions, the blood, secreted fluids, and air', and 'Internal, as the functions of the body itself, muscular exertion, thinking, emotion, and passion'. Without excitability to animate it, life ceases in the animal. Excitability may 'be too great, too small, or in just measure'. Too much excitement may lead to subsequent weakness, due to the defectiveness of the excitability. This is called 'indirect debility'. By contrast, 'direct debility' occurs when 'the exciting powers or stimulants' are withheld, following an excess of excitability. Further, 'Every power that acts on living frame, is stimulant, or produces excitement by producing excitability'. Should a carnivorous person resort to vegetarianism, weakness will ensue. This is because both types of food cause excitement, and unbalance excitability by either causing the system 'into too much motion, or causing it to sink into languor'. Changes in excitability affect the entire body because it is seated 'in the medullary portion of the nerves, and in the muscles'. Different states of excitability cannot coexist in the same body.

Brown did not define the quality of excitability, considering it *a priori*. Beddoes, however, explained it as 'a fluid lodged in a body as a reservoir', more like 'a fluid issuing from the brain as water from a spring'. In effect, the balance of excitability means good health, while debility is caused by overexcitement or under-excitement. Excitement is inversely proportional to excitability, the principle of life. The greater the excitement under stimuli, the lower the excitability, and lowered excitability means disease.

Yates and Maclean, the authors of this singular theoretical challenge, based on their practice at the General Hospital in Calcutta, to established systems of medicine, introduce their book by stating, 'The various doctrines, which have been published in the world, regarding the human body, are in general nothing more than a mere assemblage of words, without the power of conveying distinct ideas'. Medical theorists and practitioners have declined to consider the human body as subject to the same 'regular and immutable laws' as everything else in the universe. This resulted, Yates and Maclean write, in medicine being called a 'conjectural art', when in fact it is a science. They attribute to John Brown 'one of the grandest efforts of the human mind', in propounding his doctrine, which, 'although it has not yet been sanctioned by the medical schools of Britain, has, however, been very generally received in the other schools of Europe, and in America'. The Brunonian Doctrine, 'neglected from ignorance, opposed from the shame of recantation, calumniated from interest, prejudice, and passion', was undeniably logical. The authors, following 'the right path of medical investigation', deviated in several details from Brown's assertions. These included the finding that 'diseases of excessive excitement cannot exist', since these are in fact diseases of indirect debility. In fact, the authors felt that almost all the diseases ranked as those of direct debility by Brunonian practitioners, were those of indirect debility. The third area in which the authors claimed some distinction was the treatment of diseases of indirect debility.

Still more interestingly, the authors claimed that their experience in India gave them an advantage in studying the Brunonian Doctrine, since 'In climates and countries, where the transition from health to disease, and from disease to death, is always alarmingly rapid, and health always precarious, the knowledge of a doctrine, which reduces the practice of medicine to a degree hitherto unknown, cannot but be attended with great and evident advantages'. As most of the diseases of India required the application of stimulants, the authors classed them as ailments of indirect debility.

A study of the cases provided by both doctors demonstrates their belief in the amended application of Brunonian principles. Yates refers first to the case of Francis Lote, aged 35, who was admitted to hospital on 1 May 1796, with complaints of 'general pains all over his body, all those symptoms which indicate an exhausted constitution'. Lote came under Yates's care on 15 May, by which time he had been 'much purged and griped', and his mouth was sore with ulcers from the use of mercury. Between 15 May and 3 June, when Yates stopped attending him, Lote's 'complaints were considerably relieved, by the use of Opium'. Other doctors treated Lote until 21 August 1796, when he returned to Yates's care, in an advanced state of debility, 'with excessive purging and bloody stools'. Lote had moreover broken a clavicle due to violent vomiting induced by emetics. Between 21 August and 30 September, Yates administered Lote huge amounts of the 'Tincture of Opium', sometimes up to 400 or 500 drops every 2 hours. There was a crisis on 1 September, when Lote's pulse was at 120, and he was extremely weak due to diarrhoea, as he was passing 14 or more stools a day. Nonetheless, Yates's treatment worked and by 30 September he had only 2 stools a day, without any griping, was sleeping well, and even 'felt a returning appetite'. Yates concluded that this case 'may give some idea of the manner in which stimuli should be increased, in diseases of great exhaustion, until the quantity is ascertained, which is capable of producing the highest degree of excitement'. Yates also noted how the case had been successfully treated without further doses of mercury. The reader must note that Yates did not prescribe in the standard manner of the time, purgatives, emetics, or venesection.

Mercury, as calomel ointment, was copiously rubbed in, and opium and wine generously administered in the case of De Haes, aged 40, who was admitted to hospital on 26 August 1796, 'with dysentery of eight days standing'. He recovered a month later and Yates deduced that 'The great quantity of mercury that was used, in this case, with opium and wine, shows what a high degree of stimulant power may sometimes be required to effect a cure, in the state of exhaustion, which constitutes dysentery'. The case of Jacob Meyer, aged 35, was different. Meyer was admitted on 23 August 'with pains of the bowels and frequent stools'. He was administered increasing quantities of calomel and opium through the next 2 weeks, which did not help. The pain in his colon increased and on 9 September his pulse rose to 122, and then became imperceptible. Meyer died the following day. Yates's conclusion was that 'there can scarcely be a doubt that the colon and rectum, if not the whole abdominal viscera were in a state of local disease'. As for the huge amounts of mercury and opium (towards the end a scruple of calomel and 6 grains of opium every hour) given, Yates reminded his readers, 'that when a patient is evidently incurable, by the common practice, it becomes the duty of the practitioner to depart from it'.

Charles Maclean listed the fourth case in the series, in which the surgeon of the East Indiaman, *The Northumberland*, recounted the case of a cadet, aged 17, 'tall, of a slender make, and consumptive habit', reported sick on 13 June 1791, with feverish symptoms and 2 days' diarrhoea. He had been suffering from seasickness from the beginning of the voyage, in April. He was prescribed opium, and 'mutton or chicken broth, and sago alternately, as his fancy directed; and wine and water for drink'. On 24 June, the medicines not having been strictly taken, it became necessary to give him the bark, following which he soon recovered. The next case came from the same ship. In a bout of playfulness, an ensign climbed the mainmast on the evening of 10 June 1791 and fell asleep on the maintop. Around midnight, he fell, bouncing off an iron stanchion on the maintop, and the mizzen-stay, on to the quarterdeck. He was carried down to his cabin insensible, and bleeding from his mouth, ears, nose, and eyes. No fracture was found, and 'the whole consequences of the fall seemed to consist of contusions or concussions'. There were 4 doctors aboard ship in addition to the ship's surgeon. While the others suggested that the ensign be bled immediately, the ship's surgeon refused this on the ground that 'I was convinced of its being entirely wrong; and that I would not, even with the sanction of the majority, do what I was certain must endanger the life of my patient'. He offered any of his colleagues the charge of the patient if they disliked his treatment. None accepted. In 2 hours the ensign regained consciousness and vomited due to concussion. This, the surgeon noted in his journal, traditionally called for 'copious bloodletting'. However, he once more forbore despite knowing full well that if his patient died, he would be held guilty of professional neglect, following 'the non-observance of customary forms'. On the other hand, if the patient lived, 'after having been copiously bled, it would be in spite of the bloodletting'. The treatment included 'small opiates occasionally, wine, and nourishing food'. On the eighth day after his fall he had recovered enough to be carried out on deck in a chair. However, he lost completely the sight from one eye due to concussion. The ship's surgeon, whose thought coincided with Maclean's, concluded that in all cases of contusions or concussions, 'bloodletting is not only unnecessary but pernicious'. Still more interesting is the surgeon's comment on bloodletting which follows: 'In private practice, I fear, a mean and criminal compliance with vulgar prejudice, in order to conciliate vulgar favour, too often influences practitioners, whose better judgements would lead them to reject entirely so deplorable a remedy'.

Robert Williamson was admitted to hospital on 28 October 1796 with fever which had lasted for around 8 days, and recently worsened. His pulse was 'small', breathing laborious, and he had body-ache. He was given calomel, opium, and a blister applied to his sternum. Despite this, Williamson died early on the morning of 30 October. Maclean carried out an autopsy, and 'the thoracic viscera were found adhering to each other, in such a manner as to form one mass'. This was, Maclean wrote, a clear case of 'peripneumony'. 'Would the abstraction of blood', he asked, 'have produced a resolution of the adhesions, which were found in the thorax?' Venesection was 'a directly debilitating operation', and 'in those of indirect debility, it must increase the exhaustion'. Concluding that experience and theory never differ, Maclean said that bloodletting 'has never been useful in any one case of disease'. The patient, however, was dead, and Maclean said, 'Had it not been my wish to bring the theory and practice of this doctrine to the fullest and fairest point of discussion and experiment, this is one of those cases which I would have suppressed'. Later, in his 'Postscript', Maclean writes, 'Peripneumony, in reality, is seldom a dangerous disease, until by bloodletting and other debilitating means, inflammation and adhesion of the membranes, suppuration, and dropsy, are produced'. Robert Woodside was admitted on 24 October 1796 with 'dysentery of a fortnight's standing'. Despite the usual prescriptions of calomel, opium, mercury ointment, and blisters, Woodside got no better. He preferred to lie on the right side. On 15 November, hiccups began, which continued until he died the following day. On autopsy 'there were found several abscesses in both lobes of the liver, communicating with each other, and containing, in all, about one pound of matter, of a thick consistence and colour'.

Unlike Yates, who disdained the use of mercury, Maclean believed as strongly in it as Balfour did in the bark and sol-lunar influence. On his voyage from Bengal to England in January 1789, Maclean suffered from quotidian intermittent fever, and the usual medicines, viz. 'tartar emetic, and afterwards bark, and now and then a cathartic medicine'. None were of any use, and Maclean became weaker since the paroxysms of fever became severer, and his legs oedematous. Between 2 and 3 drachms of mercurial ointment were rubbed on his body at bedtime, and Maclean records, 'The alteration, which this single rubbing produced, was equally unexpected and salutary'. He recovered quickly, and made up his mind to apply mercury to every case of intermittent fever. The utility of mercury as a stimulant, and thence useful for indirect debilitating diseases, became obvious. Later, in September 1793, after being exposed to the sun the whole day in an open boat on the Hooghly, Maclean suddenly suffered high fever in the evening. The usual practice would have been, he writes, 'I should immediately have lost blood, taken an emetic, or purgative, and abstracted as far as possible all the usual and ordinary stimuli'. Instead, he took a pill composed of 1 grain each of opium and calomel, every hour through the night. 'By this means,' he writes, 'the excitement was supported'. His fever abated, though the next morning he found that 'a considerable stiffness, swelling, and pain' afflicted his left arm, from the shoulder down. It had turned livid in appearance, and 'rather alarming'. Maclean recalled from the position in which he had stood in the boat, that this arm had absorbed most of the sun's rays. His arm was bathed in tincture of opium and alternately rubbed with mercurial ointment, while he continued to take the pills. After he had taken 30 pills, the tissue assumed its normal colour, and all his symptoms disappeared, with the sole exception of a sore and ulcerated mouth, which bled from the gums. This too cleared in 2 days' time. Maclean felt that if he had accepted the common treatment of bleeding and purging, his case, like most cases in India, would have terminated in 'adhesions of membranes, affections of the viscera, or a very lingering recovery'. Another personal experience of the efficacy of mercury occurred when Maclean was ship's surgeon aboard the East Indiaman *The Houghton*, bound for Batavia, to protect it from the

French. A vicious form of dysentery struck the ship, and most sailors were down with diarrhoea and fever. Again Maclean employed the stimulants, calomel and opium, which were liberally used, with wine and water, to good effect.

In the final analysis, it did not matter 'Whether discoveries have been made by a man named Brown, or a man named Cullen; whether they have issued from the obscurity of a cottage, or the elevated desk of a professor', Maclean wrote. The only thing that mattered was to know 'the nature and extent of the discoveries'. If the Brunonian Doctrine was true, it behove physicians to embrace it; but if they thought it false, it equally behove them to prove it. Ultimately, it was not a question of party, rather, 'a contest between truth and error'.

One wonders at the influence of the Brunonian Doctrine in medical circles in Calcutta. Despite the fact that the Doctrine died out early in Europe, one is amazed by the presence of this kind of advanced medical theory and practice in Calcutta at the end of the 18th century.

CHAPTER SEVEN

JOHN PETER WADE, THE SURGEON HISTORIAN

Looking for John Peter Wade's grave is pointless, since he was buried in North Park Street Cemetery, which disappeared a century ago, and of which only one representative tomb remains standing. Wade was appointed Assistant Surgeon in the HEIC's service on 4 April 1784, and he died in Calcutta on 14 October 1802, aged 40. Like many of his countrymen, Wade was drawn to the people, languages, and cultures, of India. He continues to be remembered, less for his medical tracts, and more for the history of Assam he compiled during his service in that province.

James Balfour knew Wade, and as he notes in his *Treatises*, had discussed with Wade his conclusions. Wade, Balfour wrote, had served under him at Benaras from 1784 to 1786. During this period, Wade had learnt much from Balfour's successful application of his method of treatment, discussed in a previous chapter. Balfour claimed that Wade had acquired 'a competent knowledge of this practice'. This was further sharpened through practice along those lines at Chunar, in Bengal, and, still later, on board the East Indiaman that took him to Europe. While in England, Wade published a book, *Select Evidences of a Successful Method of Treating Fever and Dysentery in Bengal*, in October 1791, in which he not only disowned the sol-lunar theory but also noted the successful application of Balfour's technique of evacuating the system with calomel without mentioning its author. To Balfour, this injustice was accentuated by the fact that Wade's manuscript, submitted to the Medical Board of Bengal, contained 'acknowledgements on this subjects, respecting the author'.

Perhaps Balfour was too sensitive, since Wade had replied to the general letter that Balfour had circulated, eliciting observations of the sol-lunar effect from Europeans in India. In his letter to Balfour, written from Assam on 15 January 1794, Wade wrote that the officers of his detachment were 'unanimous in their declarations that they have either experienced this influence themselves, or have obtained a conviction of its reality from the experience of their brother officers'. He particularly included for

Balfour's consideration the testimonials of Captain Welch and Lieutenant Dick, who had reported at first-hand the effects of the full and change of the moon on their fevers. Of his own experience, Wade warily stated, 'I have not considered the results sufficiently as yet to authorise me to entertain a decided opinion on the subject'. He observed, however, that 'all febrile cases of neglect or maltreatment' recurred during the lunar cycle, which had 'a more obvious effect' on Europeans than locals. In cases of fever, which had not been neglected, Wade unhesitatingly asserted, 'I have seldom perceived any decisive proofs of the existence of this influence'. Nonetheless, in certain cases he had 'imagined' the sol-lunar influence to be at work, 'but the effects were not sufficiently obvious to produce conviction, unless in the instance of one European officer'. On the whole, Wade remained steadfast to his view that while the 'coincidences of fevers or relapses' with the lunar periods was 'an established fact', though 'the extent of this coincidence will forever prove a subject of doubt and of dispute'. To support his view, Wade provided Balfour with brief statistics related to his hospital in Assam, which show that of 665 admissions (including 303 cases of fever), 595 were discharged well. Of the deaths, 9 were from fever other than old, neglected cases, or those 'Brought from the jungles 10 or 15 days ill of fever before admission'. There were also 23 fatal cases who 'Refused or took no medicine'. While Wade used these figures to prove the limitations of the sol-lunar theory, we may use them to conclude that John Peter Wade, notwithstanding Balfour's aspersions, was an able doctor.

1791 was a fruitful year for John Wade. The good thing about long sea voyages was that they allowed the traveller, who was not unduly bothered by seasickness, to devote time uninterruptedly to writing. Hence, in 1791 Wade was able to submit to the Court of Directors *A Paper on the Prevention and Treatment of the Disorders of Seamen and Soldiers in Bengal*, in addition to the book previously mentioned, *Select Evidences of a Successful Method of Treating Fever and Dysentery in Bengal*. The latter consists of a series of case studies, drawn from Wade's practice at the hospital in Chunar.

Chunar is a town in Mirzapur district, in eastern Uttar Pradesh. It is of some historical importance to the East India Company, since its fort was briefly occupied by Raja Chait Singh, and, later, during his rebellion, by Warren Hastings. In 1763, the Raja of Benaras, Balwant Singh, aligned himself with Nawab Shuja ud Daulah of Oudh, against the Company. The Company's supremacy having been established at the Battle of Buxar in 1764, Benaras was granted to the Company by Emperor Shah Alam. The Company did not occupy Benaras, which then passed once more into the kingdom of Oudh. Benaras was a prosperous possession and the Nawab was reluctant to let go of it in 1770, when Raja Balwant Singh's elder son, Raja Chait Singh came of age and claimed his inheritance. Forceful persuasion by the Company, caused by its trade interests, made the Nawab recognise Raja Chait Singh as ruler of Benaras in 1773. Raja Chait Singh resented the nominal suzerainty of the Nawab, and the Nawab was glad to pass Benaras to the Company's direct administration in 1775. As an 'ally' to the Company, with an English Resident posted in Benaras to 'advise' him, Raja Chait Singh was required to finance the Company's garrison there, and also provide troops to fight the Company's battles. He refused to do this and conspired against the Company with other similarly disaffected persons, as a result of which he was arrested in 1781. Raja Chait Singh escaped confinement and took to the field. Defeated by the Company's troops within weeks, Raja Chait Singh fled first to Oudh and then to Gwalior, where he died in 1810. Raja Mahip Narayan Singh had succeeded Chait Singh, in 1781 with the Company's support. He too was unable to satisfy the Company's demands, and was deposed in 1794, after which Benaras was governed directly by the Company. On 19 September 1781, Warren Hastings concluded a treaty with the vizier of Oudh, Faizullah Khan. One of the accusations against Warren Hastings at his trial was that he had accepted a bribe of £160,000 for this treaty.

Warren Hastings found Chunar Fort pleasantly located, and in his preface to *Select Evidences*, Wade, who went there in 1787, briefly describes the place. 'Chunar has been long esteemed a very unhealthy situation', Wade wrote, 'perhaps an injustice'. The weather was better than 'in the lower country of Bengal', since the ground was stony, as 'In the rainy season the water soon runs off into the Ganges, and leaves it drier'. The fort and town were bounded by the river on one side, and stony hills on the other. Typically, the hot season commenced in March, and intensified until the arrival of the rains in July. The monsoon abated in October, with the gradual incursion of the cold season.

The hospital was 'raised considerably above the level of the ground, and built in a very open and elevated situation'. 'From the nature of the edifice', Wade wrote, 'it was not possible to prevent a very free ventilation at all seasons'. All the cases studied in his treatise were admitted to the general hospital at Chunar, and the details of most cases were generally 'written at the bed of the patient'. From the beginning of 1788, most patients admitted to the general hospital at Chunar were convalescents. There are other interesting details about doctors' practices during this time. They visited their patients at sunrise, which was between 6 and 7 in the morning.

Very significantly, Wade remarked that the phases of the moon were not marked at Chunar, but later added, before publication, 'from a London almanac', on the presumption that 'the difference is not so considerable as to render a greater degree of accuracy necessary'. Of nearly 400 cases of fever and dysentery, only 2 died, he wrote. Wade also noted, 'It is to be presumed that these cases may provide a body of evidence, by which the system of lunar influence in Fevers may be judged'. On reading the book, however, it becomes clear that some of the cases were not fully studied since their care was taken over by other doctors.

The first case that draws interest is that of Osborne, aged 50, who was admitted on 13 March 1787, with 'violent fever', 'severe colic', and 'spasmodic cough'. After 5 days of purging, during which 'His evacuations by stool continue abundant', and he was given 20 drops of laudanum at bedtime, his fever was gone, and his cough reduced. On the morning of 18 March he was found, presumably by Wade during his morning visit, to be drunk. Wade ordered the immediate administration of 3 grains of tartar emetic, and after these had worked, Osborne was discharged for drunkenness. Osborne was readmitted on 20 March with fever, a worsened cough, 'great difficulty of breathing', 'pain in the region of the liver', and 'hardness in the region of the bladder'. Purging was freely used and 8 ounces of blood taken. By 22 March his abdominal pain and hardness disappeared, as did his fever. He was able to breathe easily. From 24 March he was diagnosed with 'obstructed liver' and given 10 grains of 'mercurial laxative pill' every night. Finally, on 30 March he was transferred to the care of another doctor.

Another case was that of Eshurwood, aged 27, who was admitted on 24 February 1787, with 'low continued fever, with exacerbations every evening', which had weakened him. After admission, Eshurwood was allowed 7 glasses of wine a day and 'middle diet'. The usual array of purgatives was applied to no effect and his alcohol consumption was reduced to 2 glasses daily and a 'low diet'. Eshurwood seemed to recover until 9 March, when there was a regression. All the purgatives were stopped and he was given small doses of tartar emetic 'until it shall have operated well by vomit'. At this point Wade discovered that Eshurwood had been previously admitted to hospital and 'subjected to a considerable degree of salivation', presumably by the use of mercurial compounds. Eshurwood would not disclose the complaint for which this treatment had been applied. This led Wade to guess that Eshurwood suffered from 'visceral obstruction, and vitiation of the various secretions', for 'his evacuations are always particularly offensive'. On 18 March Eshurwood's tongue was foul and Wade suspected that he had been secretly drinking during the night. The bombardment of purgatives and emetics continued, with mercurial fever pills, which soon resulted in a sore mouth. Wade reported him to be free of fever on 30 March, but we do not get to know more about Eshurwood, since he passed into the care of another physician the next day.

Adams, aged 26, was admitted on 21 March 1787, with "severe pains 'in all his bones', accompanied with a very considerable degree of fever". 2 days later, he was much better, the fever having abated, and 'very little of the pains in his bones'. He had been administered purgatives and he had 'evacuated much putrid, bilious matters by stool'. On 25 March Adams was discharged.

The use of purgatives and emetics in combination with mercurial pills and ointment, form the basis of almost all cases recorded by Wade. The treatment was universally applied, whether for gonorrhoea, or 'ophthalmia'. Hopkins, age unrecorded, was admitted to hospital on 6 June 1787 with fever. The usual treatment, including the bark, followed until the fever abated on 20 June, when he 'complained of gonorrhoea, for which he remained in the hospital till the 24th, when he was discharged, free from all complaint'. Similarly, Frampton, aged 20, was admitted on 10 June with fever and gonorrhoea. Purgatives and emetics removed the fever by 12 June, but the venereal disease continued, for which Wade prescribed, 'Let him use the usual injection for the gonorrhoea six times every day'. Frampton's injections continued until 20 June, when Wade recorded, 'his gonorrhoea has entirely disappeared, with its several symptoms', and ordered his discharge.

John Guest was admitted to hospital on 12 March 1789, and the following morning Wade, the examining doctor, recorded that Guest 'Has been afflicted with ophthalmia for a week, which grows worse in the daytime'. Guest was put on a diet of sago, and the usual course of emetics and purgatives. 2 days later Wade ordered the application of 'the saturnine lotion', presumably Goulard's 'Extract of Saturn', or lead subacetate. By 17 March his eyes were better, but he ordered the application 4 leeches to each temple, and blistering in the nape of the neck. On 22 March, the records note, 'He had only two or three stools yesterday; his eyes are greatly better'. Guest was discharged as 'perfectly free of all complaint' on 25 March. Lead subacetate was used again in the case of Michael Keys, aged 68, who reported to the hospital almost exactly a year later, on 10 March 1790, with 'feverishness and slight ophthalmia'. Once more, the same course of purging accompanied by the application of 'Vegeto-mineral Water' (lead subacetate, shaken in distilled water and brandy), led to his discharge on 21 March.

John Anson, hospitalised on 5 September 1789, was afflicted with 'excruciating pain in his ear'. Wade ordered 15 leeches to be applied around the ear, and 'Warm milk and water to be injected into it frequently', in addition to the usual purgatives. On 7 September, a blister was applied behind the affected ear. Nonetheless, on 10 September he was feverish, and his ear very painful. To Wade, the answer lay in exciting vomit, to which end Anson was given emetic tartar and ipecac. The following day's report reads, 'He vomited very well'. This had some effect on the ear, since the same report states, 'The earache is most severe every evening; it was much easier last night'. The emetic having appeared the cure, it was continued the following day, and Anson discharged well on 13 September.

Venesection was freely used on occasion. Howell, aged 54, was admitted on 4 March 1787, with 'hoarseness', 'difficulty in breathing', pain in his joints, 'particularly his wrists', and a 'high degree of fever'. Wade's prescription was, 'Eight ounces of blood to be immediately taken from him'. Purging and the use of emetics were ordered as usual, with further instructions, issued on 8 March, for 'The wrist to be rubbed with a warm and dry hand for half an hour twice a day'. For his throat, Howell was to use a flannel to cover it, and gargle with a 'pectoral decoction, with a little of the spirit of sal ammoniac in it'. By 13 March he was 'nearly well', and on 16 March he was 'Discharged perfectly well'.

Similarly, Handley, aged 21, was admitted on 10 May 1787, possibly for fever. He came under Wade's supervision on 1 June. By this time he was feverish all day, and suffering from headache and thirst. He had been put on a 'milk diet' and allowed 3 glasses of wine daily, as a result of which he was 'considerably debilitated'. Wade stopped the milk and wine and as usual put the patient on the 'low' diet. Then he renewed the use of purgatives and emetics, with the addition of castor oil and infusions of senna, which operated 'freely', undoubtedly to the great discomfort of the patient. On 7 June the fever returned with 'slight shivering' and the bark was given every 2 hours. 11 days later, Wade recorded, 'The mercurial laxative keeps his body open – Eight ounces of the decoction of the bark, with one drachm of elixir of vitriol to be taken daily'. Despite the heavy use of mercury, Wade seemed rather surprised to note that 'His mouth is not sore' on 20 June. However, he was coughing 'a little' and there was blood in his spittle. Wade checked Handley's pulse, found it 'quicker and smarter than usual', and directed, 'Ten ounces of blood to be taken from him immediately'. Handley had no return of the fever after 23 June, and he was allowed the 'middle' diet, along with 2 glasses of wine daily. The mercurial laxative, with vitriol, the bark, and castor oil, was continued. On

28 June he experienced tenesmus, which must have been painful, and he was administered a clyster of 'forty drops of laudanum in six ounces of rice-water' at bedtime. 2 days later, Handley again seemed to be free of fever but he was too weak to be discharged. As his appetite had returned, further hospitalisation was ordered, during which he continued with the mercurial laxative, vitriol, and the bark. Handley presumably went out of Wade's care at this time, since the latter's record ends with the note that Handley was to stay in hospital 'till he acquire more strength'.

Not everyone wanted to undergo the long, wearying, and excruciating, process of bowel evacuations and vomiting many times a day. Decruse, 20, was admitted on 22 May 1787. He came under Wade's care on 1 June, and was recorded as being on a 'middle diet' with 2 glasses of wine daily. Decruse continued to suffer from fever with fits of shivering, and was prescribed the 'low diet' along with purgatives including castor oil. The next day, though evacuated, he complained of 'a violent pain in the front part of his head'. To address this, 8 leeches, 4 to each temple, were ordered to be applied. On 3 June, Decruse had no fever, and reported the headache gone. Wade noted, 'He would not permit the leeches to be applied'. The purging continued 'copiously', and on the evening of 8 June Decruse requested to be discharged. Since he had no fever, the request was granted, and 'recommended for an exemption for three days from duty'. Decruse's profession is nowhere mentioned in Wade's records. In any case, Decruse was readmitted on 10 June, the fever having returned almost immediately upon discharge. The fever worsened by 12 June, and he was prescribed the usual purgative pills and salts. Additionally, he was ordered 3 clysters [glisters / enemas] during the day. Wade records on 13 June, 'He refused to take the clysters, and was with great difficulty prevailed upon to take the solution, which, however, operated well'. The purging was intensified, with the addition of an infusion of senna [powder of dried leaves of *Senna Alexandrina*]. The bark was also given, and Decruse finally discharged fit on 20 June.

Decruse's case may be compared to another, D L Win [? the name is recorded as DLWIN], who had been admitted on 23 May 1787, and came into Wade's care on 1 June. D L Win was recorded as suffering from continued fever, with pain in the regions of the stomach and liver, and frequent retching and vomiting. Wade removed him from the 'middle diet', which included 2 glasses of wine, and put him onto a diet of sago. However, the purgatives offered no relief, and on 2 June Wade recorded that D L Win had had no stools. In keeping with medical practice of the time, Wade strove to clear the system by prescribing half a grain of tartar emetic, 'with forty drops of laudanum to an ounce of water'. This did not help and at 7 pm, the patient was 'in a cold sweat and very faint', as a result of which he was given a warm bath, followed by the same draught as before. Since there was no improvement at 9 pm, Wade ordered the administration of 2 grains of 'solid opium'. 2 hours later, the patient was 'much easier in every respect'. On 3 June the patient was faint, and, strangely, clysters were ordered to empty the bowels. At 11 am, Wade wrote, 'The vomiting has been incessant and violent since the morning visit', which is not surprising considering the amount of emetics administered. The answer to this was the immediate use of a clyster, and 40 drops of laudanum 'to be taken every hour in an effervescent neutral mixture'. On 4 June the patient was unchanged, 'His skin is hot and dry, and his pulse extremely quick, yet somewhat stronger'. To Wade the enhanced and combined use of purgative and emetic seemed to be the immediate answer. He ordered 2 teaspoonfuls of emetic tartar every 10 minutes 'until he begin to vomit freely'. To ensure this, the steward of the hospital was required to tickle his throat with a feather and, after the vomiting had cleared the stomach, give him 30 drops of laudanum in half an ounce of water. The vomit elicited 'a most extraordinary quantity of bile and some other matters'. D L Win, however, continued to decline, despite further warm baths, 'blisters to the head and thighs', and bottles of warm water, presumably applied to the feet, and died on the morning of 5 June.

Another astounding case is that of William Earle, who was first admitted on 9 April 1788, with high fever 'and a flux' for several days. The remedy was a 'solution of salts to be taken, so as to purge copiously', which was given on 10 April. The purge having worked, Earle was 'much better of the fever and flux', and so the next day an emetic was administered. This was followed on 12 and 13 April by further and vigorous purging. Earle was discharged fit on 15 April. Another William Earl, probably the same person, given the erratic printing of the time, aged 53, was admitted on 14 September 1789, with fever accompanied by shivering, and 'great frequency and heat of stools, with griping and straining'. Castor oil was at once given, which worked, and this was followed by a cocktail of tartar emetic, calomel, and infusion of senna. This led to a considerable increase in stools, 'of a better colour, and with less straining'. The fever returned twice over the next 2 days, and as usual, the purging was reinforced through the addition of 2 ounces of castor oil. On 20 September, Wade recorded, 'The fever, griping, and straining, have entirely vanished'. 3 days later Earl was discharged, 'free from all complaint'.

In 1791, Wade presented to the Court of Directors *A Paper on the Prevention and Treatment of the Disorders of Seamen and Soldiers in Bengal*, which he published the following year. Wade presents the necessity for his book by stating that 'The information … to be procured from books, respecting the health and diseases of Europeans in Bengal, is neither ample nor satisfactory'. Though admitting that a few authors had written on the subject, Wade is unkind in adding that 'it was perhaps to be wished, as far as regards the treatment that still less had appeared'. In what is almost certainly a snide cut at Balfour, Wade says that the tendency of such prescribed treatment 'affords not only the best apology, but the best argument also, for obtruding on the attention of the honourable company's medical servants a few cursory remarks on the subject'. These remarks are, however, far from being cursory. Wade drew upon his experience in Bengal to present, to the medical fraternity in England, a textbook of practical medicine. In so doing, he fearlessly trod over traditionally accepted medical hypotheses.

One of the 'forcible and serious' bases of medical studies in European universities, Wade wrote, was 'that fatal and impalpable agent in the excitement of fevers, which is called CONTAGION'. The young practitioner lived in fear of it, 'particularly in warm climates, which are supposed to be more favourable to its reception'. Voyages to and from India, and 'a long residence in Bengal' [he had been there only 6 years and at the time the two-monsoon rule was still popularly believed in], had quietened his apprehensions about contagion, and 'shook his faith on this subject'. This was because 'to the perfect conviction of his own judgement', he had not seen, 'either in or out of hospitals, a single instance of contagion'. The fear of contagion, however, was a cause for panic, especially aboard ship, due to 'the terror attending the idea of a contagious disease' within a closed space. Wade's first instruction to the surgeon was 'to be particularly cautious how he encourages an opinion' on contagious fevers, 'unless on the most positive evidence, which is not furnished by any combination of circumstances aboard an Indiaman'. A practical aspect of this was that the patient's messmates, who would otherwise have helped nurse him, would 'assiduously avoid exposure to a supposed contagion', and thereby also avoid 'rendering them numerous little offices, which, after all, may prove of more consequence in the cure of their disorders than medicine itself'. The possibility of contagion aboard a ship would also alarm a port's medical officer, who would then order the ship to keep to sea.

Wade had been allowed to go home on sick certificate. Despite this, 'The sick were always examined before breakfast, on an empty stomach, and an open skin, with a constant feverishness, the remains of a former fever, and affection of the liver'. His medical duties thus exhausted him completely, and 'An hour's repose' revived him, and thus provided 'the most unequivocal personal evidence of the absence of contagion'. Rather than contagion, 'miasma, or marsh effluvia', was in Wade's opinion, a more potent cause for disease in Bengal. 'In the season of the periodical rains', he writes, 'or at their termination, which is the only unhealthy part of the year in any place in India', the swampy areas 'alone might be deemed adequate to the excitement of the diseases in question'.

Another reason for disease and death almost immediately following a safe voyage and landing in Calcutta was 'The elevation of spirits', and the 'emancipation from every restraint of diet'. 'The very change of air', Wade reasoned, was enough to enhance appetites, so that people ate and drank with no consideration for possible ill effects. In particular, they disregarded 'the dreadful effects of strong liquors', which had been rationed aboard ship, but were plentiful in Calcutta. These liquors were 'of the very worst and most inflammatory kind'. Other temptations frequently indulged in by sailors and passengers soon after arrival at Calcutta included 'an unrestrained indulgence of the passions with women', which generally encouraged 'a total neglect of personal cleanliness'. The local climate brought about 'profuse sweating from the great heat and a suppression of the insensible perspiration by an alternation or coincidence of hot and of wet weather'.

While Wade's strictures could be imposed on passengers, sailors claimed their traditional right to their drams. Hence Wade recognised the fact that sailors 'will remain for many days extremely ill, and perhaps dangerously so, than be deprived of their liquor'. Very diffidently Wade declared to the Directors 'his humble belief that the daily allowance of liquor on board of Indiamen, in its most favourable view, is at least unnecessary and useless'. In fact, this tradition, Wade argued, encouraged a habit, which might have been avoided. In cold climates, he asserted, 'strong liquors are so far from providing a protection against cold and wet, the consequent inflammatory diseases of the season, or even the scurvy, that their ultimate effects are to furnish a disposition to be affected by all these'. In hot climates strong drinks wreaked havoc on the body: 'Their immediate action is to increase the prevailing distress from the heat; to induce or confirm a costive habit, the febrile source of most of the diseases of warm climates; to create a disposition to be affected by bad air, by marsh effluvia, or by contagion, if such be supposed to exist'. Wade's tirade against the quantities of strong drinks quaffed by Europeans in Bengal derived not from reasoning alone but 'decided experience and a long attention to this subject', through 'extensive practice among the soldiery of Bengal'.

Rubbishing the excuse that alcohol improved the taste of stale water on ships, Wade wrote that Indiamen were notably famous for 'provisions of every kind, especially this very article', that is, good water. This was because the Company's ships sailed with 'the most abundant supplies of water, taken from the River Ganges, beyond the reach of the tide'. In his opinion as a doctor, 'No water in the world can excel that of the River Ganges, when collected and preserved with due attention'. Similarly, the waters of Bombay, St Helena, and Madras, were 'probably superior to any in Great Britain'. 'In reality', Wade concluded, 'were an allowance of spirits in any instance indispensably necessary to sailors, foreign ships would labour under very great disadvantages'.

Foreign ships sailing to and from India had other advantages in matter of diet and health. The better health enjoyed by their sailors derived from the 'sparing allowance of salted provisions' aboard ship, in favour of 'Farinaceous vegetables'. Wade laments the predilection for English sailors to consume huge quantities of salt meat in particular. Such a diet is specially unsuited for the tropics, 'where large quantities even of the best and freshest animal food are in the highest possible degree inimical to health', leading 'to costiveness, to all bilious complaints, to affections of the liver, to dysentery'. Taking a lesson from locals, Wade concluded that in the warm climates people were accustomed to retain health through 'the use of vegetable diet'. Not only in warm climates, 'the most athletic part of mankind, the peasantry all over Europe, excepting England, in some measure live, thrive, and grow strong on a diet almost entirely exclusive of animal food'. Two-thirds of the world, he wrote, lived on a vegetable diet. Diets heavily dependent on animal food imparted no especial physical strength. In fact, such diets derived from 'thinly populated' and 'uncivilised' countries, 'where vegetation is not abundant, and where animal food affords the only source of half-starved existence'. One wonders how the Directors of the Company took this last statement.

The English sailor, Wade said, was the most unclean species of his profession, seldom thinking of a 'change of linen, were he not occasionally compelled to it by being wetted to the skin', besides which 'their heads remain long strangers to the comb, their beards to the razor, and their faces to cold water'. This was distinctly unhealthful, since 'it cannot be supposed that the general prevalence of vegetable diet and frequent bathing amongst rational creatures in tropical countries is the mere effect of accident and not the result of reason and experience'. To this Wade added the issue of physical exercise, which he admits would not have been the case in 'colder climates, on more boisterous and inconstant seas, and in more variable weather'. In the case of East Indiamen, however, 'during the prevalence of trade winds, and nearly on all occasions, a ship's crew may indulge in very enervating habits of laziness', which is removed only by 'the compulsion of authority'.

At this point in the book Wade surprisingly breaks out in praise of the slave traders, who used dancing to keep their slaves healthy. This discordant, indeed irritating, note worsens when Wade waxes about the 'personal cleanliness of the slaves' and 'the neatness of their accommodations', which rival the cleanliness of an officer's cabin on an East Indiaman. Slave trade was common in Wade's time, and like most of his contemporaries, Wade, despite his medical education, does not pause to consider the moral aspects of human trafficking. It does not strike him that the slaves would hardly have wished to dance, considering the position they were in, and would be, for the rest of their lives.

However, Wade next proceeds through a very modern discussion of the usefulness of good ventilation aboard ship. While this is of little immediate interest to us, it is interesting to note that he urges the patient to move even though suffering from fever, rather than lying down. This, he says, is a 'mistaken indulgence to the sick'. Equally important for the doctor was to see the patient move, for 'A surgeon may acquire more knowledge of the state of his patient from a view of his countenance, and his general appearance, than from the most distinct answers to the most sagacious questions he may propose'

In discussing the fevers of Bengal, Wade dismisses contemporary theories of the origins of fevers in Bengal by claiming that all such afflictions 'originate, in those latitudes, from the bowels and their contents', as a result of which the most effective cure was purging. Surging ahead in this belief, Wade declares that all fevers in Bengal, as well as other afflictions, such as gout, arise from the same cause. Further, all ailments of children come from irregularities in the bowels as well.

We get an idea of how medicine was practiced in Bengal, when Wade informs us of the way in which fevers insidiously impersonate one another: 'But when the bilious fever is disguised under doubtful appearance, or to speak more properly, when the foul contents of the stomach and intestines excites appearances which impersonate the putrid, the inflammatory, or the nervous fever, and their several modifications, the evacuations are generally restricted to a vomit and a laxative medicine, perhaps a single repetition of the latter with occasional glisters, succeeded by diaphoretics, vigorous antiseptics, corroborants, cordials, stimulants, opiates, and death!' The worst offender, Wade asserted, was wine, 'that favourite corroborant, cordial, and stimulant', which was widely dispensed at the hospitals in Bengal. He later states that 'It required the hand of government in Bengal to restrain the libations in the hospitals within narrower limits'. Experience had demonstrated beyond doubt that in Bengal wine 'is very ill adapted to any period of any fever in those latitudes, when the treatment has been proper in other respects'. The local soldiery, who were in his charge in Bengal, were not allowed by their religious prejudices to consume alcohol. This confirmed him in his belief of the needlessness of wine as a cure. 'No doubt', he wrote, 'the mischief occasioned by wines is in proportion to the quantity of spirit in each'. Nonetheless, Wade judged that 'Claret may possibly have the advantage of port and Madeira, and hock may be still less detrimental than the first'.

Like wine, Wade dismissed opium, whose copious use was common in all ailments at the time. He considered most medical writers to be writing 'for' practice, rather than 'from' it, as it should be. As such, he was able, from his own experience, 'to give a pretty positive assurance, that its exhibition will, with the exception of very few instances, be found extremely mischievous, even in combination with antimonials'. Nevertheless, he admitted that if one was to choose between opium and wine, 'Wine of every kind would seem to deserve a preference to bark and opium, as it is not attended with effects equally permanent in suppressing the secretions of the bowels'.

Wade begins his theory of therapy by rejecting diuretics and blisters. The latter, he wrote, only caused pain and increased febrile symptoms, concluding 'that they have any other influence on the general system, except what proceeds from the pain they occasion, is very doubtful'. Further, the possibility of blisters removing fevers 'appears utterly impossible'; rather, 'they have often been the instruments of much mischief'.

Wade only gave a qualified approval to the bark, whose utility in 'remittent, intermittent, and continued' fevers he admitted, and he was of the opinion that 'During the first stages of every kind [of fever], before evacuations, powerful in proportion to the violence of the symptoms, have taken place, its exhibition is in direct contradiction to the nature of the appearances, and to every indication of cure, and consequently, must always be improper, and often fatal'. Only after the system had been properly purged, and the bowels restored to normalcy, could be bark be used.

Giving Brunonian medical theory short shrift, Wade wrote, 'it is hoped that the number of his [Dr Brown's] disciples, or the prevalence of his method of treatment, is entirely confined to those gentlemen, who, like Dr

Brown, have had little opportunity of exercising the practice on any but themselves'. 'This gentleman's tenets', he continued, 'demanded particular notice here, as several addresses, attributed to surgeons of the honourable company's ships, and recommendatory of Dr Brown's practice, were published in the newspapers in Calcutta, during the years 1788 and 1789'. Other competing theories of treating fevers were equally dismissible. 'Is a fever', asked Wade, 'like a nuisance in the street, which may be equally removed in every opposite direction of the compass, removable from the constitution by a contrariety of means?'

Fevers in Bengal had typical symptoms, 'The full, strong, rapid pulse, the red eyes, bloated and florid countenance, burning skin, high-coloured urine, parched tongue', and occurred during the summer, 'in the season of the hot winds' and 'in constitutions habituated to excesses'. Wade strongly advised against the use of venesection in these fevers, since bloodletting quickly led to profuse sweating. However, it debilitated the patient, and 'This deceitful interval of ease, which succeeds this operation, soon vanishes; the fever rekindles, probably with redoubled fury, and finds the patient much less capable of resistance to its violence, exhausted by the bleeding, and by the excessive discharges from the skin, which have been imprudently prolonged by various means'. Considering that most of these fevers commenced from 'a high degree of inflammation from the region of the liver' subsequent to the accumulation of 'the foul contents of the stomach, duodenum, etc', the best means immediately available to the physician, was the evacuation of the bowels. This would help preserve the patient's strength to battle the ailment. Venesection, Wade particularly noted, was harmful in the case of puerperal fever, in which it has 'often proved fatal', since this fever, like most other fevers of the region, arises from the same cause, viz. costiveness of the bowels. As is well known, puerperal fever was considered fatal for long. Wade propounded in his book that this fever, 'which a celebrated professor of midwifery in the University of Edinburgh deemed absolutely incurable, may be prevented invariably by effectual evacuations from the intestines after delivery'.

Wade goes on stressing the importance of his belief in this matter through his work, affirming 'that the foul contents of the stomach or intestines are capable of exciting the cuticular secretions morbidly; that in the instances of spontaneous sweats described by authors, which have not proved beneficial, these have probably been the exciting causes, and, in conjunction with malpractice, have had a share in all forced sweats; that from the entire expulsion of these from the body, or their removal from the neighbourhood of the stomach, all sweats of a favourable termination, and such as have been esteemed critical, have flowed'. Consequently, he thundered, 'the whole tribe of sudorifics should be exploded from practice in Bengal'.

Alongside evacuations, Wade emphasised the application of antimonials, which, in prescribed doses, would produce and support a tendency to vomit for some time before the actual evacuation takes place'. This means of treatment, nonetheless, required that 'the antimonials should be joined with some purgative medicines, principally in a liquid vehicle, to give the matters a final tendency downwards, through their natural channel'. Dependence on emetics alone would serve 'to destroy the remaining strength of the patient'. Wade chose to apologise for seeming to deride emetics, seeking that medical readers of his treatise should consider this 'apparent disrespect' merely an endeavour 'to procure precedence to a more natural and more powerful means' of effecting a cure.

Aware that his treatise had long 'exceeded the limits which were at first prescribed to it', Wade nonetheless felt that it was necessary for him to proceed to a discussion of his advocacy of purging as a means of effective cure in Bengal fevers, 'the treatment of fevers by active purges'. He began by dismissing the use of glisters, which he said had little more than local use, despite which physicians depended heavily on them. But 'the reliance which practitioners have misplaced on their evacuating powers has often rendered them instruments of destruction, notwithstanding their general insignificancy in these complaints'. He goes on to scathingly criticise his professional brethren, saying that 'the practice of gentlemen in Bengal, at least in some fevers, is deficient rather in the extent than in the nature of the means'. He divides them into two classes, attributing to the first group, consisting of 'the most experienced', this deficiency. The second group comprises physicians and surgeons 'who trust to information acquired from books and lectures'. The members of this latter group 'crawl on in a blind routine, proceed greater lengths in error, and misapply means altogether'. By 'means', Wade means that the first group, through experience of the problems caused by the climate of Bengal, carry out 'the gentle exhibition of evacuants', while the second is characterised by 'the total, or nearly total, omission of them', which is a fatal error. While the first group is doubly informed, both through practice and reading, the latter is smugly ensconced in limited knowledge, unwilling to learn from the members of the first group, since their opinions often remained 'unsupported by the glare of reputation'. 'What sentence shall we be compelled to pass', asks Wade, 'on doctrines and practices nearly the reverse, though promulgated by men esteemed the greatest lights, but in this sentence the *ignes fatui* of their profession, when those opinions are deemed applicable to the treatment of fevers in Bengal?' 'Shall we permit our judgment to be blinded', he continues, 'our experience to be entirely discredited, and our lives to be sacrificed to the fame which blazons the volumes of several authors, whose treatises are in every gentleman's possession, and whose practice, of course, as generally as their names are known?' Many of these writers have never approached Bengal 'except in contemplation', while others have deemed a few months' stay 'sufficient to give a stamp of authority to their writings'. Such treatises 'have led to the destruction of thousands'. This type of writing does not 'appear to deserve credit for more than a good intention, industry, and stone-blind experience'. The worst are those, who 'recommend a practice, the mortal tendency of which will appear from the broad evidence of their own writings'. Age, Wade thundered, is not proof of experience. 'God knows', he wrote, 'it is not necessary to proceed the length of India in quest of instances to corroborate this suspicion'. It was obvious that observation and judgment had nothing to do with age and experience in the case of medical practice in India, where, 'a practitioner of any age, who possesses those qualities in a much more confined sphere of practice, will become an experienced physician without a wrinkle'. In thus categorising and critiquing his seniors, Wade knows that he shall stand accused of presumption. His only wish was that such reproach should not affect 'the general adoption of the practice recommended in these sheets'. Only if such general adoption of the recommendations he had made were spurned, would he regret all he had written about his colleagues.

'The necessity of purging', Wade wrote, 'is not restricted to any species of fever, but affects every set of symptoms usually denominated fever, in proportion to the multiplicity and dangerous tendency of those symptoms'. Had purgatives been effectively used, writes Wade, 'We may suspect that what is generally understood by the appellation of putrid fever, under the various forms and circumstances of ship, hospital, jail, puerperal, jungle, pucca, and hill fever, would never have existed [*sic*] the terror of mankind'. The use of purgatives at the first sign of indisposition, 'will infallibly prevent the approach of dangerous symptoms, particularly those called putrid and, at their height, will always save, and generally cure, the patient'. Often, in serious cases, the purgatives required the assistance of emetics for speedy evacuation. While discoursing on the comparative qualities of the saline and oily purgatives, Wade comments that the observation of intestinal mucus in faeces is a certain means of assessing the utility of the purgative. 'That the cause of the protraction of fevers is often connected with the state of the mucus, as well as some of the other secretions, appears from the immediate cessation of all the symptoms on a copious discharge', he wrote, stating further that 'the mucus is often vitiated in a most extraordinary manner', for which 'the sense of the observer will afford ample testimony'. However, the condition of intestinal mucus was never studied by those whom Wade calls medical gentlemen with 'extreme delicacy'. These delicate persons would miss every sign of the progress of the disease by avoiding such examinations.

Wade recommended the use of calomel, not in the usually prescribed dose of two or three grains, which he deemed as adequate 'to remove the complaint altogether, in slighter cases, by copious evacuations'. Fevers in Bengal necessitated doses of up to ten grains of calomel, 'and after intervals so short, as would terrify most of the faculty, even in India, and appear to practitioners in Europe necessarily fatal'. To remove its worst effects, calomel should be administered in combination with liquid purgatives, at night, in order to procure evacuations early in the morning or through the day. 'These doses may and should be repeated every second night', he wrote. The 'pressure of the symptoms' might require these doses to be repeated every night, 'as long as anything offensive remains to be discharged from the bowels'. Wade drove home his point by stating that 'Forty grains or more of calomel, with a larger quantity of the mercurial laxative pill, have been exhibited with innocency, and with great benefit, in this manner, in the course of five or six days'.

Mercury given in such high doses was bound have ill effects, which often led the physician to the conclusion that the patient was declining, when the reality was otherwise. 'The formation, or discharge of the bile, which has been suppressed, deficient, or irregular for a long time', Wade said, 'will not unfrequently be attended with severe symptoms of dysentery and fever'. These were favourable symptoms, and required the doctor to prescribe 'frequent changes of situation and air, with a diet of mild vegetables and water only, and frequent exercise of the gentler kind'. The best was for the convalescent to undertake a sea voyage, with the same diet. It was of especial importance 'that fish of every kind, as well as all animal food, to the utter exclusion of chicken broth, should be prohibited during the existence of lurking symptoms of fever, however trifling it may appear'. Moreover, fresh vegetables were 'frequently inapplicable to the purposes of diet in fevers; so that farinaceous aliment alone, or with mild and ripe fruits, would seem to be best adapted to every period of these disorders'.

Wade next takes up the lunar influence on fevers, though a little hesitantly. 'The operation of this influence', he writes, 'however, is by no means equally remarkable through all seasons of the year'. He follows this up by saying that the unhealthy seasons were those when this influence was most felt, and then changes tack to point out that observation demonstrates 'that the season of the rains, or the termination of the periodical rains, is particularly favourable to the production of fevers, fluxes, and other disorders'. He then brings the two theories together to suggest that the lunar influence is at its height during these periods, and needed to be addressed by the physician, who needed to remember that 'The principal prophylactic is intestinal evacuations before the different periods of the moon'. However, Wade was clearly doubtful of this theory, for he follows it up with another statement in which a similar contradiction is noticeable. Wade writes, 'In recent fevers, it is *imagined* this influence will be very obscure at all seasons of the year' [my emphasis] and no special precautions were needed. 'In fevers of great length', Wade continues, '*which never occur, but from mismanagement, it might possibly be improper to treat it with entire neglect*' [my emphasis]. Wade closes his discussion on the lunar influence by stating that the effects of this on fevers had best be 'abandoned' to the 'ultimate decision' of readers, 'as may esteem the subject of sufficient importance to deserve a particular scrutiny'.

Wade was not impervious to making a name by publishing, for he added, perhaps a little hastily, to his treatise, an article on dysentery that he had published in Bengal in 1789, 'with some trifling alterations'. It was obvious he would not be returning to England for some time again, so he wished to make his book as substantial as possible. Wade never returned home.

Wade begins his discussion of dysentery by saying that medical practitioners in the Company's service would be glad to know that both dysentery and fever can be cured, since their pay did not depend on the number of patients. This is a significant statement, for it at once creates a division between those engaged in private practice in Bengal and those in the Company's service. It seems to imply that the private practitioners, whose incomes depended entirely on the number of patients they attended, were unscrupulous. They would not be gladdened by the news that Wade had to offer regarding the treatment of dysentery. On the other hand, the salaried physicians and surgeons, who were indifferent about the number of patients they saw, were more willing to invest time in reading what Wade had to say. Thus Wade referred to 'the ingenuity as well as the leisure of the medical gentlemen in the honourable Company's service'. The Company's doctors were willing to observe, judge, and even evolve new methods of treatment, which the private practitioners were possibly averse to.

In Bengal, Wade writes, 'any distinction between diarrhoea and dysentery will in general be found unnecessary, if not pernicious'.

Recalling Dr Thomas Sydenham's (1624-1689) famous identification of 'dysenteric fever', Wade reminded his readers that 'the dysentery is a fever of the intestines'. This definition should at once make all clear to discerning doctor, in that it should 'suggest an argument in favour of the little diversity of treatment requisite in fevers and fluxes'. This being enough to proceed upon, Wade stated that 'venesection is utterly inapplicable to any stage of this distemper'. Sudorifics were 'greatly detrimental', unless used in moderation towards the termination of the disease. Similarly, 'The efficacy of ipecancuan [*sic*], to the exception of its emetic powers, is too questionable to authorise any reliance on its virtues, in these complaints'. Wade then dismisses as 'alexipharmacs', 'those multifarious compounds of dispensaries'. He called it 'a word of little meaning, and medicines of little use'. In fact, the treatment of dysentery had showed how 'Technical expressions of undeterminate, or of no meaning, have at all times proved the resource of ignorant men, and may have occasionally misled the most enlightened'. Demonstrating what this meant, he wrote, 'When a vague suspicion of *relaxation*, *atony*, *putridity*, has glanced on the practitioner's imagination, a ready expedient has presented the numerous lists of *corroborants*, *tonics*, and *antisceptics*' [Wade's italics]. 'In this strange nomenclature', Wade wrote, 'bark has always obtained the first place', both in Europe and in India. When the patient has been unable to sustain the bark, nature 'has been soothed into a temporary acquiescence by the addition of opium'. Equally bad is the prescription of wine, which was often done because dysentery was accompanied by great lassitude and 'depression of spirits'. Wade drew upon his practice in hospitals for European soldiers in Bengal to conclude that 'patients of every denomination crave an allowance of wine with utmost earnestness'. Those who are 'sober and prudent', 'conceal and preserve their allowances, until an opportunity occur, to dispose of the accumulated treasure to their own pecuniary advantage, and the great detriment of the purchaser'. So great is this dependence on wine that 'scarcely one man in one hundred possesses the resolution or the honesty to acknowledge that it has proved in any degree prejudicial to his disorder'. In fact, 'The exhibition of these fatally vigorous medicines has been the offspring of a jargon (excuse the term) which has long filled the pages of authors'. In particular, the symptom of '*relaxation*' was considered to be associated with 'most disorders in Bengal', which necessitated the issuance of wine to counteract it. While the Company, on the recommendation of its doctors, who did not have to depend on the number of patients for their salaries, had stopped the allowance of liquor in hospitals in Bengal by order, private practitioners sought their patients' favour by prescribing it. When these private practitioners saw that the wine would often 'go sour and return from the stomach', or cause 'cardialgia, and other disagreeable sensations'. The private practitioners would then substitute wine with spirits mixed with 'various proportions of water', and thus enhance the ill effects of the disorders. 'This mischievous beverage', Wade said, 'is also dictated by a fancied relaxation', which was of no consequence to the private practitioner.

Wade's own preferred method of treatment involved the use of calomel with liquid laxatives, supported by mild emetics. He warned the doctor that the use of calomel, laxatives, and emetics, would make the patient appear more ill, whereas in reality 'the patient will ultimately be found to acquire strength'. Chronic fluxes were, like fevers of long standing, the ill consequences of bad doctoring, 'occasioned by neglect, or what is still more pernicious, the unskilful treatment of preceding disorders'. Here too 'unless in the very last stage', a large dose of calomel would cure, administered if necessary with opium.

In the next chapter, Wade addresses the ailments of the liver, whose successful treatment, he says, 'has long been understood in the honourable Company's settlements in the East Indies, and perhaps there only'. 'It was formerly, in Europe', wrote wade, 'pretty much the practice to suppose every disease, curable by mercury, connected with a venereal taint'. 'In this respect', he continued, 'liver has supplanted the lues venerea in India, and with great propriety, for every purpose of practice'. Due to the fact that mercury was the proven drug to treat diseases of the liver, Wade pointed out that 'It is certainly no very incontrovertible statement to say, that because mercury has been found of almost certain efficacy in affected liver, and has proved successful in a great variety of other diseases, that these diseases must necessarily have been the liver'. The only true means of proving this was through post-mortem examinations, which, however, given the heat of the climate and the rapid putrefaction of the body, tended to be fallacious. Nonetheless, 'when dissection exhibits the viscus in question, deranged in its form, substance, size, or even offices, beyond all expectation, and almost beyond conception', its involvement cannot be questioned any longer. However nebulous this evidence might have appeared to European medical thought, to the English doctor in India it indisputably established the connection between the liver and 'all complaints in those countries'. Wade admitted that he had attended few autopsies, but those few had provided him with ample information, which, when shared with colleagues, showed that their observations had been the same.

'On all occasions, when the secretion of bile is morbidly increased, diminished, or irregular, it is clear', Wade wrote, 'that the viscus has not its natural action'. In effect, 'the liver should be suspected under every derangement of the secretions of any of the bowels'. This connected the liver to all complaints typical of Bengal: 'in old pains, general or local, which are not decidedly venereal; inmost, or in all, cuticular affections; and in all obstinate complaints of the head, chest, and abdomen'. Exploring uncharted territory, Wade was unsure of his conclusions, but he listed the symptoms of the ailment popularly termed in Bengal and indeed the rest of India, '*The Bile*' [his emphasis]. These symptoms, which Wade recollected from his own medical experience, include: 'Frequent and severe thirst, if this be referable to the head; a bitter, or other unpleasant tastes in the mouth; foetid breath, especially in the morning; various discolouration of the countenance; sometimes yellow, sometimes extremely free from all yellow tinge, pale, but not clear, often of a deadly leaden colour, sometimes of a copper tinge, on some occasions a kind of mixture of all these in various proportions; frequent flushing of the whole face, or of particular parts only, especially of a circumscribed spot in one or both cheeks; partial sweats of the head, sometimes of the forehead only; frequent giddiness, or confusion, on stooping particularly; sense of weight in the head, sometimes approaching a degree of pain, especially on rising suddenly, or on rising on the toes, and falling on the heels again with a jerk; frequent drowsiness; mouth generally foul and covered with viscid secretions; the sauces particularly foul and often foetid; the gums and other parts of the mouth liable to frequent ulcerations, which are extremely painful when touched, but not otherwise; the gums sometimes sufficiently firm, at other times apparently deficient in firmness and colour; the teeth also less white, and much more difficult to keep clean, subject to frequent aching, and to become carious; the salivary secretions irregular; the tongue very seldom perfectly clear, but of all degrees and complexions of foulness, though generally moist, sometimes, however, very dry after sleeping, and subject to ulcerations like the other parts of the mouth; a remarkable degree of continued inaptitude to continued motion in the lower jaw, particularly evinced in chewing; the eyes sometimes yellow, generally muddy, and on some occasions perfectly free from all tinge, clear, but not vividly clear as in health, and sometimes of a slight bluish cast; vision not quite so perfect as in health, especially after looking for any time at one object; in some instances, a general greasiness of the face, and a glassy appearance of the eyes; stuffing of the nose and other catarrhal symptoms, sometimes a discharge of blood without any apparent cause'.

The Bile was not always connected to a permanent and irreversible affliction of the liver, but 'almost always a pretty certain attendant on fixed derangement of the liver'. Even afflictions of the lungs were linked to the liver. Asthma, cough, 'suffocation, increased, sudden, quick, difficult, laborious respiration', 'difficulty of laying on one or both sides, and sometimes of a recumbent posture altogether, though not often in chronic cases, chiefly, however, in the last stages', 'a sense of stricture about the pharynx', 'sometimes a slight degree of difficulty in swallowing', 'a degree of hoarseness or various changes in the voice', all indicated that the physician ought to 'have the liver in view'. Wade goes on to examine the involvement of the liver in dysentery, as studied through the contents and quality of the stools, and in vomit, again through its contents, along with other symptoms such as 'a fixed pain in the pit of the stomach', 'unpleasant heat in the stomach on swallowing wine, spices, and other things', 'shooting pain through the regions of the stomach and spleen, or from the epigastrium to the back', and 'pain from wind occasionally', besides 'cardialgia' and other similar pains though to emanate from the stomach.

'It is very remarkable', noted Wade, 'that in the most decided affections of the liver, there is often neither pain nor uncommon sensation of any kind', other than in acute cases, when there is both pain and swelling. The patient most commonly experiences 'A sense of some fullness and an uneasy sensation, constant or occasional'. If pain is felt, 'It is most generally obtuse, and very obscure, sometimes recurring after brisk motion and after meals only, sometimes permanent'. This pain is usually felt 'pretty high up under the ribs'. 'The pain is not uncommonly felt only on the left side', noted Wade, 'and indeed the liver, in a morbid state, far on that side sometimes'. While there is sometimes no pain at all, at other times the abdomen is tense 'and extremely painful to the touch'. In particular, the 'region of the bladder is often much affected, and the urine exhibits every variety of condition; it is sometimes exactly as in health, or of a beer colour, or pale, clear, in small quantities, white, muddy, experiencing sudden alterations, like Madeira wine, difficult, hot with straining, suppressed, like muddy porter, greatly tinged with bile, or totally free, and all the intermediate stages thin and watery, sometimes foetid, sometimes apparently purulent, much sediment, or none, perfectly clear or much clouded, depositions of various kinds, sometimes bloody'. Additionally, the spleen is 'obstinately enlarged', and prolapsed ani are common, along with 'violent haemorrhages', often not related to piles. 'Dropsy, in all its forms', Wade noted, 'is very frequent', besides flatulence, hiccups, and 'violent eructations'. Strangely, Wade recorded that jaundice occurred 'in slighter degrees, very frequently', and that 'violent jaundice' was not 'a very common disorder in India'. 'There is not one form of fever', he concludes, 'but what has occasionally been found connected with the liver'. This conclusion is followed by Wade's own experience. 'During the rainy season of the year 1789', he wrote, 'several cases of the yellow fever, as described by West India practitioners, and by Doctor Lind, occurred in the general hospital at Calcutta'. The afflicted had, 'previously to the attack, inhabited the low, damp, arched ways of the fort'. In all these patients, 'the skin was particularly suffused with yellow', the stools were 'black and putrid', and they vomited 'lumps of black bile'. One of the doctors related how he had successfully treated similar cases with mercury when faced with 30 patients suffering similarly during a voyage to India. He had dissected the first one who died, and had found an alarming enlargement of the liver. The rest recovered with mercury. Following his experience, the first patient who died in Calcutta was opened, and his liver too was found to be 'astonishingly enlarged', in fact so much that 'the lungs, in the right cavity of the thorax, were compressed by the enlargement of the liver, into a very small and hard mass', despite which the patient does not seem to have complained of difficulty in breathing. The finding of the post-mortem in Calcutta being similar to that described by the ship's surgeon, mercury was at once prescribed: 'The mercurial inunction, without intermission, was applied to every part of the skin where absorption could be expected to take place, and continued until the mouth began to affected, when every symptom of the disorder vanished'. Additionally, laxatives and gentle emetics 'were occasionally exhibited, with great relief to the patient'. After the fever had been reduced, wine was given to the patients, which 'was thought to relieve very effectually the oppression and anxiety about the praecordia, to enable the patient to support the constant exhibition of purgatives'. Further and more importantly, 'The bark was entirely neglected, unless as a strengthener after every symptom of the disease had vanished'.

Often in Bengal, Wade recorded that mercury, 'in the various forms of ointment, calomel, and mercurial pill', though prescribed to the patient seemed to have no effect either on the disease or even the salivary glands. In venereal cases, this 'inertness of the medicine' was attributed to the debility of the patient. Wade pointed out that even in cases of debility and advanced disease, the salivary glands showed the effect of mercury, which left only one possible answer, which was that in Bengal the patients suffering from the liver 'may have deceived the practitioner'. 'These deceptions', he continued, 'are very frequent in Bengal, where the practitioner's attendance is held of less value, as of no expense to the patient'. Besides, not every doctor believed in the efficacy of medicine, and there existed some doubts about its ill effects on the body. Wade dismissed these worries, arguing contrarily. 'It may be said', he wrote, 'that this drug will increase the debility, and tend to render the salutary efforts of nature less powerful; but those who have much experience of its use in warm climates, are well assured that its effects on no occasion are so considerable in this respect, as have been generally apprehended; that it has even a contrary tendency, if fullness and strength of pulse may be allowed to stand as proofs of it'. Mercury needed to be used wisely, in combination with medicines other than opium. The only alternative for treating an abscess of the liver, at a regrettably advanced stage of the disorder, was to operate, when 'a bold incision will often rescue the patient from inevitable death'.

Besides mercury, diet was a vital adjunct to the liver. Should a patient listen to medical advice such as that given by 'one of the oldest professor in the university of Edinburgh', and consume porter and beefsteaks, 'certainly no means could save the patient'. If the patient wished to avoid relapses, which was very frequent, 'a spare and vegetable diet' was advised, and 'fermented or spirituous liquor of any kind' prohibited, for life. Wade ended his book with a copy of a letter written him by Dr Paisley, of Fort St George, who famously attended on Lord Pigot, in which the symptoms and cures of many cases of liver are discussed in detail.

One cannot help wonder what John Peter Wade died of. Was he attended by colleagues who shared his views, or did he order his own treatment? The argument, as always, must have raged between venesection, the bark, mercury, opium, laxatives, and emetics, as well as the phases of the moon. Clearly this severely limited pharmacopeia was insufficient to save the life of this brilliant young doctor, who had the courage to question his seniors and their personal theories on the diseases of Bengal.

CHAPTER EIGHT

JAMES JOHNSON AND THE INFLUENCE OF THE TROPICS ON EUROPEAN CONSTITUTIONS

James Johnson's work, *The Influence of Tropical Climates on European Constitutions, Being a Treatise on the Principal Diseases incidental to Europeans in the East and West Indies, and Coast of Africa*, became one of the few determining textbooks on tropical diseases, long before the term came into medical use. It first appeared in 1813 when, as Johnson wrote in the preface of the third edition, it was 'published chiefly at the Author's own risk and expense, for he could find no Bookseller to undertake it', after which its popularity and relevance ensured the appearance of 5 editions.

Johnson, born in the parish of Ballinderry, county Derry, Ireland, in February 1777 or 1778, belonged to a time when apprenticeship to a surgeon was a perfectly legitimate way to enter the medical profession. Orphaned early in childhood, Johnson passed an examination in the classics in Dublin, and was apprenticed at 15 to a surgeon-apothecary, Mr Young, at Portglenone, in county Antrim. He spent 2 years there, followed by 2 more years at Belfast as apprentice to Mr Bankhead, after which he went to London to pass his medical examinations. Having no money or relatives and friends in London, he became apprentice to an apothecary, and used the little spare time he had to prepare for his surgeon's examination by studying hard and occasionally attending lectures on anatomy and surgery. In 1798 Johnson passed the examination of Surgeons' Hall, and was appointed surgeon's mate aboard the naval ship, *Mercury* in May of the same year. There was a great demand for surgeons and surgeons' mates aboard naval and merchant vessels, since it had been made illegal by 26 George 3 cap 80 (1786) for any vessel to leave port without a surgeon or surgeon's mate. He sailed to Newfoundland and Nova Scotia, but at the same time persisted with his studies, gaining practical experience whenever the ship docked, by going ashore to visit naval hospitals. The captain of the *Mercury* connived in Johnson's long absence in London for some months towards the end of 1799. In 1800, Johnson again cleared an examination at Surgeons' Hall. Through the patronage of the same captain, Captain Rogers, Johnson was promoted to full surgeon and appointed to the sloop, *Cynthia*, in February 1800. The ship soon sailed for Egypt, where Napoleon had landed in 1798 with a considerable army. Napoleon left Egypt in August 1799, but the French army remained as a constant reminder to the English of their control over the land route to India.

Johnson fell ill while in the Mediterranean, and he was admitted to the naval hospital in Gibraltar. Towards the close of 1800, Johnson returned to London, and resumed his study of anatomy and surgery. In May 1801, having run out of money, he applied once more for a surgeon's post on a naval ship. He was appointed to the sloop, Driver. However, peace came in 1802, and Johnson lost his livelihood. Luck and hard work paid off, and Johnson was appointed to the frigate Caroline, which sailed for the East in May 1803. He spent the next 3 years aboard this ship, and returned to England in 1806, having voyaged to India and China. . Though Johnson was in India for only a short while, his travels in the East provided him with considerable professional experience. Having made some prize-money on this voyage, Johnson enrolled as a student at Guy's and St Thomas's Hospital. Appointed to a land establishment, he looked after prisoners of war at Plymouth and Portsmouth. Soon he was appointed to the man-of-war, Valiant, on which he served for 5 years, seeing a lot of active service.

In the introduction to his treatise, Johnson posits what might be called the 'Three Winter' rule for persons from tropical lands visiting England. Children from Africa 'brought over by the Sierra Leone Company for education, seldom survived the third year in this country'. They got through the first winter, drooped through the second, and succumbed to the third. For the European in the tropics, in addition to the monsoon, there was the heat, which in some parts of the colonies never gave way to winter, or even mildness. This made the issue of perspiration controversial. Should perspiration be checked or allowed? If checked, the body would suffer, for thirst would increase, and the lowering of temperature lay the body open to chills taken from even the slightest sea breeze, and if allowed to flow, would lead to debility. Johnson wrote, 'We are no sooner beneath a vertical sun, than we begin, as may naturally he supposed, to experience the disagreeable sensation of unaccustomed warmth; and as the temperature of the atmosphere, even in the shade, now advances within tenor twelve degrees to that of the blood, and in the sun very generally exceeds it, the heat perpetually generated in the body, cannot be so rapidly abstracted, as hitherto, by the surrounding air, and would, of course, soon accumulate so as to destroy the functions of life itself, did not Nature immediately open the sluices of the skin, and by a flow of perspiration, reduce the temperature of the body to its original standard'. From this point on, Johnson refused to follow the physiology of perspiration any further, as being of little 'practical importance'. Nonetheless, he rejected the use of porter or other wines for checking the perspiration, since the drinker, getting thirstier, would not stop short of intoxication, by which time the suddenly lowered body temperature would have allowed incipient sickness to develop. Johnson sided with water due to which, he said, the external surface of the body immediately sympathizing with the internal surface of the stomach, relaxes, and a mild perspiration breaks out, which reduces the temperature to its natural standard'.

Johnson's own preference was for the theory of sympathies between parts and organs of the body. In this case the main sympathy was between the external surface of the body and the alimentary canal. Thus when cold drinks were imbibed, the sympathetic tendency was from the inner lining of the stomach to the surface of the skin, making it susceptible to chills. If water had been merely applied to the skin, thirst would have been assuaged by a sympathetic reversal. Similarly when perspiration was allowed to flow unchecked, it caused a sympathetic 'loss of tone' in the stomach, leading to 'that anorexia, or diminution of appetite, which we seldom fail to experience on entering the tropics, or, indeed, during hot weather in England'. Johnson knew the uselessness of trying to get Europeans in India, particularly in Bengal, to drink more water, since alcohol consumption was encouraged by 'high authority' as 'not only innocent, but salutary'. Besides, 'The probability of future suffering will rarely deter the European from indulging in present gratifications'. Hence instead of adapting their plethoric European constitutions to tropical heat, Europeans goaded the stomach 'an organ already debilitated', by drinking alcohol. Speaking from personal experience, Johnson noted how it was the usual practice for Europeans to come in perspiring from physical exertion in the tropical sun, and with 'the extreme vessels relaxed, we find, on sitting down to table, our appetites entirely gone, until we take a glass of wine, or other stimulating fluid, to excite the energy of the stomach'. 'Under such circumstances of artificial or forced relish for food', he felt, 'it is not to be wondered at, that the digestion should be incomplete, and that the intestines should suffer from the passage of badly concocted aliment'. Instead, 'an hour's cool repose before dinner' was preferable, 'and if on commencing our repast, we find we cannot eat without drinking', it was nature's warning against eating at all.

Axiomatically, diseased livers were most commonly found in Europeans in India, as compared to the locals, the cause of which was put down to the Europeans' 'richness of food, tenseness of fibre, grossness of diet, and rapidity of circulation'. Johnson, however, found at work a strong sympathy, 'hitherto unnoticed', between biliary secretion and perspiration, which he named the 'Cutaneo-hepatic sympathy'. Increased perspiration in the tropics was a sure index to increased flow of bile from the liver, and any attempt to check perspiration also checked hepatic secretion, resulting in disease. It was common to see Europeans in Bengal coming in from work in the hot sun, perspiring freely, and then checking the sweat by drinking cold liquors. At the beginning the excitement caused by alcohol improves appetite through an increased biliary flow and all seems to be well with, however, the incipient atony secretly increasing until it strikes suddenly, to deleterious effect. What actually happens, Johnson tells us, is that the biliary secretion is at first increased but fails over time, until it is too late. Johnson observed from personal experience that in vitiated bile,' attendant on hurried secretion, both the colour and taste are surprisingly altered; since it occasionally assumes all the shades between a deep bottle green and jet black; possessing, at one time, an acidity that sets the teeth on edge; at other times, and indeed more frequently, an acrimony that seems absolutely to corrode the stomach and fauces, as it passes off by vomiting, and when directed downwards, can be compared to nothing more appropriate than the sensation which one would expect from boiling lead flowing through the intestines'.

Johnson, again speaking from personal experience, listed the symptoms associated with the 'first effects' of decreased hepatic function: 'Irregularity in the bowels; general languor of body and mind; slight nausea, especially in the morning, when we attempt to brush our teeth; a yellowish fur about the back part of the tongue; unpleasant taste in the mouth, on getting out of bed; a tinge in the eyes and complexion, from absorption of bile; the urine high coloured, and a slight irritation in passing it; the appetite impaired, and easily turned against fat or oily victuals'. Disregard of these warnings would lead to nausea and 'sickness at the stomach', diarrhoea, and costiveness, depending on the exciting causes. These, in turn, 'pave the way for serious derangement in the biliary and digestive organs', unless aggressively counteracted by temperance and medical measures.

He then goes on to mention other problems endemic to tropical lands, which were not addressed by any of the previous writers of medical texts that we have perused. These include the irritation caused by 'prickly heat', and insects like mosquitoes and cockroaches. 'Prickly heat', or 'Lichens tropicus', Johnson says, is 'a very troublesome visitor, from which few

Europeans escape'. 'Many a time', he writes, 'have I been forced to spring from table and abandon the repast which I had scarcely touched, to writhe about in the open air, for a quarter of an hour: and often have I returned to the charge, with no better success, against my ignoble opponent!' He had been so afflicted with this soon after arrival in India that for some weeks he could not sleep for more than an hour at a stretch at night, before he was forced to leave the bed, and 'if there were any water at hand, to sluice it over me, for the purpose of allaying the inexpressible irritation!' This gave only temporary relief, since the discomfort soon recurred, to still greater effect. In one of the first descriptions of 'prickly heat', Johnson puts his personal experience of it to good use: 'It is usually, but not invariably accompanied by an eruption of vivid, red pimples, not larger in general, than a pin's head, which spread over the breast, arms, thighs, neck, and occasionally along the forehead, close to the hair'. In the heat, 'the pimples become elevated, so as to be very distinctly seen, and but too sensibly felt'. When one sat quietly in cool comfort, these irritating pimples often disappeared, returning with activity in the heat, and also with the drinking of beverages that warmed the body, like tea, soup, and wine. Johnson tried various means of treating himself for 'prickly heat', including hair powder, lime juice, and many other 'external applications', to no effect. However, he discovered that 'until the constitution got assimilated to the climate', the only means of lessening its violence included wearing light clothes, eating and drinking lightly, avoiding the sun, ensuring 'open bowels', and, 'last, not least, a determined resolution to resist with stoical apathy its first attacks'. The last was the hardest, and Johnson had discovered that 'if we can only muster up fortitude enough to bear with patience the first few minutes of the assault, without being roused into motion, the enemy, like the foiled tiger, will generally sneak off, and leave us victorious for the time'.

These practical tips on surviving the tropics dispensed, Johnson moved on to a discussion on fevers. Asserting his independence from established theory, Johnson writes that he will not apply the term idiopathic to fevers, since in his mind all fevers were associated to inflammation and congestion. In this sense, although he was writing in the second decade of the nineteenth century, Johnson appears to have moved closer to the later identification of fever as a symptom of underlying disease. He divided the causes of fever into two main groups, the 'predisponent' and the 'exciting'. The predisposing factors were 'innumerable', while the exciting causes were only two, 'human and marsh effluvia'. The predisposing causes include 'plethora', 'inanition from excessive evacuations', 'the depressing passions', 'excess, whether in eating drinking, gratification of the sensual passions', 'mental or corporeal exertions', 'extremes of atmospheric heat and cold, especially alternations of these or of heat and moisture', and, finally, 'sol-lunar influence'. This last predisposing cause derives from James Balfour's prolific writing on the particular effect of the phases of the moon on fevers in the tropics, discussed in an earlier chapter, and rejected by John Wade. The sol-lunar influence in fevers was then a new hypothesis, and quite sensibly, Johnson added that with its exception, each of the other predisposing factors could, when present in a very high degree, induce fever independently.

Taking up typhoid fever as an example of human effluvium or 'contagion', Johnson showed common-sense in stating that 'It does not appear to be much under the control of the seasons, since a full dose of it will produce the specific effect at any time of the year'. 'Of what this contagious matter consists', he wrote, 'we are totally ignorant, as it is perfectly incognizable by the senses, and incapable of being submitted to chemical analysis'. He surmised that the contagion consisted of 'a fruitful source for the dissemination of the disease by means of fomites, a form in which the mutter of contagion is eminently powerful'. These 'fomites' were to be found in the exhalations of the sick, dissipated by the free circulation of air in the summer, while the closeness of winter particularly 'the confined air of small apartments of the poor', helped condense them so that they stuck to the sick persons' bedding and personal belongings. Not everyone was affected by the 'febrific effluvia'. The eruption of disease required 'seldom less than fourteen, or more than sixty days between the receipt of the infection and the unfolding of the fever', which was preceded by a period when 'many doses of the poison' were received by the patient, aided by the operation of the predisposing factors. Johnson also rejected the term 'marsh' for 'vegeto-animal effluvium or miasma' since he observed that 'these febrific exhalations arise from the summits of mountains as well as from the surfaces of swamps'. The two main causes of fever operated differently, human effluvia affecting the nervous system, while marsh effluvia ruined the circulation. Beyond this, Johnson did not have anything to offer, saying 'The nature or essence of many of these causes themselves is also totally beyond our comprehension'.

Moving through a discussion of the common remedies for fevers, including venesection, whose use Johnson recommended at the height of the fever to relieve the patient, he begins discussing the 'Endemic Fever of Bengal' also called the 'Marsh Remittent Fever'. Commonly seen in the 'small portion of the Hooghly, between Calcutta and Kedgeree', a route used by all European ships, an average of 300 European sailors died annually of it. Johnson had seen a similar fever at work around Cairo, and in Georgia, where its ravages reduced the span of life to a maximum of 40 to 50 years. In Europe, the marshes around Walcheren had the same effect on its inhabitants. Johnson criticised the Bengal government for 'the apathy or impolicy, which still allows Diamond Harbour, the principal anchorage of our Indiamen, to continue backed and flanked by woods, jungles, and marshes, to the annual destruction of one-fourth of the crews of such ships as load and unload at this place'. Johnson dismissed the theory that the impenetrable jungles protected the harbour, asking that the jungle be cleared along a radius of 6 miles in Diamond Harbour. The draining or opening of Diamond Point to the movement of the tide would be of equal help in removing the cause of this fever. Until this was done, the lives of sailors could be preserved by docking ships at Sagar Roads, further from the shore, rather than at Kulpi or Kedgeree.

In Bengal, Johnson says, the flooding of the Ganges in the rainy season 'keeps the plains of Bengal overflowed from the latter end of July till the middle of October', because a slight rise of the land at the point where the great river meets the Bay of Bengal checks it from bearing the excess water at once into the sea. Instead, the swollen river slowly empties itself through a number of distributaries. Hence during the rainy season, 'noted cities, populous villages, exalted mosques, and stupendous pagodas, are seen just above the level of this temporary ocean, surrounded by innumerable boats, now the habitations of domesticated animals'. The water stood, in Johnson's time, between 10 and 30 feet high, and the course of the river was only marked by the water, which flowed down it at about 4 miles an hour, while in the flooded areas, it crawled at half a mile or a mile an hour. Through November and December, the flooded areas dry up, leaving 'a number of miry and slimy marshes to the action of a still powerful sun, when those who are in their neighbourhood, are sure to come in for a share of remittents and intermittents'. While one cause of death was 'the intense heat of the sun in June and July', to Johnson's mind it was nothing compared to 'a sudden and premature cessation of the rains', when 'an immense surface of slime and feculence is all at once exposed to the rays of a vertical sun'. 'The consequence is', Johnson continued, 'that the profuse exhalation of miasmata spreads pestilence and death in every direction; while famine, from the rice being left dry before it has attained maturity, completes the dreadful catastrophe!'

As a result, 'the country for some way round Calcutta, being in most places rather above the level of high water mark, become, during the rainy season, an immense woody and jungly marsh, neither perfectly overflowed, nor yet quite dry in a word, presenting a surface as well supplied with animal and vegetable matters in a state of decomposition, and combining all the other circumstances necessary for giving miasmata their full influence on the human body'. In the inundated districts, Johnson noted, 'The inhabitants and domestic animals ... are all this time cooped up in a state of ennui or torpor, which to an active European would be dreadful, had he not a number of mental, as well as corporeal resources for beguiling the tedious hours'. Bu in Calcutta and Diamond Harbour there was work to be done, and both locals and Europeans were exposed to the marsh remittent fever, to which was added the predisposing factors of rain, dew, heat, and intemperance.

For the young and inexperienced doctor, as Johnson was, when he went to Calcutta, 'arriving at an unhealthy spot in a foreign climate, unfortified by experience, unaided by advice, and, as is too frequently the case, but scantily supplied with books, containing local accounts of the country and its prevailing diseases' was fraught with great anxiety and distress. The young medical practitioner could only be 'agitated and alarmed by the mortality around him'.

Johnson reached Calcutta in September 1803, having made very good time, since the voyage took only 3 months. As soon as they began sailing up the Hooghly from Diamond Harbour, the marsh remittent fever made its appearance among the crew. Johnson resorted to reading treatises by James Clarke (1737-1819), and James Lind (1716-94), in order to combat it. However, Johnson wrote, 'a very few trials convinced me I had calculated without my host, and that I must use other weapons than those furnished me by Drs. Lind and Clarke, if I meant to be victorious in the contest'. Clarke's description of the fever was accurate, in that the 2 main symptoms described by him almost never failed to catch Johnson's notice, 'oppression of the praecordia', and excruciating pain in the stomach and head. Lind, had never been to India and depended on secondary sources, and so mentioned neither of these symptoms, but referred to the vomiting of bile. His own experiences made Johnson add delirium as one of the first symptoms of this fever, which he frequently found present, especially 'among young men who were employed in boats' since this exposed them particularly to the marsh effluvia. Other symptoms, which Johnson noted, included visceral obstruction, dysentery, and 'a yellowish suffusion on the skin'. Death usually occurred between the third and seventh days, though life was occasionally prolonged to the fifteenth or twentieth day. The fever had been found by Clarke, who experienced it in India, to have 3 stages. The first stage was one when the pulse was weak but rapid at 130, and the patient agonised with acute pain in the stomach and head, with vomiting. The second stage was the remission, occurring 12 0r 14 hours after the first stage, when the fever abated with perspiration, and the pulse fell to

90. The patient, however, felt very weak, and complained of pain in the stomach. This remission was brief, and was followed by the second attack of the fever, which returned more intensely. The final stage was the cold one, when the skin became moist and clammy; the pulse weak; the tongue was encrusted and black; while the vomiting continued. If the patient was not treated during the first stage of the fever, death was inevitable. Johnson was called in to treat a young man in the third or cold stage, and though an emetic brought about a remission, the fever soon returned. Johnson, "with an air of confidence, began to 'throw in' the bark: quite sanguine in my expectations of soon checking this formidable disease'. The vomiting became violent, and though he 'tried to push on the bark through the paroxysm, by the aid of opium', every draught was cast out. Johnson felt helpless. 'The plain truth was', he wrote 9 years later, 'that I knew not what to do; for the sudden and unexpected failure of that medicine on which I was taught to depend, completely embarrassed me; and before I could make up my mind to any feasible plan of treatment, my patient died, on the third day of his illness, perfectly yellow vomiting to the last, a dark fluid resembling vitiated bile, and exhibiting an awful specimen of the effects which a Bengal fever is capable of producing'. His experience was very common among European doctors practicing in Bengal, though few admitted it. Of particular significance was the deep sense of failure, worsened by helplessness. European medical theory and practice had failed to save European lives, ravaged by a disease few medical men in Europe had cared to think, or write, about.

Johnson dissected the body to obtain some clue that would help him grapple with the disease later. He wrote, 'On laying open the abdomen I was surprised to find the liver so gorged, as it were, with blood, that it actually fell to pieces on handling it'. Further, 'it appeared as if the greater number of the vessels had been broken down, and almost the whole of the interior structure converted into a mass of extravasation'. Made still more aware of his 'folly', and the 'oversight' of his teachers, he found some solace in the fact that James Clarke had only published accounts of 2 unsuccessful cases, 'without a single dissection'.

Soon Johnson had other cases, down with the same fever. He decided on venesection as a pre-emptive to purging and emetics, and must confess it was with a trembling arm and palpitating heart, that I first opened a vein, expecting every instant to see my patient die under my hands'. The patient seemed relieved by the bleeding. However, this did not cure him, since the fever returned with fury, and through it, Johnson carried out evacuations. The patient recovered, and Johnson was convinced that 'the evacuating plan' was the best. This he applied 'with a high hand'. Later, of course,

Johnson realised that he had been lucky,' for my patients, a great majority of them were fresh from Europe and high in health and strength; these recovered wonderfully, after bleeding and evacuations, though not always'. He noted, however, that the crew also included sailors, who had been pressed into service as soon as they had returned home from a previous voyage to India. In addition to suffering from the influence of the climate, the condition of these sailors was worsened by 'depressing passions', and 'galling disappointment'. These needed a different mode of treatment, which involved early evacuations, and the use of means to remove the 'congestions from the head and liver'. In fact, he felt that 'most of those, who were of a timid disposition, and easily alarmed at the prevalence of the endemic diseases of the country, fell under their influence sooner than those of a contrary temperament'. Nonetheless, Johnson wrote that he committed 'many glaring blunders', and drew 'false conclusions' until he 'arrived at anything like a steady and successful method of checking this Herculean endemic'.

The first symptom, Johnson said, was pain in the stomach, and vomiting. The patient would, at this stage, be made comfortable through bleeding, 'But the trifling manner in which it is too often performed, when it is ventured on at all, does more harm than good'. Johnson's dictum was, 'Bleed boldly and decisively till the head and praecordia are relieved, or draw no blood whatever'. During venesection, 'a scruple of calomel', given with a grain, or half a grain of opium, 'will act like a charm on the stomach'. However, in Europe there were doubts about how much calomel could be given without any danger to a patient. Johnson drew on the experiences of his brother officers, and said that in India, 'twenty grains of calomel will act as a sedative, and so far from griping and producing hypercatharsis, it will sooth uneasiness, and rather constipate than purge'. In a few hours, the calomel could be followed up with any purgative, whose actions would reveal to the doctor 'a most copious discharge of intolerably foetid, bilious, and feculent matter, to the unspeakable relief of the head and epigastrium'. The second dictum thus became, 'The more copious the catharsis, the less danger there will be of the return of vomiting'. Any returns of the symptoms of the first stage should invigorate the doctor to use bloodletting without hesitation. In fact, the medical practitioner must never allow 'Those bugbears, debility and putrescency', which 'still paralyse the arms of medical men in hot climates ... particularly where the subject is lately from Europe and not broken down by the climate'. Johnson exhorted the use of the jugular vein for bloodletting to relieve headache.

This treatment was to be followed by 5 to 10 grains of calomel, combined if needed with half a grain of opium, given every 4 to 6 hours until all symptoms disappeared. This was, Johnson claimed, the sine qua non 'in the medical treatment of this fever, as well as many other fevers in the East'. He had also learnt that in the Bengal marsh remittent fever, emetics had to be avoided, since they would exacerbate gastric irritability, which was one of the major symptoms of this disease. In some cases the symptoms disappeared with the effective use of purgatives, and Johnson was 'tempted to follow them up, and try if they might not supersede the necessity of impregnating the system with mercury'. But he soon knew better, because he lost a patient in this experiment. If the patient found it difficult to swallow mercurial pills, the alternative was to use mercurial ointment. As soon as salivation was seen, which happened usually by the third day, the doctor could be sure of having 'secured' the patient. If there was no abatement of the symptoms by the third, fourth, or fifth day, every passing day made it more difficult for the patient to survive. In such cases, Johnson used increased doses of calomel, at more frequent intervals, bolstered by the application of mercurial ointment, until some positive symptoms, like 'mild and uniform diaphoresis, a refreshing sleep, and the appearance of natural stools' were seen. However, the use of mercury made the mouth sore, and soon the patient complained of the inability to eat.

Besides these prophylactic measures, Johnson suggested that patients be moved to the airiest, and coolest part of the ship or building, the feet be immersed in warm water; the head shaved, and placed in an elevated position, and constantly applied with folds of cloth dipped in vinegar and artificially cooled water. This 'cold affusion' derived from the practice of the locals who, when assailed by this fever, drank water copiously, and applied wetted cloths to their heads'. Wine and bark were to be used only in cases of 'protracted convalescence'. Nonetheless, acknowledging James Balfour's experience, Johnson places his method of treatment, independent of the sol-lunar influence, of using bark and calomel towards the end of the section, as another way of addressing the fever. Of the sol-lunar influence, Johnson was convinced. He had himself experienced its effect in Calcutta. At the full and change of the moon, he used to be 'affected with tremor, a sense of weakness, and sometimes a dimness of vision about mid-day, succeeded by a certain quickness and irritability of pulse, which would continue for an hour or two'. Johnson was so acutely aware of this that he kept himself as quiet and cool as possible at those times, for the least exertion, especially in the sun, exacerbated the problem. This was the reason most Europeans in Bengal complained of 'faintness' around noon. For Johnson, a cold bath at this time worked wonders. However, the influence of the moon around midnight could not be avoided, for it woke him from sleep, 'disturbed with dreams, and a feverish heat', until 2 in the morning, when sleep would return.

With the approach of the cold season, Johnson wrote, 'the fever changes from an almost continued to a plainly remittent, and finally, in December, to an intermittent form'. 'From this time', he continued, 'for two or three months, the climate of Bengal is cool and delightful; the only diseases being visceral obstructions, the sequels of the preceding endemic'. Like the other medical writers, whose works have been discussed in this book, James Johnson too observed the locals and learnt from them. The locals, he saw, were able to withstand this fever due to 'the assimilation of their constitutions to the climate, their singularly abstemious habits, and various other causes'. In them, the fever changed character, and turned from remittent to intermittent 'but often of great obstinacy'. The local medicines used included the 'black purging salt', the 'Bit-Noben, or Cala Neemuck, a solution of which in water is certainly one of the most nauseous potations that can well be conceived, having an abominable taste, and a flavour resembling rotten eggs, or sulphuretted hydrogen gas'. The bowels having been purged, 'the kernel of a seed, produced by a low, creeping kind of cow-itch, (*Caesalpina Bonducella*,) called by the natives, Kaut-Kullagee, or Catcaranja Nut, is taken to complete the cure'. This kernel is very bitter, but 'possesses the tonic or febrifuge powers of Peruvian bark, in a very high degree'. Many European practitioners thought highly of it because it did not carry the same side-effects, like constipation. Rather, it additionally acted as a mild laxative. Another medicine often used by the locals was the decoction of 'Cherettah', 'a species of gentian, indigenous in the mountainous countries north of the Ganges, and is to be procured in every bazaar throughout Bengal'. Johnson was sure that Cherettah would, 'at no distant period, supersede entirely the bark, to which it seems infinitely preferable in a hot climate'.

Johnson drew upon his own experience to explain his view that the vegeto-animal miasmata, which caused the fever, 'descended with the dews'. In October 1805, he had travelled from Madras to Calcutta aboard a merchantman. He was sitting late on the deck soon after the ship arrived in the Ganges, and lay anchored a mile from the shore. There was 'not a breath of wind moving in any direction', and as the dews began to fall, 'I perceived, all at once, a faint, heavy odour, to account for which I was much puzzled, as there was no breeze to waft any exhalation from the adjacent shores'. Soon he felt 'a sense of faintness, giddiness, and at length, nausea'. I immediately went below', he said, 'not a little alarmed, and fully persuaded that I was seized with the fever, whose effects I had so much reason to dread'. Below decks, he drank some warm water to clear the stomach, and followed it up with 'a dose of calomel and opium', and the next morning, some castor oil. While 'no further symptoms of fever occurred', he felt an unusual lassitude and depression of spirits for some days after reaching Calcutta.

The way to avoid these miasmata was to travel in the jungles and marshes at 'that point of time at which we are least likely to meet those miasms, whether in their ascending or descending state'. 'This period', Johnson felt, 'seems to extend from three to six o'clock in the afternoon; that is, after the greatest heat of the earth and air, and, consequently, the greatest evaporation; and before the condensation and return of such exhalations as rose during the day, and which combine with those still issuing from the heated soil, for some time after sunset'. The usual shipboard practice of using the cool of the morning and evening for wooding, watering, and other shore duties was therefore wrong.

The condition of the plethoric European landing in Bengal bore no comparison with the situation in the West Indies, where the same fever existed. In the West Indies, 'they are destitute of many powerful shields which are pretty generally interposed between Europeans of the east and the burning climate'. These 'powerful shields' include the palankeen, the budgerow, the punkha, and 'the light, elegant, and cool vestments', in addition to the retinue of servants, who saved Europeans from exertion. This was not 'Asiatic effeminacy', insisted Johnson, but a necessary aid or 'salutary precautions' for survival. The passions were also catered to, for the European soldier was permitted to 'intermarry with the native Hindostannee nymph; and, whether married or not, he has generally a domiciliated *chere amie*, who cooks, washes, and performs every menial drudgery for *massa*, in health, besides becoming an invaluable nurse when he is overtaken by sickness'.

These comforts notwithstanding, Johnson soon fell seriously ill. A few weeks after he had arrived in Bengal, Johnson went with a group of fellow officers to hunt and see the country around Kedgeree. The day was a very warm one with a 'broiling sun', and the ground was 'half inundated'. Johnson and his friends 'waded and rambled about, through marshes, jungles, and paddy fields' the whole day, supported by refreshments from a basket. Returning in the evening, 'to the bank of the Ganges, at a place appointed, we found that the boat could not approach the shore, the water was so shoally; we therefore dashed into the river, and waded off to where the boat lay at a grapnel'. With a strong tide against them, it took 2 hours to reach the ship, during which time the officers sat in the boat 'dripping wet and shivering with cold'. Johnson, tired out by the day's activity, should have slept well; his sleep, however, was disturbed, and he felt chills coming on 'alternated with flushes of heat'. On waking, all seemed normal, though by dinner, 'I had no appetite; and soon afterwards I felt uneasiness in my bowels'. 'As the evening advanced', he recorded, he was stricken by increasingly frequent 'calls to stool, with griping, and some tenesmus', during which only some mucus was evacuated. Soon fever came, and the spasms were so bad that by 11 pm, Johnson 'could scarcely leave the commode'. He spent a very miserable night, with no relief from the tenesmus, and the frequent stools, his mind giving way to delirium whenever he lay down. There was no medical assistance to hand, and he had taken 'a dose of salts' in the evening, which only carried out some 'feculences', and caused 'a momentary lull' to the constant urge to relieve himself. Early the next morning, 'a medical gentleman belonging to an East Indiaman, visited me, and found me in a very bad way'. Johnson had high fever, and was frequently passing blood. He was first bled, and given castor oil. A few hours later, he took the first dose of 6 grains of calomel with 1 grain of opium, the medications to be repeated every 5 hours. Johnson was also prescribed 'emollient injections' to help ease the tenesmus. These were of course rectal injections. The medicines helped a little, but fever raged, as did great thirst, and a restlessness which, when not lulled by opium, led to delirium. The calls to stool continued, during which nothing but mucus and blood came. The delirious bouts, Johnson later recalled, 'the phantoms that haunted my imagination were worse than all my corporeal sufferings, which were, in themselves, indescribably tormenting'. By the following day Johnson was very weak. The tenesmus continued, and he was so debilitated that he could not make the effort to leave the commode. He yearned for even momentary relief. The medications were now being given every 4 hours, and mercurial ointment was being rubbed into his skin. Additionally, he was taking a dose of castor oil daily, 'which brought off a trifling feculence, with inconsiderable relief'. The fever raged higher than before, with a 'hot, dry, constricted skin'. As night came on, Johnson became anxious about whether he would be able to survive another night of such pain and unease. His doctor assured him that he would recover as soon as salivation showed that the mercury was working.

Indeed, as night came on, Johnson's symptoms worsened, and he became sure that he would die unless he did something to bring on salivation as quickly as possible. To this end, he asked his assistant to give him 'a scruple of calomel'. He had been told that excessive use of mercury had bad effects but in his own case he found that, to the contrary, the additional dose 'rather lulled the tormina'. This, however, was temporary, and the fever and tenesmus continued such that soon Johnson looked forward to death as the only available means of release. Though extremely weak, he survived the night, and repeated the scruple of calomel at 4 am. Finally, at 8 am he fell, 'for the first time, into a profound and refreshing sleep, which lasted till near midnight, when I awoke'. For a while he lay still, he said, afraid to move. There was no pain, and his skin was covered with a warm perspiration. Soon he felt a call to stool, which depressed him, for he thought it showed the return of the tenesmus. To his delight, however, Johnson found that the stool, brought out 'copious, feculent, bilious' matter with no tenesmus. On getting into bed again, he found that his gums were swollen, and that he was salivating freely. These were symptoms of mercurial action, and he was going to live. He stopped taking mercury and, being young, quickly recovered.

This was an example of the dysentery typical to tropical countries, and later study only reconfirmed to Johnson their 'remote causes'. These were 'atmospherical vicissitudes', caused by 'Perspiration and biliary secretion being in excess during the intense heat of the day', checked suddenly by 'the damp chills of the night'. The treatment, as exemplified by his own experience, involved the administration of 24, 36, or 48 grains of calomel, with an anodyne and a diaphoretic, at intervals of 3, 4, or 6 hours, depending on the seriousness of the case. This could be supported by evacuations using castor oil, and the bodily pain suffused using 2 to 4 grains of opium. As listed by Johnson, the other surgeons 'in that quarter', i.e. Bengal, all used the same pharmacopeia, with some differences in their combination only. Their main aim was to use mercury to achieve 'ptyalism', whose appearance informed them that the patient was out of immediate danger. His own brush with dysentery convinced Johnson of the efficacy of mercury, which he thenceforth used on some occasions in similar 'scruple doses', administered 2, 3, or even 4 times a day, to push on boldly for 'ptyalism'. On one or two occasions, the bad effect of excessive mercury made itself felt through nausea, which was quickly removed by administering opium with a diaphoretic.

Johnson was also aware that mercury provided only a temporary cure. 'Those', he wrote, 'who have had most experience in hot climates, best known the melancholy fact, that in every repetition of dysentery, and after every successive year of our residence between the tropics, we find the remedy has greater and greater difficulty in conquering the disease'. As the intervals between attacks of dysentery reduced, 'we find it a very tedious process to bring the mouth affected with mercury; and, what is still worse, the check thus given to the complaint is only temporary ; for soon after the influence of the medicine wears off, our patient returns upon our hands as bad as ever'. Finally, 'the system absolutely refuses all impregnation from mercury: and we have the mortification to see our patient waste away, and die'. The only certain cure was an immediate change of climate, which was not in the power of doctors to give. In fact, most of those who spent long years in tropical lands, returned home with chronic dysentery.

There are other points, which Johnson interestingly makes, in relation to dysentery. For instance, he points to patience as the greatest virtue of those ill with dysentery. Writing from personal experience, Johnson said that calls to stool had to be disobeyed as much as possible. Movement was debilitating, as was the straining that accompanied the tenesmus, particularly since the stools brought away little more than blood and mucus. The patient had to give the medications the opportunity to work. To help the patient sustain these urges, warm baths and fomentations to the abdomen were advised. Similarly, on recovery, the patient was urged to keep for a while to an 'unirritating and farinaceous' diet, such as sago, arrowroot, and rice. 'A very excellent dish for chronic dysentrics', he wrote, highly relished by the patient, 'is flour and milk, well boiled together, which with a very little sugar and spice'. Too often, however, 'the appetite too often outstrips the digestion, and so do chylification and sanguification exceed the various excretions, so as to occasion a dangerous inequilibrium between assimilation and secretion', resulting in fatal relapse. It was necessary, therefore, for the patient to follow medical advice closely, and with fortitude.

The final section of Johnson's book addresses 'Tropical Hygiene or, Hints for the Preservation of Health in all Hot Climates'. The usual advice given to all Europeans on arrival in India, and other hot climates, is 'to observe and imitate the conduct of our own countrymen long resident in the climate'. 'This', commented Johnson, 'is certainly the most practicable; but, in my opinion, it is not the safest plan', because 'that residence alone confers on them immunities and privileges, of which it would be death for us, in many instances, to claim a participation, before the period of our probation has expired'. For the stranger, then, there were 2 cardinal rules, temperance and coolness. The latter was most important, and in fact included the latter. For this reason, 'coolness' was regarded as 'the grand principle of Inter-tropical Hygiene'. Here too moderation was the essential perquisite, for heat was the predisposing factor for diseases in the tropics, accentuated by cold. The 'great object is to moderate, by all possible means, the heat, and habituate ourselves from the beginning to the impressions of cold'. This was also 'the grand secret of counteracting the influence of tropical climates on European constitutions'. To this end, while in India, it was necessary to observe, and learn from, the practices of 'the ancient and civilised race of Hindoos'.

Johnson particularly noted the dress of the Bengal dandy or waterman, who dressed only in a loincloth, 'passed between the thighs, and fastened before and behind to a piece of stout packthread, that encircles the waist'. The remaining part of his body uncovered, the waterman worked for hours at the oars of the budgerow, 'in the scorching noontide heat, till perspiration issues from every pore, he darts overboard, when necessary, with the track-rope on his shoulder, and wades through puddles and marshes this moment up to the middle, or the shoulders in water the next, in the open air, with a rapid evaporation from the whole surface of his body'. Equally admirable was the way in which he exposed his skin to the high sun, 'a deluge of rain, or a piercing north-wester, with equal indifference', and 'All this, too, on a scanty meal of rice, being seldom paid more than three pence per day board wages!'

The skin of these hardy persons seemed to Johnson to exude an 'oily and tenacious' perspiration, different from that seen in Europeans. In fact, oil, which was 'assiduously and regularly rubbed' over the whole body by all classes of locals preserved the softness of the skin, and 'a moderate, equable flow of perspiration'. Further, Johnson noted the use by all classes of locals, of the turban and the cummerbund, the former to protect the head from the direct rays of the sun, and the latter 'preserving the important viscera of the abdomen from the deleterious impressions of cold'. The light, flowing cotton clothes used by the richer persons, were 'for ornament than use'. The European was urged to learn from these local customs, and cover the head with a large, cotton handkerchief, preferably wetted, folded and tucked into the hat, and wear 'a fine shawl' in place of the cummerbund. This last 'should never be neglected, especially by those who have been some time in the country, or whose bowels are in any degree tender'. The European was advised to avoid the sun at the hottest time of day, when, if it was essential to go out, Johnson urged the use of an umbrella.

The European was urged to abandon linen for cotton, 'which from it slowness as a conductor of heat is admirably adapted for the tropics'. Similarly, 'When a vicissitude takes place, and the atmospherical temperature sinks suddenly far below that of the body, the cotton, still faithful to its trust, abstracts more slowly the heat from our bodies, and thus preserves a more steady equilibrium there'. 'To all these must be added', Johnson said, 'the facility with which it absorbs the perspiration; while linen would feel quite wet, and during the exposure to a breeze under such circumstances, would often occasion a shiver, and be followed by dangerous consequences'. Ever observant, Johnson also noted that 'The musical ladies of India are not unacquainted with this secret, since they take care to keep their pianos well covered with blankets in the hot season, to defend them from the heat, and prevent their warping'. Many of the English preferred flannel, which appeared to Johnson to be inferior to cotton, since it was heavier, conducted heat much more slowly, and was unpleasant on the skin since it caused friction.

Prejudices among Europeans blinded them to the benefits of local customs, such as the one in the upper provinces of Bengal, 'where the summer is intensely hot, and the winter sharp, the dress of native shepherds, who are exposed to all weather, consists in a blanket gathered in at one end, which goes over the head, the rest hanging down on all sides like a cloak'. Of all customs, the worst was the insistence on uniforms 'on almost all public occasions, and in all formal parties, under a burning sky'. There were officers, who paid no heed to the climate, and insisted on dressing formally on all occasions, which led Johnson to observe, 'It is certainly laughable, or rather pitiable enough, to behold, for some time after each fresh importation from Europe, a number of griffinish sticklers for decorum, whom no persuasions can induce to cast their exuviae, even in the most affable company, pinioned, as it were, in their stiff habiliments, while the streams of perspiration that issue from every pore, and ooze through various angles of their dress'. The host or hostess would often give the youth no encouragement to dine in shirtsleeves, leaving him to suffer silently from prickly heat and perspiration at the table and, later, 'the raw, chilling vapours of the night, on his way home'.

Cloth and bleaching being cheap in Bengal, 'The European, contemplating, with great satisfaction the multitude of changes he has thus cheaply amassed, and calculating the very reasonable terms of ablution, determines to enjoy in its fullest extent a luxury, which he deems both salutary and grateful, independently of all considerations respecting appearance'. 'It is therefore', Johnson continued, 'very common to see him shift his linen three or four times a-day'. However, this was an injurious practice, since the perspiration, 'already in excess', was 'powerfully solicited', and thus 'morbidly increased, instead of being restrained'. The usual practice of the griffin was to consign shirts wet with perspiration to the dhobi's care without a further thought. Johnson, however, reasoned that 'It should not, therefore, be consigned to the wash, but carefully dried, and worn again, once, or even twice; and that, too, without the smallest infringement on the laws of personal cleanliness, but with the most salutary effect on the health'. By this practice the wearer would need only one shirt a day, since 'It is astonishing how much less exhausting is the linen, which has been once or twice impregnated with the fluid of perspiration, than that which is fresh from the mangle'. Here too Johnson spoke from personal experience, since he had lost his stock of shirts during a voyage from Trincomalee, and learnt from necessity the utility of this practice.

The newly arrived European was urged to consume more vegetables than meat, not because it was more easily digested, but because it excites less commotion in the system during that process, and is not so apt to induce plethora afterwards'. 'Almost the whole of the upper classes are absolutely FALSTAFFS, he noted, 'and often have I been puzzled to know how some of them cold stow themselves away in a palankeen, and still more so, how their bearers could trot along under the pressure of such human porpoises'. In fact, 'the Hindostanee fops, (and most of the superior orders are such,) pride themselves above all things, on rotundity of corporation, and particularly on the magnitude of their heads'. This was accomplished by the use of ghee, 'a kind of semi-liquid butter, made by evaporating the aqueous part from the rich milk of the buffalo', and indolence. Thus, there was little difference between Europeans who gorged on meat to death, and those who swilled ghee, since both made their way 'by the same short routes of apoplexy, and other fashionable near cuts to heaven'.

On the other hand, the hardiness of the 'palankeen bearers, coolies, dandies, hircarrahs', was admirable, for they underwent 'three times as much fatigue, under a burning sky, as would kill an Englishman outright'. These persons, though they lived abstemiously on very simple diets, were addicted to 'bang, toddy, arrack, opium, and other inebriating materials, which all countries produce, in some shape or other'. Despite their hardihood, Johnson did not find robustness in these persons, but commented on how they had no stamina to bear illness, and succumbed rapidly to them.

Indians generally breakfasted very early in the morning, soon after sunrise, a practice which was impossible for the European to follow. Also, the locals breakfasted heavily, in most cases eating nothing else until sunset. Europeans also sat to breakfast tables loaded with viands of meat, fish, and eggs, with relish, thinking falsely that a good appetite meant good health 'but the stomach, though it may relish, is seldom equal to the digestion of such alimentary substances as those allude to, where a sound night's rest has hardly ever been procured'. The newly arrived European in Bengal was adjoined 'to content himself with plain breakfasts of bread and butter, with tea or coffee; and avoid indulging in meat, fish, eggs, or buttered toast'. To drive home his point, Johnson gave the example of a ship's purser he knew, who revelled in prodigious breakfasts, heavy drinking, and neglecting every adage for good health in the tropics. He had survived the West Indies, and the greater part of his tour of the East Indies, until he died from the enormity of his last breakfast, of which 'The prominent articles were, four hard-boiled eggs, two dried fishes, two plates of rice, with chillies, condiments, and a proportionate allowance of bread, butter, coffee'. No sooner had he finished this gargantuan repast, he was taken ill, in which condition he spent several days, in agony, for his system defied all efforts at evacuation by the attending surgeon 'till a few hours before his death, when mortification relaxed all strictures'.

The local midday meal, the tiffin, was laudatory, and Johnson wrote, 'The tiffin, at one o'clock, consisting of light curries, or the like, with a glass or two of wine, and some fruit, is a natural, a necessary, and a salutary repast'. This should logically have led to a balanced dinner, but Europeans in Bengal ate heavy meals after sundown. Enjoying themselves in the cool, they made this the most important social event of the day, and so 'savoury viands - the stimulating wines of the evening feast, prolonged by the fascination of social converse, greatly exacerbate the nocturnal paroxysm of fever imposed on us by the hand of nature, and break with feverish dreams, the hours which should be dedicated to repose!' The newcomer to Bengal should 'beware of indulging in this second and unnecessary dinner, particularly during the period of his probation; but will rather be satisfied with the meridian repast, as the principal meal, when tea or coffee, at six or seven o'clock in the evening, will be found a grateful refreshment'.

Local fruits were enticing, but usual medical advice indicated avoidance by Europeans, since they were suspected to be the cause of dysentery. Johnson did not find any evidence of his in his own experience of eating local fruits, like the mango, which were plentifully available. If fruits caused dysentery, he reasoned, it was because 'the intestines are already in an irritable state, from irregular or vitiated secretions of bile, they certainly tend to increase that irritability, and consequently predispose to the complaint in question'. The local fruits included mango, shaddock, pineapple, and plantain. Mangoes, though delectable, were not free of medical suspicion, since they were believed to cause Europeans to break out in 'a plentiful crop of pustules, or even boils'. In fact, one of Johnson's patients died of addiction to 'an unrestrained indulgence in fruit, particularly mangoes'. Johnson claimed that this ill-effect of eating mangoes was well-known in India. Pineapples were similarly not 'the safest fruit to make too free with at first'. Shaddocks were more preferable, especially in hot weather, 'from their subacid and cooling juice, so well adapted to allay the unpleasant sensation of thirst'. Bananas also were useful, since they were 'wholesome and nutritious, especially when frittered'. Indian spices, the primary reason for the arrival of English traders in India, were to be avoided until 'those ulterior periods of our residence in hot climates, when the tone of the constitution is lowered, and the stomach participates in the general relaxation', when their use proved 'safe and salutary'.

One of the banes of Europeans living in India, particularly Bengal, was their predilection for wine. For Johnson, water was the only necessary liquid refreshment, since its use led directly to his cardinal principle for health in the tropics, the need to keep the body cool. 'But no', he said, 'a wretched, sensual theory has spread from the vulgar to many in the profession, (who ought to know better,) that since the heat of the climate occasions a profuse perspiration, and consequently renders that discharge the more liable to a sudden check, we are to aid and assist these natural causes by the use of gently stimulating liquids, and, of course, increase those very effects which we pretend to obviate!' Johnson claimed that this was medical advice given out 40 years previously, and that it had since gone out of fashion. No European of any social standing would be seen indulging in 'gently stimulating liquids' between meals. The griffin was particularly warned off calling for 'brandy-shrub- pauny'. The reasoning for this was that in local culture, intoxication was proscribed. An inebriated European would thus only ruin 'the European character in the eyes of those natives, whom it was desirable at all times to impress with a deep sense of our superiority'. Such temperance was not the case in the West Indies, he wrote. In fact, 'the general temperance in this respect, which now characterises the Anglo-Asiatic circles of society, as contrasted with Anglo-West-Indian manners, must utterly confound those fine-spun theories, which the votaries of porter-cup, sangaree, and other gently stimulating liquids, have invented'.

Brunonian medical theory advocated the use of stimulating liquids, but Johnson lost no time in sarcastically negating it: 'I can conceive only one plausible argument which the trans-Atlantic Brunonian can adduce, in support of his doctrine after the unwelcome denouement which I have brought forward respecting oriental customs ; namely, that as the range of atmospheric heat, in the West Indies, is several degrees below that of the East, it may be necessary to counterbalance this deficit of external heat, by the more assiduous application of internal stimulus!' Even aboard East Indiamen, captains did not allow decanters to circulate the table more than half a dozen times at dinner, and twice during the 'frugal' supper.

This, however, was not a true picture of European society in India, as Johnson was forced to admit, stating that "at each of the presidencies, there may he found several individuals of the old bacchanalian school, whose wit, humour, or vocal powers, are sometimes courted, on particular occasions, to 'set the table in a roar'". This was hardly to be wondered at, since 'It might appear very reasonable, that in a climate where ennui reigns triumphant and an unaccountable languor pervades both mind and body we should cheer our drooping spirits with the mirth-inspiring bowl'. Johnson followed this up with a personal anecdote from the time he was on convalescent leave on Prince of Wales's Island [Penang]. One evening he dined with several gentlemen there, one of whom 'was remarkable for his convivial talents and flow of spirits'. Johnson, who had expected his flow of wit to flag the more he drank, was surprised to see him 'maintain a uniform level, after many younger heroes had bowed to the rosy god'. Johnson talked to him and discovered that 'he had drunk nothing but water for many years in India; that in consequence his health was excellent his spirits free his mental faculties unclouded, although far advanced on time's list'.

The newcomer was urged not to drink more than 4 glasses at mealtimes, and never 'admit it to his lips between meals, unless excessive fatigue and thirst render drink indispensable, when cold water might be injurious'. A very refreshing liquid in the warm countries was coconut milk. It was accused of producing 'bowel complaints', which Johnson dismissed. 'It was my favourite beverage', he said, 'and never did I feel in my own person or perceive in others, the slightest inconvenience from indulging in this most delicious liquid'. It was necessary, however, that it 'be fresh-drawn, limpid, sweet, and never drunk after the deposit on the inside of the shell begins to assume the form of a consistent crust'.

Johnson then recounted a unique event, when a Lieutenant Britton, of the Royal Marines, 'a very fine young gentleman, had heated and fatigued himself, by driving about the streets and bazaars of Calcutta, in the autumn of 1803, in which state, he had the imprudence to swallow an ice-cream, for the purpose of allaying his thirst'. Britton died aboard ship en route to Madras, under Johnson's care. Johnson recalled that 'He died in dreadful agonies, flying from one part of the ship to another, for relief from the dyspnoea and oppression on his chest', and reasoned that his slaking his thirst with an ice-cream caused 'inflammation about the fauces, which subsequently spread down along the membrane lining the trachea, to the lungs, producing symptoms exactly resembling croup'.

The need for exercise was explained following a very devious argument. 'Perspiration and certain secretions, (the biliary, for instance,)',

Johnson wrote, 'being already in excess, in equatorial regions, a perseverance in our customary European exercises, would prove highly injurious, and often does so, by greatly aggravating the natural effects of climate'. However, exercise was necessary, for 'this excess very soon leads to debility and diminished action, in the functions alluded to, with a corresponding inequilibrium of the blood, so it is necessary to counteract these, by such active or passive exercise as the climate will admit, at particular periods of the day or year; a discrimination imperiously demanded, if we mean to preserve our health'. Knowledge of the time for exercise could be observed through local customs, when at the hottest time of day even the ubiquitous adjutant bird of Bengal, spent hours soaring in the higher reaches of the sky, and the locals stayed in their homes, sheltering from the sun and drinking copiously of cool water and sherbets. After sunset, in the cool of the evening, 'Then it is, that the esplanade at Calcutta, and the Mount road near Madras, pour on the astonished eye of the stranger a vast assemblage of all nations, casts, and complexions, comprehending an endless and unequalled variety of costume and character, hurrying to and fro, in all kinds of vehicles as well as on foot, enjoying the refreshing air of the evening!' This was a common scene in the cool season too. During the rains, however, hot land-winds prostrated the Europeans, 'Perspiration being then profuse, the most trifling exertion is followed by languor and lassitude'. The European, 'Cooped up behind a tatty, or lolling about under a punkha … can neither amuse his mind, nor exercise his body', which led to an oppressive tedium.

One popular form of exercise in the tropics was dancing. Johnson did not approve of this, saying 'It might seem ill-natured if I animadverted on the custom of my fair countrywomen, who show off with such éclat, at the Pantheon in Madras, regardless of all thermo metrical indications'. He followed it up with the strange observation that dancing 'does not appear to agree so well with married ladies as with virgins, whatever may be the reason'.

'Gestation in a palankeen', he wrote, 'is a species of passive exercise exceedingly well adapted to a tropical climate'. Its use was evident from 'The languid circulation of the blood in those who have been long resident there, is pointedly evinced by the inclination which everyone feels for raising the lower extremities on a parallel with the body, when at rest; and this object is completely attained in the palankeen, which indeed renders it a peculiarly agreeable vehicle'. Massage, or shampooing, was another similar form of mild exercise suited to India, in which 'the gentle pressure and friction of a soft hand, over the surface of the body, but particularly the limbs, invigorate the circulation after fatigue, and excite the insensible cuticular secretion'.

From exercise Johnson moves over to the design of houses in the tropics. Considering European houses in India better constructed to deal with the heat than those in the West Indies, Johnson points out their advantages. 'As there is no dread of earthquakes or hurricanes, in the former place', he wrote, 'the dwellings are solid the apartments lofty the windows large, and the floors, in general, composed of terras, which being often sprinkled with water, is cool to the feet, and diffuses an agreeable refrigeration through the room'. The deep verandahs, typical of European dwellings in the East, 'ward off the glare of the sun, and reflected heat, (an important consideration,) by day, and afford a most pleasant retreat in the evening, for enjoying the cool air'. Johnson only wished that these verandahs to extended all around the house.

Of still greater utility were the 'tatties, which are affixed to the doors and other apertures, in the hot season, and kept constantly wet by bheesties, or water-carriers, whereby the breeze is cooled by evaporation, in its passage through the humid grass, of which the tatty is constructed, prove a very salutary and grateful defence against the hot land-winds ; since this simple expedient makes a difference of twenty or thirty degrees, between the bheesty's and the European's side of the tatty!' Another utility in India was the punkha which, 'suspended from the lofty ceilings of the Eastern rooms, and kept waving overhead, especially during our repasts, is a very necessary piece'.

Europeans in India also needed to see the way in which locals built their houses in the simplest way possible, and avoided both heat and glare, and learn from them. The first noticeable matter was that 'His habitation has very few apertures, and those high up'. The next characteristic was unpleasant to Europeans, but quite effective, 'His floor, and the inside of the walls, are moistened two or three times a-day, with a solution of cow-dung in water, which, however disagreeable to the olfactories of a European, keeps the interior of the dwelling as cool as it is dark'. And within this dark and cool dwelling, the local 'sits on his mat, enjoying his aqueous, but salutary beverage; and with such simple means and materials, counteracts the heat of the climate more effectually than the European, in his superb and costly edifice'. At other places, similar ingenuity was seen at work, as in Benaras, where houses were 6 stories high, 'with small windows', and stood on streets 'so extremely narrow' that the sun had little access to them.

Smoking, through the use of the hookah, was not necessarily a bad thing, for 'the practice is very general among Europeans and Natives, and seems to spring from that listlessness and want of mental energy, so predominant in the character both of sojourners and permanent inhabitants of sultry latitudes'. Johnson's verdict on it was 'the custom may not be insalutary at certain seasons of the year, in particular places, where marshy or other deleterious exhalations abound; and as it is often a succedaneum for more dangerous indulgences, it is best, perhaps, to pass it over with little comment'. 'Yet', he added, 'it has ever appeared to me a degrading habit, for a gentleman to become a slave to his hookah; and it is beyond endurance, to see a great, lusty hookah-burdaar, insinuate the pipe of his long snake into the delicate hand of a European lady, after dinner, who plies the machine with as much glee'.

Another subject of medical discussion was the cold bath. Johnson felt that a cold bath was not necessarily dangerous, other than 'where visceral obstructions obtained, I cannot conceive why it should be denied to almost all, except females, in hot climates'. For Johnson, 'wide experience' had settled the point, that in the East, 'the Native arid European the old and the young the male and the female, resort to the BATH, as the greatest luxury and the best preservative of health'. The best example was the buffalo, whose instinct led it to the use of the bath in hot weather. 'In the middle or hot period of the day', he wrote, 'these animals repair to pools or marshes, and wading in, either stand or lie down there, with every part except the nose immersed in water; or, where there is not water, in the mud'. Buffaloes were so possessive of their cool haunts that Johnson found it necessary to warn European against approaching them, particularly if dressed in red coats, which was 'a very unfortunate dress at such critical rencontres, as the animals in question have a decided antipathy to that colour'. Soon a few of them, on noticing the intruder, would begin to snort and advance in irritation, when the European was advised to beat 'the most rapid retreat to a place of safety'. The cold bath steeled the constitution to the 'atmospheric vicissitudes' that caused disease. The use of the cold bath, then', he wrote, 'should be regularly and daily persevered in, from the moment we enter the tropics; and when, from long residence there, the functions above alluded to begin to be irregular and defective, instead of in excess, we may prudently veer round, by degrees, to the tepid bath, which will be found a most valuable part of Tropical Hygiene among the seasoned Europeans'. Europeans generally preferred to bathe soon after rising in the morning, and before dinner. a cold bath in the morning 'powerfully obviates that train of nervous symptoms, so universally complained of by our countrymen between the tropics'. 'Before dinner it is salutary', he added, 'apparently from that connexion which subsists between the external surface and the stomach, in consequence of which the tone of the latter is increased, and the disagreeable sensation of thirst removed, that might otherwise induce to too much potation during the repast'.

This took Johnson to the subject of sleep. In the tropical countries, particularly India, 'disturbed repose' was common. But 'Whatever we detract from the period of our natural sleep, will assuredly be deducted in the end, from the natural range of our existence, independently of the predisposition to disease'. The newly arrived European in Bengal expected a refreshing sleep after sunset, but this was in vain, since 'A new host of foes instantly appear in arms to annoy us! mosquitoes, ants, and cock-roaches, lead on the insect tribes the bat wheels in aerial circuits over our heads on which he sometimes condescends to alight, without ceremony while the snake patrols about, in the purlieus of our apartment: coils himself up under our beds, or even deigns to become our bedfellow without waiting the formality of an invitation'. He even recounts a horrific case in which a snake was discovered coiled between two sleeping infants. 'It is said', he added, 'that if a chaffing-dish, filled with clear, live embers, be quietly placed on the floor of a room, in such emergency, the reptiles will repair to it; especially if some new milk be also left near the chaffing-dish'.

While looking for 'cool repose at night', the European was warned against sleeping in the open, on account of 'rains, heavy dews, or exhalations from contiguous marshes, woods, or jungles'. 'But', he wrote, drawing on personal experience, 'pending the hot and dry season in Bengal, and almost always on the Coromandel coast, except during the hot laud-winds, or at the change of the monsoons, we may indulge, not only with safety, but with infinite advantage, in the seemingly dangerous luxury of sleeping abroad in the open air'. Since this opinion clashed with his previous assertion that the European ought to avoid the dew, which bore disease-causing 'atmospherical vicissitudes', Johnson wrote that he felt 'The truth is, however, that while the custom of sleeping in the open air steels the human frame against these same effects, it is, in reality, attended with less exposure to sudden atmospherical transitions than the opposite plan'. Consequently, 'those who exclude themselves from the breath of heaven, whether from necessity or inclination, become languid, from the continued operation of heat, and the want of repose'. So, when exposed suddenly to the 'atmospherical vicissitudes', they at once fall ill.

Other rules, to be followed, included retiring to bed by 10 pm, and rising at daylight, 'to enjoy the cool, the fragrant, and salubrious breath of morn'. The bedclothes used by Europeans were unhealthy, and the indigenous practice of using a bed 'consists of more than a mat', with a 'piece of calico wrapped round him'. 'Indeed', Johnson said, 'a thin hair mattress, with a sheet and palampore, are the only requisites, independently of the thin gauze or mosquito curtains, which defend us from insects'.

A common sleep disorder among Europeans in the tropical countries seems to have been the 'Incubus', or nightmare. 'One of the symptoms almost inseparable from the disease is this', Johnson wrote, 'that the patient appears to himself to be kept down upon the back by some external force; and as, at the moment of recovering the power of volition, a great confusion of ideas prevails, a person may easily imagine that he has recovered himself by some effort of his own, by turning from his back to his side'. This disease 'has its seat in the digestive organs, and that nightmare originates in defective digestion, whereby the food which should be converted into good chyle, is transformed into a half-digested mass of acid matter, which is productive of heart-burn, eructations, flatulence, gripes, with the whole train of dyspeptic and hypochondriacal complaints'. The best medicine for this was a scruple of 'the carbonate of soda, taken in a little ale or porter'. 'This medicine', he explained, 'not only neutralizes any acid in the first passages, but likewise brings away by stool, vast quantities of viscid slimy matter, so acrid as to burn and excoriate the parts it touches'. Nonetheless, the 'propensity to acidify remains for a long time in the stomach, and requires great attention to diet and regimen'. In Bengal, 'cucumbers, nuts, apples, and flatulent kinds of food, are the articles most likely to bring on nightmare'. Additionally, intemperance, and 'pastry, fat, greasy, and salted meat, are to be avoided'. Moderate exercise was advised, and 'sedentary employments, intense study, and late hours' exacerbated nightmares caused by acidity and costiveness.

The final, and very brief, section was addressed to sexual relations between Europeans and local women. The cause for this seemed to Johnson to be 'The monotony of life, and the apathy of mind, so conspicuous among Europeans in hot climates, together with the obstacles to matrimony, too often lead to vicious and immoral connexions with Native females, which speedily sap the foundation of principles imbibed in early youth, and involve a train of consequences, not seldom embarrassing, if not embittering every subsequent period of life'.

CHAPTER NINE

WILLIAM TWINING, FROM NOVA SCOTIA TO CALCUTTA

There is no doubt that living in India carried with it a higher mortality rate for the English since it brought to them new – unknown to contemporary European medicine – diseases. This created a demand for specialised knowledge of such disease and hence, for textbooks of tropical medicine. One such work is William Twining's *Clinical Illustrations of the More Important Diseases of Bengal with the Results of an Inquiry into their Pathology and Treatment*, 1832. We get to know about William Twining's life from two sources, *The Bengal Obituary* (1848; 1851), and the *Supplement to Some Facts in the History of the Twining family* (1893). The latter, a far more reliable source, takes some information from the former, corrects it, and adds to it, thus rounding off very well the remarkable biography of this doctor. Its information is corroborated by *The Twining Family* (1905). He was born in Nova Scotia, and not in Wales as is tentatively stated by the *Bengal Obituary* of 1848, although he was Welsh by origin. His father, the Revd William Twining (1750 – 1827) migrated from Pembrokeshire to Halifax, Nova Scotia, after 1770. William Twining was born to the Revd William and his wife, Sarah Weeks, at Halifax in 1790, the eldest of three sons. Twining attended St Guy's Hospital in 1808, and is indeed unique in that he joined the army as a surgeon, and saw action all through the Napoleonic Wars, first in Portugal, and later also at Waterloo. In 1817 he married Martha Montgomery, and their daughter, Ellen, was Twining's only child. Subsequently he came as surgeon with Sir Edward Paget in 1823, when the new commander of the East India Company's army in Bengal. On resigning from the army, he was appointed Senior Permanent Resident at the Presidency General Hospital, Calcutta. He held this position until he died. The manner of his death is related in some detail in both the *Supplement* and the *Obituary*. On 19 August 1835, his coach hit a buggy, overturning it as well as the passenger in it, who fractured his thigh. Twining rushed to his aid, and in lifting him to a palanquin, he (Twining) felt something snap within his chest. Both accounts refer to a possible rupture in a major blood vessel. He fell ill at once, and died on 25 August. His wife and daughter were then in England, and Twining had planned on joining them soon there. He lies buried in South Park Street cemetery. In the memorial plaque in St John's Church, Calcutta, Twining is given the qualification of CRCLS, which probably makes him a licentiate, while on the front page of his book, he is proclaimed an MRCS, London.

Twining begins his tome with the 'dysentery of Bengal', which he considers many time more acute than 'that which we designate by the same name in England'. In Bengal, 'We find dysentery occurring here at all seasons of the year, but it is more frequent and more severe during the rains, and at the commencement of the cold weather; or from the beginning of June to the end of December'. In particular, Europeans lately arrived in India after a quick passage, were the worst affected by dysentery. Putting the cause of dysentery to intemperance was incorrect, for Twining found it equally acute in persons 'of the most exemplary temperance and regularity of living'. Twining correctly traced dysentery to 'Bad water, and unwholesome food', even as he questioned the popular theory among his colleagues that dysentery originated from diseased livers. Since he worked in a large hospital, Twining was able to carry out post-mortem dissections on Europeans and locals who died of dysentery there. Their livers showed no signs of disease. In fact, the hakims, or local physicians, 'assert that dysentery arises generally from the same causes as fever, viz. high temperature and humidity; exposure to changes of weather; fatigue, and privations'.

This dysentery struck with 'common evacuations', which soon gave way to copious and fluid stools. This was followed by griping pain in the belly, and tenesmus. The symptoms would worsen with great rapidity until 'until the evacuations consist entirely of blood and slime, or of bloody water, like the washings of raw meat'. 'In three or four days', Twining continued, 'the stools have a horrid odour of putrid blood'. The patient's body also exuded a 'foetid, cadaverous exhalation'. These odours, accompanied by a rapid pulse, and hiccups, indicated approaching death. Fever was often absent through the entire course of the disease, and the tongue was seen as moist and clear. Twining was a believer in the bold use of venesection, and he advised that a patient suffering from severe acute dysentery be bled 2-3 times, at intervals of 8-12 hours, from the arm, and 'to take as much blood each time as shall decidedly reduce, and permanently keep down any frequency and hardness of the pulse that may exist'. 12-16 leeches were to be applied to the parts of the abdomen, which were painful. After the first bleeding, the patient was to be given a dose of castor oil. After it had worked, ipecacuanha powder, with gentian, and mercurial pills, was to be administered. In a few days, Twining advised the administration of 'a drachm of sulphur, mixed with half an ounce of mucilage, and one ounce cinnamon water, to be taken in the morning early'. Rectal ulcers were to be treated by injections of up to 30 grains of sugar of lead [lead acetate]. The diet of the patient was of the greatest importance, since it was necessary to keep the colon as empty as possible to help healing. One wonders how the patient bore the enormous loss of blood on a diet of 'tea, barley-water, and thin sago', given in a coffee cupful, every 6 hours! To slake the patient's thirst, a cold wine-glassful of 'a weak infusion of chamomile flowers' could be allowed, every 2 hours. Errors in allowing the patient all types of food would lead to quick and fatal relapses. 'As a common domestic remedy for slight cases', Twining wrote, 'I have often advised with success, an infusion of two drachms of ipecacuanha root, with half a drachm of fresh ginger root sliced, in a pint of boiling water: of which, when cold and strained, a table spoonful is directed to be taken every half hour; and no food or drink used except a teacupful of tepid barley water three times a day'.

To use mercury until it caused salivation, accompanied by a sore mouth, was needless in Twining's opinion. 'Extensive experience, has established the efficacy of ipecacuanha, in the dysentery of Europeans in Bengal; whether they be recent arrivals, or old residents'. Children, as young as under 2 years of age, were subjected to the same medicines: 'For patients under two years of age, I usually give ipecacuanha, extract of gentian, and blue pill, each half a grain, night and morning (the pill being mixed in syrup): or, calomel and ipecacuanha each half a grain, hydrargyrus cum creta, four grains, night and morning; and a small dose of castor oil, or of compound powder of jalap, daily at noon'. Calomel was also not suitable for treating dysentery in Bengal. In any case, it was essential for patients to seek medical assistance at the earliest, since dysentery could quickly turn fatal.

The case of John Wilson, 31, who had been in India only 6 months, shows how treatment had not undergone any significant and effective change. Wilson, 'much emaciated', was admitted to the Presidency General Hospital on 1 April 1831. He had been sick for the previous 70 days. For the last 39 days previous to admission, he had been dysenteric. He went to stool around 14 times in 24 hours, and his belly was flat, 'and much retracted'. Pressure on the caecum caused pain. Wilson was administered leeches, magnesium sulphate, jalap, cold enemas, mercurial pills, gentian, lead acetate, cinnamon extract, and sulphur, for over 3 weeks. Attempts were made to revive his health by improving his diet from tea, bread, and sago, to soup and wine. It was all in vain, for Wilson died on the afternoon of 24 April. Post-mortem examination revealed nothing more than 'some old adhesions' in the right side of the chest, and numerous ulcers in the intestine, and ascending and descending colons. It never occurred to Twining that Wilson might have died of medical care.

The case of Thomas Sweeney shows the limitations of available medical treatment. The medicines could only be repeated. Sweeney was 29, was a soldier, and was sent to hospital on 4 November 1830 from the ship on which he had just arrived from Madras. The voyage had taken 22 days, 15 of which Sweeney had spent with dysentery. The ship's surgeon had bled him once, and treated him with mercury such that his mouth was sore, and his gums ulcerated. When admitted to hospital, Sweeney was going 37 times to stool every 24 hours. He was passing little more than blood and mucus. There was little use in employing mercury again, so Sweeney sustained repeated purges with jalap, alongside the use of ipecacuanha, until 15 November, when he was discharged fit. That same day, Sergeant Avery, aged 37, who had recently arrived from England, was admitted to hospital with the same complaint. Avery too had been given calomel for the last 7 days, due to which his mouth was very sore. The medicines prescribed included jalap, gentian, and ipecacuanha, until 28 November, when he too was discharged.

Twining identified what he called the dysentery of the rectum, 'in which the rectum and lower portion of the colon only are affected'. The symptoms of the disease include 'almost incessant calls to stool, with dreadful tenesmus and straining, the evacuations are not generally very scanty, but they consist of viscid tenacious mucus, that adheres strongly to the bottom of the stool-pan'. A variation of the disease was called the 'white flux', he added, when it became chronic, and led to evacuations of white mucus 'resembling mucilage of gum tragacanth mixed with chalk'. A frequent complication was an inflammation of the bladder, which led to strangury, when the patient strained to urinate, but without any relief. Twining advised the application of leeches to the anus. Ipecacuanha was of little use in this case, but compound of colocynth, mercury, and laudanum worked. Stubborn cases could be helped by injecting Goulard's Water into the rectum.

The severe acute dysentery of Bengal also led to inflammations of the caecum. Twining presented the case of Moffett, aged 33, of 'dark complexion and red face, subject to bilious and febrile attacks, in consequence of intemperance in drink'. Moffett had been in Bengal for 2 years, and worked as a clerk in an office. He was admitted to the Presidency General Hospital on the evening of 19 July 1831, for dysentery of 5 days' standing, during which he had been to stool around 30 times every 24 hours. He also had mild fever. The usual treatment of bleeding, mercurial pills, and purgatives, was used. The patient seemed to rally on 22 July, but there was a painful and troublesome tumescence of the caecum, which persisted despite the application of 10 leeches for 3 days. The next day the tumefaction had increased, the belly was hot, and the patient feverish. His pulse was at 120, and he occasionally lapsed into delirium. The application of a blister over the caecum did not help. The tumefaction increased, fever rose, and Moffett became completely delirious. No other means of medical intervention being available other than the continued application of leeches, Moffett died at 4 am on 24 July. Autopsy revealed 'Numerous deep and large sloughing ulcers' in the caecum.

Another similar case, successfully treated, gives us an idea of the paucity of medical assistance in Bengal. The patient here was aged 23, and employed as a merchant 160 miles upriver from Calcutta. Of 'active habits', this youth was afflicted with dysentery on 26 September 1830. Since no European doctor was locally available, he tried to treat himself by taking purgative salts in the morning, and 'weak brandy and water at bedtime'. This was of no use, and as soon as he realised he was getting no better, he took boat to Calcutta. This journey took a week, during which 'he suffered extreme misery from the constant tenesmus, and frequent calls to stool'. Nauseated by all food, he subsisted on tea for 7 days, as a result of which his purging lessened, though tenesmus forced him to the commode 10 times a day, which yielded mucus with some blood in it. Reaching Calcutta on the morning of 5 October, he went to a friend's house where, since he was feeling faint, he was persuaded to eat a little rice and fish. Since he had eaten for the first time in many days, this led to distension of the belly, and Twining was called in to see him. It was noon by the time Twining answered the call. He found that the young man was suffering from a tumefaction 'in the right iliac region'. Twining at once bled him, and administered the usual medicines, including calomel, colocynth, mercurial pills, and ipecacuanha, assisted by the application of leeches to caecum. The tumefaction increased over the next few days, and fomentations and poultices were applied. The patient was sore in the mouth by 8 October, though the tumefaction had reduced. The mercurial pills were continued, and the diet, hitherto consisting of tea and 2 ounces of bread a day with a cup of arrowroot, was improved by the addition of milk to the arrowroot. On 19 October, Twining noted that the induration of the caecum remained. A blister was applied over the caecum, to be kept open for 10 days, and the diet improved still further to include soup, bread, sago, and milk. The patient recovered by the end of the month. One can only imagine his sufferings.

While the youth and circumstance of this patient aided his recovery, James Post, aged 20, a recruit of HM 16th Lancers, was taken to hospital for dysentery on arrival at Calcutta, on 14 November 1830. He had been dysenteric for 14 days, and had been given so much calomel during this period that his mouth was very sore. Pressure over the abdomen was painful and, strangely, calomel was continued. Additionally, Post was bled immediately after admission. Jalap was added as purgative, and Post continued to suffer until 17 November, 'when this patient was seized with Cholera, marked by deadly coldness of the skin, sinking of pulse, and watery stools; which symptoms continued till he died at 2 A. M. next morning'. Post-mortem dissection revealed the sad fact that James Post had died due to poor medical treatment. The stomach and small intestines were distended with gas, and the caecum was 'distended with flatus'. The only medical curiosity was an abscess, 'found outside and behind the caecum, but not communicating with its cavity: a round earthy mass, larger than the stone of an olive, was found in the centre of the abscess'. This, while potentially dangerous, does not seem to have been a direct cause of death.

Another young man who suffered similarly was Neville, also aged 20. Neville had arrived sick in Bengal, in June 1828. Twining notes, 'He suffered from low spirits while on board ship, and had pain in the region of the liver during the greater part of the voyage from England, for which he was bled, blistered on the side, and took calomel'. Soon after arrival, Neville was struck down by fever and cramps in the feet. 16 leeches were applied to his temple, but they provided no relief. Calomel and extract of colocynth were also useless, though they purged him 'freely'. Soon the fever rose, and he had bloodshot eyes and 'hot forehead'. The calomel and leeching continued, until the fever abated. Before long, however, dysentery struck, 'attended with pain under the right false-ribs, which was increased by pressure, or by the erect posture, and by raising the hand over the head; he had a troublesome cough, and full inspiration gave pain in the right side of chest, and at the region of gall-bladder'. The fever returned in force, and Twining noted that 'This young man had, during the greater part of his illness, a flushed face, and more fever than dysenteric patients in Bengal generally suffered'. 'He was bled', Twining continued, 'and leeches applied in large numbers: also mercury again used to salivation, under the impression that hepatic abscess was impending'. Neville began sinking, despite medical care by Twining, and the 'assiduous attention' of another doctor, 'many years in this climate'. Within days Neville had 'the incessant desire to remain on the stool, and voided nothing but blood, which exhaled a horrid putrid odour'. Soon he was exhausted, and died. He had been in Bengal only 2 months. Nothing more significant than ulcers in the caecum and colon were found, and these most likely were due to the heavy and prolonged doses of mercury he had been given. Twining wrote of a third young man, also recently arrived from England, who similarly became dysenteric. This case was complicated by an intussusception, which was not discovered until autopsy.

William Brown, a sailor, aged 23, became dysenteric aboard ship, which was at harbour in Calcutta. On 9 October 1829, Brown was taken to the hospital since he had been ill for the previous 3 weeks, without any regular treatment. He was bled, and given the usual medicines, including calomel, which reduced the fever, until the caecum became inflamed. At this point, his doctor, who, so Twining tells us, was fully convinced that the disease arose from the liver, began giving him calomel in very high doses. The following day, Brown died, and the autopsy showed that intussusception of the ileum was the cause of death, besides the usual ulcerations in the caecum and colon, which were probably caused by calomel.

One may consider the case of J Balmain, a sailor aged 17, who was admitted to hospital on 21 August 1830, after 4 days' dysentery, which the ship's surgeon was unable to treat with calomel, laudanum, and castor oil. On admission, Balmain was bled 'from the arm as freely, and repeatedly, as his strength would admit'. Then, he was given the usual 'antiphlogistic regimen' for dysentery. On 25 August, the patient appeared to be sinking, due to which he was given the most astounding combination of drugs: senna, as compound and tincture, magnesium sulphate, and quinine sulphate. The next day, there was a 'horrid putrid odour' from his body, though he seemed to be a little easier. That day, the same medicines were given again, with horrific results, for the following day, at 8 am, Balmain passed, 'per anum, with some pus and bloody ichor', 'a tube of small intestine, five inches long, and some fragments of equal length'. This tube, Twining noted, 'appeared to consist of the whole of the coats of the small intestine inverted, and on its surface some sloughing ulcers were very distinct'. The medicines were continued, and by 29 August, Balmain had passed more bits of intestine. He was allowed back on board ship on 16 September. Though Balmain was 'very weak and emaciated' when released, Twining felt that his youth and voracious appetite would help him recover quickly. Twining asserted the importance of using quinine in 'desperate cases', in which the sloughing of intestinal mucous membrane was seen. Usually, he wrote, these cases were fatal.

While severe acute dysentery was seen in persons recently arrived from England, chronic dysentery was common among Europeans long resident in India. In these patients, who are usually debilitated, fever does not accompany the frequent watery stools. The medical aim was to procure a regular and uniform secretion from the mucous membrane of the intestines, by the influence of mild purgatives; and by such remedies as have the property of restoring the capillary circulation to a healthy state, and moderating profuse discharges'. So the patient was advised jalap or castor oil, following which extract of gentian, ipecacuanha, mercurial ['blue'] pills, and a daily drachm of sulphur. For the latter, small doses of a mild purgative, like ipecac, were recommended. A suitable diet was essential for complete recovery. This special diet included 'sago, gruel, or other farinaceous food, four times a day; in quantity not exceeding 6 oz. each time; two ounces of milk may be added to the breakfast and supper, and one ounce of wine to the mid-day meal'.

One sufferer of chronic dysentery was Mrs Costello, aged 19. She had been dysenteric for a month previously, and had been passing blood during the previous 6 days. She was admitted to the Presidency General Hospital on 25 September 1830 in a serious condition, especially because she was nursing her 11-month-old child. The night before, even as she breast-fed the child, she had taken a large dose of laudanum. To present-day parents, this is shocking. The purges were administered, and on 27 September she was ordered to wean her 'stout child', and 'in consequence the breasts are now painful, and her head is hot'. Since Mrs Costello began taking mercurial pills from 26 September, this order was quite proper. She was discharged cured from hospital on 11 October. Twining asked his readers to note that 'recovery was owing to the medicine and not to the cessation of nursing her child, though that circumstance may have contributed to the restoration of her strength'.

In relation to chronic dysentery in locals, Twining wrote, 'My own practice, as well as frequent communication on this subject, with hakims or native physicians, leaves me no room to doubt, that with some slight modifications, the same plan of treatment advised in the foregoing pages, is exceedingly successful in the Dysentery of natives of India'. Venesection was not prescribed for them, and the medicines were reduced to half the measures usually given to Europeans. As for diet, Twining observed that 'The natives of Bengal are so scrupulously attentive to propriety in diet, when they are ill, that we have no difficulty in restraining them to as small quantity of food as may be consistent with the cure of their diseases'.

Twining relates a very interesting anecdote about how he treated a local girl, afflicted with dysentery. She was 11 years old, and 'rather small for that age'. Twining was called out to see her at 10pm on 2 December 1830, because she had not responded to treatment by 'some of the best native practitioners'. 'I found her in great agony', he wrote, 'passing small quantities of blood and slime by stool every five minutes; the belly tense, and thirst extreme; tongue white, dry, and very little loaded; pulse rapid and small, slight morbid heat of surface'. He prescribed the usual, ipecacuanha, extract of gentian, and mercurial pills, to be administered at midnight, and 4 am. To help matters along, he also prescribed jalap. When he saw the child again at 10 am the next morning, she was 'crying aloud with pain, and had been very little better all night'. Nonetheless, the jalap had worked, and she had passed copious stools, including some 'dark faeces'. The same medicines were ordered to be given, at 3 pm, and 6 pm. Twining visited the patient at 9 pm, and 'was assured she had been crying vehemently, ever since the morning visit'. The pain was unabated, and the pills had led to nausea. The medicine was reduced to 2 pills every 3 hours, and a small quantity of Goulard's ointment was to be introduced rectally every 4 hours. On 4 December, the child was better, so the treatment continued, with the pills ordered at 4 pm and 8 pm. Over the next few days she recovered completely. Had it been a European child, Twining would have applied leeches to the region of the caecum and the sigmoid flexure. 'This child', he added, 'belonged to a respectable family, and had suffered no sort of privation; her friends considered her past recovery when I was sent for, and her state was such on the morning of 3d December, that I hardly expected to find her alive in the evening'. Post-parturition dysentery was common among local women, he noted, since 'The high temperature in which the lying-in-room of native women is kept, for many days after parturition, may occasion some peculiarity in the Dysentery which happens to them, of which we are not well able to judge, as European medical men are seldom called to such cases'

Local diet for dysentrics included 'a sort of gruel called in the Bengalee language *coee munda*' [his italics]. 'The coee, or parched paddy, is prepared constantly in all the bazaars', he explained, 'by placing the unhusked rice on heated sand, until each grain swells and bursts, forming a large irregular white morsel, which is very light, and would not be recognised as a grain of rice by those who had not seen it prepared'. This was considered 'very light food', and always recommended by locals for dysentery.

Twining was called in, on 24 January 1831, to see a young local woman, aged 19, 'of an opulent family', who was stricken with dysentery.

She had a child, aged 3 months, whom she was unable to nurse due to her illness. In fact, her dysentery had begun 5 months before her child was born. 'She had been carefully treated by hakims or native physicians', he found, 'but continued gradually to get worse'. Twining found her emaciated, with a total loss of appetite. Her illness made her pass 8 to 9 watery stools daily. The same medicines were given, and the woman recovered rapidly.

Diseases of the hepatic system also depended on the length of the European patient's stay in India. Writing from experience, Twining theorised that in persons recently arrived, the gall bladder was most often found to be distended with bile, while it was smaller in size than usual in those who had resided for long in India. 'The causes of Inflammation and Abscess of the Liver in Bengal', he wrote, 'appear to be a humid atmosphere, and high temperature during the day, followed by cold nights: the more superficial acute inflammation certainly occurs most frequently during the dry hot months of April and May; while we observe the inflammatory congestion, with tendency to central abscess, more commonly taking place towards the latter end of the rains; and at the beginning of the cold season, when considerable diurnal changes of temperature happen'. Most cases of 'inflammatory congestion with tendency to central abscess' occurred 'during the two first months of the cold season, from 10th November to 10th January'. The cause for this was 'Habitual plethora, and superabundance of stimulant food, beyond the real wants of the constitution doubtless keep the greater number of Europeans in India, in an almost perpetual state of proclivity to inflammatory and suppurative disease of the liver'. The cold season encouraged this tendency. As always, the treatment of hepatic ailments followed the same theory as used for other diseases, 'to diminish the quantity of circulating fluid, and permanently to subdue the action of the heart and arteries; and by abstaining from food, and taking very little drink, at the same time that we use purgatives; to keep the system so empty and low, that absorption shall be performed with activity'. This meant aggressive venesection and the simultaneous use of purgatives. 'It is very rarely requisite to bleed from the arm oftener in the worst cases', wrote Twining, 'than twice or three times on the first day, and once on the second day: after which leeches must be repeated every forenoon, until the pain and fullness of the liver, with other symptoms of hepatic disease, are removed reducing the number of leeches to 10, or 6, as the patient's strength fails; and as the progressive subsidence of disease may permit'. Mercury was the only effective drug available, and Twining advised its moderate use in cases of liver disease. Blisters, if used with discretion, also helped.

A 'small but muscular' man, aged 20, resident in India for 4 years as an employee of a mercantile house, consulted Twining on the evening of 12 June 1830, 'on account of acute pain in the region of the liver, which affected respiration, and prevented his lying on the left side'. 'He ascribed his illness to a bruise on the liver', noted Twining, 'by a fall 19 days previously, and he had been gradually getting worse for four days'. Twining immediately bled him, removing 20 ounces, and then applied leeches for further depletion. He was prescribed calomel and jalap, and his diet was restricted to some bread and tea. The leeching and purging continued until 16 June, by which time he had apparently recovered. However, 'On the 20th June, he felt a slight return of pain in the region of the liver, which was increased on the 21st, and then he applied again for advice'. Again there was a fullness and 'morbid sensibility' in the region of the liver. At the same time, he was weak due to the recent and vigorous application of 'antiphlogistic treatment'. Nonetheless, he was purged again, and given more calomel, with leeching. 'By these means the pain in side and tumefaction of the liver were subdued', Twining tells us, 'and he soon afterwards proceeded to sea; but was repeatedly leeched, and blistered during the voyage; he has since recovered robust health'.

An interesting case is that of Henry Weager, aged 55, resident in India for 39 years, 'of active habits and temperate'. He was admitted to hospital at 1 pm on 11 July 1827, since he had been suffering from pain in the region of the liver for 10 days previously. The usual treatment was given, until he had recovered, 2 weeks later. This was not the end of Weager's story. He left for Europe after his recovery, but returned to Bengal in 1830, 'suffering from a large Cancer of the left side of the face and orbit, of which he died on the 20th April 1831'.

Another clinical illustration was the case of a second 'small but muscular' man, aged 24, who sent for Twining on 4 November 1827, because he had suffered an attack of fever. The patient had been living in Bengal for the last 2 ½ years, and was engaged in trade. His symptoms initially were 'head-ache, great anxiety, and the tongue exceedingly loaded with grey mucus'. A regimen of calomel and the usual purgatives, accompanied by venesection restored his health in a week's time. However, the patient called Twining in again on 22 November, because of 'a swelling in the pit of the stomach'. 'I was truly shocked on observing the extent and prominence of this tumour', Twining records, 'which had arisen in the course of a few days, and though not previously evident externally, I had no doubt must have commenced insidiously during the fever, if not previously'. This swelling 'occupied the epigastre, extending towards the left, it was very prominent anteriorly, and must have extended through the whole left lobe of the liver, as it received a strong impulse from the action of the heart'. This was the left lobe of the liver, and pressure on it caused pain. The patient was otherwise generally in good health. So, assigning the cause of this enlargement to 'tardy convalescence', Twining vigorously repeated the previous treatment, with venesection, purgatives, and mercurial pills. Further, 'He was directed to remain on his couch, observing the utmost quiescence, avoiding conversation, or anything that might in the slightest degree quickens the pulse'. The commode was placed close to his couch, and when he wished to use it, a servant was to help him sit. The patient was not allowed any solid food until the tumefaction had been reduced. A cup of tea was permitted at morning and night, and a tablespoonful of plain water every half an hour. Liquor was disallowed. There was no improvement for a week, and Twining began to wonder if the patient would be able to withstand further treatment. A blister was applied to the epigastre on 29 November, and 2 ounces of bread permitted, with the tea. On 6 December Twining noted a distinct reduction in the size of the tumour, though the patient showed no effect of mercury. Ordering the rubbing of a mercurial ointment 'over the right side of the chest and belly', Twining allowed him 'With a view of affording more nourishment, without producing redundancy of fluids or much excitement in the system, a boiled egg, and some salt was allowed once a day, without any increase in quantity of bread'. The fact is, the patient was very weak, and becoming weaker through daily leeching. On 11 December, Twining noted that the tumour was much decreased and so ordered the continuation of the ointment, while leaving off the mercurial pills and other medicines. The patient's mouth still showed no effect of mercury. The quantity of bread was increased, and he was allowed a teacupful of soup with it. The ointment was continued until 19 December, though pills of scammony and colocynth were continued for another 6 weeks. The patient eventually recovered fully. There were many remarkable points to this unique case. 'When I first saw the tumefaction at epigastre and towards the left lobe of the liver', Twining recalled, 'I did not think myself justified in giving his friends any hope that an abscess of the liver could be prevented'. In fact, he had never before treated a case 'so far advanced as this'. Further, he found it remarkable that 'all the mercury taken, caused no sign of salivation'. The same patient had to take a course of calomel 3 years later, when a far lesser dose, of 2 grains every night for 8 doses, caused a sore mouth.

Observation XXVIII studies the case of a 51-year-old man, resident in India for 26 years, who 'enjoyed almost uninterrupted good health, attending diligently his business, in an office', until 1830, when 'domestic calamities' impaired his appetite and slowed the bowels. However, he continued with his work without seeking medical advice. Then, on the morning of 2 December 1830, he felt sick due to a sudden and severe pain in the epigastre soon after breakfast, and vomited. He treated himself with laudanum and aromatic spirit of ammonia in tepid water. Twining saw him 2 hours later. The patient had recently undergone a severe family crisis, and so Twining 'was anxious if possible to avoid a debilitating plan of treatment; therefore ordered a purgative enema to be given, and repeated in an hour'. By 10 am the following morning mercury caused the patient to freely salivate. Nonetheless, the patient continued to suffer nausea and felt fullness in the region of the liver. By 9 December, the symptoms had abated, and the patient soon recovered completely.

D Dominique, a 'stout' French sailor aged 44, 'a hard-working man, of regular habits, and good conduct', was admitted to the hospital on 4 December 1830, because he had been ill aboard ship since 27 November, during which time treatment by the ship's surgeon had failed to cure him. Twining was amazed that his naval colleague had applied 40 leeches and bled Dominique 8 ounces from the arm. The usual purgatives and mercurials were used, but they only succeeded in depressing the patient, who declared on 13 December that 'he was determined not to die of debility, and that unless unrestricted quantity of food were allowed, he had resolved to procure it'. Soon came 'the first unfavourable symptom which arose from improper diet, was a return of cough; then gradually increasing emaciation, and a sharpness of visage; followed by dysenteric symptoms, with blood in the stools'. Dominique became still more depressed, and sank faster, even as he continued to refuse medicines. He died on 8 January 1831.

On 9 October 1829, one Mr Hollman visited Twining for some medicines for headache and cold that he presumed he had contracted by getting his feet wet in the course of his work, which was the superintendence 'of a place that was not laborious, but required his being out early in the mornings, and he frequently got his feet wet, in the dew on the grass'. Hollman was 37, and had been 18 years in India. He opted not to be bled, and so Twining suggested 30 leeches to the liver, since there was fullness at the epigastre, along with daily doses of calomel and extract of colocynth until the ailment passed. Twining later learnt that Hollman had applied only 20 leeches, and took the medicine only twice. Certain that 'he had no fear of liver disease, and felt no pain in the side' Hollman applied the leeches to his temple, since he was equally sure that all he had was a cold. 2 days after his first visit to Twining, Hollman felt better, and resumed work. On 16 October, Hollman had a severe return of fever, which made him consult Twining again. Treatment resumed in vain. Though mercury soon affected his mouth, Hollman did not respond favourably to the medicine, and died on 12 November 1830. Twining attributed this death to the patient's wilfulness. 'He had an idea that at his time of life, and after so many years residence', Twining wrote, 'in India, with sober habits of living, he was not liable to liver disease; therefore he would not at any time, submit to be bled: and after applying leeches once to his head, he attended to his daily business'. 'He never acknowledged any pain on pressure at the epigastre', Twining continued, 'but it is hardly possible to believe that so much superficial inflammation at the convex surface of the liver, with fullness at epigastre, could have existed without morbid sensibility on pressure'. Maybe Hollman, like Dominique, was doubtful about the efficacy of contemporary medical treatment.

The next illustration involved a professional colleague, who had arrived in Calcutta in August 1827. 'He was habitually temperate in eating and drinking', Twining recalled, 'but utterly careless of his health in every other respect'. Used to field sports in England, he 'tried the same amusements here, in the most imprudent manner; going out many miles before day-light, in the cold foggy mornings of November, and often riding and walking till near mid-day, when the sun was very hot: going sometimes half the day without food'. He disregarded several attacks of slight fever towards the end of November, treating himself with saline purges, and continued with his sporting activities. At the beginning of December, the fever returned with intensity. Twining sounds rather amused by his colleague's naiveté, when he recounts that a persistent low fever, 'did not prevent his persisting to go out as usual: and he took some hot brandy and water at night, to check a troublesome purging'. On 14 December, this gentleman consulted Twining, who discovered 'pain under the right false ribs that was increased by pressure: there was evident enlargement of the liver'. On 16 December, Twining noted that his colleague continued to 'suffer from anxiety, and his strength was much reduced'. That day, Twining concluded, 'there is reason to fear that the acute disease in the liver is not removed'. On 18 December, the application of camphorated mercurial ointment was ordered, but to little effect, since 'The circumscribed tumour of liver slowly increased; and in a few days dysenteric symptoms became very distressing'. This made it 'too evident that an extensive abscess existed'. Since the patient was unresponsive to treatment, he was ordered to sea on 13 February 1828, and Twining was later informed that his colleague had died aboard ship on 25 February. In addition to his patient's neglect of the first attacks of fever, Twining also attributed his death 'to his eating soup during the use of active antiphlogistic remedies, when he should have lived on bread and water'. In other words, as a doctor he should have known better.

'Some persons lose their health in Bengal in a very gradual manner, becoming emaciated, and having returns of fever for a few days, once in two or three weeks', Twining wrote, after which 'they then suffer from slight pyrexia almost every day, attended with more or less of diarrhoea, and followed after some weeks by hectic, and quick pulse: they very often die from abscess of the liver, which is attended with little pain during its progress'. Enlargement of the liver was also common 'in children below the age of four years' in Bengal. 'But', Twining noted, 'the most frequent enlargement of the liver in subjects of this tender age, comes on slowly, attended with emaciation and occasional slight returns of fever; these children are pale, and frequently have Diarrhoea, with some cough; and in the majority of cases, the enlargement of the liver is not very palpable, until the constitution is much impaired'. The prognosis was poor, since the most that could be done, was to apply middle-sized leeches to the epigastre, 'followed by a small blister', and a course of mild purgatives, just enough for 4 stools a day, using jalap, scammony, and calomel. Experience had taught Twining that in half the children afflicted with liver disease, mercury was harmful. The child's body was to be kept cool and comfortable and, as a last measure, 'a voyage to Europe should be enjoined in all cases where that is practicable'. Twining was convinced that acute liver disease was uncommon among locals.

Another ailment, to which European children in Bengal were particularly susceptible, was disease of the spleen. 'The disease is far more distressing to children', Twining wrote, adding that 'in them, if careful attention to diet, and correct medical treatment be omitted ; the enlargement of the spleen, and corresponding decay of the general health are in most cases progressive, and they sink into a state of marasmus'. 'I have observed', he continued, 'he disease in its severest form to come on after Fevers, affecting the children of wealthy Europeans who lived in every comfort, and were attended with the greatest care'. In children, however, enlarged spleens were idiopathic, and characteristic of feeble and undernourished constitutions, compounded by 'by the combined influence of a damp climate, variable temperature, want of exercise, unsuitable clothing'. 'During the slow and silent influence of long continued grief, and distress of mind', Twining stated, 'the secretions generally appear to be perverted, the cutaneous circulation becomes languid, healthy transpiration obstructed, and then we often find enlargement of the spleen take place in Bengal'. In fact, enlarged spleens were common throughout Bengal: 'The tumefaction of the spleen occasionally comes on very suddenly, in the course of remittent Fevers, in Bengal; and in a few days the enlargement can be seen as well as felt, extending far below the cartilages of the left false ribs'. A doctor in Calcutta would see several cases of unusually enlarged spleen. In these extreme cases, 'the diseased spleen fills more than half the belly, extending to the right of the navel, while its lower extremity reaches the left iliac region'. Twining's formula for treating this ailment included jalap, ginger powder, supertartarate of potassium, ferrous sulphate, and tincture of senna. The dose for adults was 1 ½ ounces at 6 am and 11 am daily, to be reduced for children to such proportions 'so as to produce not less than three, and not more than four stools daily'. This medicine acted, Twining claimed, as 'purgative, tonic, and diuretic'. During treatment, patients 'must live on tea, bread, sago, gruel, and chicken broth, or kid soup in very small quantity'. 'But in the more chronic cases, where we must patiently wait for slower changes in the constitution, and the gradual removal of the enlargement of the spleen', wrote Twining, 'the mixture is given once daily, in the morning; and in such dose as to act less powerfully, only twice a day: it is then not inconsistent to allow some roasted or boiled meat, and curry'. In many cases Twining had recommended the drinking of water' which has been used for cooling heated iron at a blacksmith's forge'. If allowed to stand and cool for a while, this water became perfectly transparent, and hardly carried any odour or taste.

Nussevun was 3, and the daughter of one of Twining's servants. She was taken to his care on 26 June 1831 'suffering from Fever of 11 days duration'. 'The eyes were heavy and watery', Twining noted, 'the head was hot, belly tumid and elastic, spleen large and rounded, so that it could be distinctly felt two fingers breadth below the cartilages of the left false ribs, and extending half way from the ribs to the umbilicus'. She was bled using 2 leeches over the spleen, and mildly purged that day and the following day. On 28 June, Twining commenced dosing her with his Spleen Mixture. On 14 July Nussevun was declared fit.

John O'Brien was also aged 3, 'a stout boy', who 'has had a paroxysm every second day' since he first suffered fever on 30 September 1826. Admitted to hospital on 10 October, John was discovered to have a 'very large and round' spleen, 'extending as low down as the navel; there is morbid sensibility on pressure being made over the left hypochondre; the skin is dry and face pale'. 'This child', Twining noted, ' had resided in a house overlooking the broad ditch of Fort William, and his illness as ascribed to a noxious exhalation from the mud of the wet ditch, from which the water had been allowed to run off at the usual time of the year; and this patient was taken ill a few days afterwards'. The Spleen Mixture worked well, and the child was discharged on 19 October. However, 'On recovery, O'Brien returned to the same residence, and was attacked on the 2nd November with tertian intermittent; the cold stage of which was severe, followed by a prolonged hot fit'. John was readmitted to hospital in the evening of 4 November, once more with an enlarged spleen. His treatment included purgatives, and 1 ounce of the Spleen Mixture, as a single dose. Additionally, he took a single dose of 2 grains of quinine. John was finally discharged well on 27 October. Of course, he returned once more to the same house. However, there was no recurrence of the disease for the next 4 years, and Twining knew that 'he became a robust active fellow, and his health during that period was always good'. Subsequently, John moved with his parents to the Upper Provinces where, to the date of Twining's writing, he had not suffered a relapse.

On 5 December 1830 Twining was consulted by a lady who had come to see him from beyond Rajmahal, around 200 miles from Calcutta. 'She was emaciated and pale', Twining found, and 'there was a livid circle round the eyelids, and the conjunctivae were pale and bloodless: her skin was dry and cool, the feet slightly oedematous; tongue white and moist, but nearly clean; pulse 94, soft and weak'. Particularly, her spleen was unusually enlarged, 'being nearly the size of a child's head, round, and very moveable, and rather lower down than a level with the umbilicus'. It was also painful on pressure. Her situation was worsened by the fact that she was in the 5th month of her 3rd pregnancy. She was immediately bled, using leeches on the spleen. Thereafter, she took, besides purgatives, magnesium sulphate and quinine. She continued with the quinine in addition to the Spleen Mixture until 10 January 1831, when she was declared well. Twining did not pursue her case, and we have no idea how the medicines affected her pregnancy. Twining, not knowing any better, did not bother about the possible impact of bleeding on the health of the foetus.

Another unusual case was that of John Brown, aged 7, 'a delicate child, of light complexion, and active habits, born in Bengal of European parents'. He was taken to hospital on 28 November 1828 due to 'general ill health and a swelling on the left side of his belly'. This was a splenetic enlargement of such size that it 'filled the whole left hypochondre, and extended laterally quite to the navel; its lower extremity reached half way from the umbilicus to the pubis: it could be plainly seen when the child was laid on his back'. It was 'rounded, hard, and firmly fixed in its place', besides being painful on pressure. John had had fever in October 1826, and his enlarged spleen was noticed during convalescence. It seems to have been thought that the tumefaction would subside over time. It did not, and the child had never gained full health since. Twining first ordered the child to be dressed in flannel. Then, meat was removed from his diet, which was to consist only of soup at dinner. This was followed up with the usual purgatives, Spleen Mixture, and quinine. The enlarged spleen was leeched. The child soon grew weaker, and on 5 December 'a very small quantity of vegetable curry with rice, and toasted bread', was allowed for dinner. By 20 December, the spleen was much reduced. However, the child was fretful and, as often happened with leeches, the bites became infected. In order to build up his strength, Twining improved his diet, by allowing some roasted or broiled chicken every 2nd day; alternately with a kid or fish-curry; and vinegar is offered with his food whenever he will take it'. To raise his spirits, the child was also permitted, daily with his dinner, 'Half a glass of port wine … diluted with twice the amount of water'. On 2 March 1829, Twining recorded, 'The child has become stout and fat, and has a healthy complexion', and from that date, medication was stopped. Interestingly, Twining followed this case through to 6 December 1831, when he noted, 'health has been completely restored, and he is now the most active and healthy boy in Calcutta'.

Peter Crawley, also 7, of Calcutta, had the same ailment, and he was treated similarly. The only problem was that Peter displayed some of the side-effects of the medicines he was taking. Taken to Twining on 19 November 1830, Peter remained under treatment for a very long time. On 23 March 1831, Twining noted, 'he suffers from occasional vertigo, and has a head-ache almost every forenoon, which is ascribed to the quinine'. This is not surprising, since he had been taking quinine for over 4 months. The quinine was stopped, and the Spleen Mixture continued. Peter, however, did not improve as dramatically as John Brown. On 10 July 1831, Twining directed him to take iron filings in a teaspoonful of mustard oil. By 22 September, the spleen had reduced greatly, and Peter had gained in health. This progress was briefly interrupted by a fever in November 1831, which was treated in 4 days using an infusion of senna and quinine. 'He is now a fine healthy boy', concluded Twining, 'residing in Calcutta, and can be seen at any time'.

A lady, aged 22, and the mother of a 5-month-old child whom she could not nurse, consulted Twining on her chronic enlarged spleen on 16 December 1828. Among other things, Twining discovered that she was undergoing scanty and irregular menses. He wrote, 'She was directed to live on a small quantity of good soup, with a little broiled mutton for dinner, and to use only tea and bread, with sago, night and morning'. Then, in order not to arrest 'the feeble remains of regular menstruation', she was ordered mild leeching, 'commencing their application on the second day after the menstrual period was over, so that for the ten days prior to the menstrual period, no leeches were applied'. She was also given no medicine during her periods. She consulted Twining over the next 18 months, and on 6 March 1831, he declared her fit.

Turning to local medical practice, Twining noted that they too used the same or similar ingredients to treat splenetic enlargement, like ferrous sulphate, copper sulphate, and garlic and aloe. 'Long needles are said to be used by native practitioners', he said, 'to puncture the spleen: and if they ever penetrated to the diseased organ, and a cure succeeded, it is very probable that the successful event might be ascribable to the peritoneal inflammation excited at the diseased part'. However, he had only seen them using needles so small 'that I am quite certain the surface of the spleen was never touched in any of the operations which I witnessed'. The local practitioners were theoretically correct, and Twining used the same method to reduce enlarged spleens rapidly in several chronic cases by inserting '2, 3, or 4 needles, deeply into the substance of the spleen: the needles were introduced exactly two inches, and no unfavourable symptom has ever followed the operation; the effects were deemed by those gentlemen who witnessed these operations, useful in accelerating the absorption of the enlarged spleen'. Twining believed that 'The natives of this country generally use remedies in disease, from practical knowledge of their efficacy; without much reasoning: therefore I would not reject any of their therapeutical expedients as despicable, without an enquiry into their modus operandi and an experimental investigation of their utility'.

Mercury, used widely in Twining's time, was grievously dangerous in cases of spleen enlargement. He recounts the case of a 47-year-old man, a long-time resident of India, who came to Calcutta for a change of air because he had been suffering 'from Dysentery and remittent Fever, for several weeks, in autumn 1824; at a station which was remarkably unhealthy during that season'. He had taken calomel, which had moderately affected his mouth. When Twining was called in to see him on the morning after his arrival, he noticed that the man had an enlarged spleen, and that his 'right cheek was enormously swollen, hard, and shining'. The patient said his cheek had been affected by exposure to cold during his journey to Calcutta. Twining then noticed 'a dreadful Mercurial odour from his mouth'. There was a tumour in the cheek, which soon worsened, and 'in spite of every remedy that could be suggested, he died in six days'. A similar case was that of 'A poor man, who had been exposed in an unhealthy and low situation; suffered from remittent fever and enlarged spleen in July and August 1824'. He told Twining he had taken some calomel, though in the light of subsequent events Twining felt he might have taken more. This patient was soon afflicted with 'A dreadful salivation followed, with sloughing of the gums and destruction of the teeth, and part of the alveoli of the jaw bones'. Later, Twining wrote, 'He gave me 14 teeth, and several portions of the jaw bones: some of the latter are above two inches long'. 'This poor fellow still lives', he continued, 'a melancholy example of the baneful effects of mercury, in cases where men are labouring under the constitutional affections that generally attend vascular engorgement of the spleen'.

Cholera was one of the most dreaded diseases. Twining, like his colleagues, struggled to understand and treat this ailment, which struck suddenly, and was very often fatal. 'The invasion of Cholera most frequently appears in a violent form', he wrote, 'between the hours of 2 and 5 am'. His experience had further shown that 'The Cholera is occasionally preceded by a slight pyrexia: and it has also appeared to me, that congestive fevers do sometimes, though rarely, fall into a state of collapse resembling the low stage of this disease; not indeed very often attended with violent vomiting and cramps, but the patient suddenly becomes weak and cold; sometimes voiding one true Cholera stool: at other times, even this symptom is absent'. A 28-year-old gentleman, resident in Bengal for 5 years and previously very healthy, felt a slight uneasiness on rising on the morning of 18 March 1830. Thinking this to have been caused by indigestion, he took a dose of Epsom salts on returning from his morning ride. However, he soon began vomiting, his extremities became cold, the countenance livid, and he passed 4 stools. He thereafter sank rapidly, and died at 4 pm, only 9 hours after he had taken the salts. Another case was that of a young lady, aged 22, who had just risen from childbed, and was beginning to resume her daily routine. Her child was only 22 days old when, on 14 September 1825, the mother felt 'slightly feverish' and took 6 grains of calomel at bedtime. She rose to feed the baby at 2 am, and retired to bed. Soon after 3 am, 'soon after three o'clock a profuse purging of dark fluid took place; some of the evacuations passed in bed, and those that were last voided, were a pale-grey water; there was neither vomiting nor spasms; the hands and feet became cold'. At 4.45 am, she died. 'This woman was living in tolerable comfort in an upper-roomed house', Twining commented, 'had not been down stairs since her confinement; and the friends asserted, that she had not been imprudent in diet, or in any other respect'. Correctly pointing to a possible cause, he also noted that 'Cholera of a severe description was at this time frequent among the natives, in the immediate vicinity of this person's house'. The third demonstrative case was again of a woman aged 26, 'stout and healthy', who fell ill at 3 pm on 2 September 1825. 'This person had been quite well', Twining recounted, 'up to the moment of the attack: ate her tiffin as usual, and was afterwards occupied in arranging books in the library, standing on a chair to place those on the upper shelves'. She thought that the spasm of sickness came from her 'reaching too high' while arranging the books. Cholera struck with violence, and she was beyond recovery by 5 pm.

Twining had also noticed that when cholera epidemics were raging, giving 'drastic purgatives' brought on the disease in persons who might otherwise have escaped it. 'The experience of many years has so far confirmed this opinion', he wrote, 'that we usually are cautious in ordering either jalap or salts in the Hospital, when we have many patients with Cholera under treatment here; or when that disease is prevailing in the town; and at such times it is deemed hazardous to give a patient any medicine likely to act on the bowels, between 2 and 5 a. m.: therefore we have usually, if possible, avoided giving even to febrile cases on those occasions, calomel and colocynth, at bed time'. Despite his own studies in the pathophysiology of cholera, Twining, like his colleagues across the world of the time, concluded that 'The cause of the more frequent appearance of Cholera for some years past, is unknown; and we are unacquainted with any circumstances which are sure to produce the disease, or by avoidance of which, residents in India can be certain of always escaping its attack'. It attacked all, particularly if they were wealthy, and lived in comfort, 'exempt from any species of privation', and 'avoiding excesses of any sort'. In fact, these persons were struck down by the most fatal form of cholera. Observation also proved that 'the disease prevails most, among those who reside in low and ill-ventilated situations, exposed to humid atmosphere and sudden changes of weather ; who are frequently using ill-cooked or bad food ; and who indulge in eating cold or unripe fruits: more especially if they be at the time exposed to fatigue and unusual privations'. Especially susceptible were debilitated persons, and those who newly arrived from Europe. 'Cholera in India may be ascribed to a distempered state of the atmosphere, he wrote, 'which we have no means of appreciating, except by its effects: as we judge of the presence of malaria, in the case of intermittent Fevers'. It was difficult for physicians to collate symptoms specific to cholera. Twining wrote, 'If the diseases which are acknowledged to be Cholera, were so ranged on a scale as to place those cases which have most affinity, together; and those most dissimilar, at a distance: we should find one end of this scale occupied by diseases in which the actions of the constitution are distinctly febrile, and in many of them the evidence of local inflammation is strong and unequivocal, as in the most intense examples of gastro-enteritis'. 'Between these two extremes, every possible variety exists', he continued. Treatment was mainly supportive, and consisted of venesection to relieve feverishness and spasms. Calomel, blue pill, and opium, could be administered, with caution. Thin gruel of arrowroot or sago, such as could be retained by the stomach, was advisable. Opium worked better in desperate cases. Twining stated that 'Two grains of opium in a pill sometimes arrest the most formidable symptoms'. 'If we are so fortunate as to arrest the progress of symptoms threatening sudden death', he continued, 'the patient generally sleeps for some hours'. Thereafter, 'The subsidence of urgent symptoms should make us satisfied to wait for three or four hours; and then we must give some aperient medicine every four hours, until the bowels are made to act moderately'. Convalescence had to be carefully supervised. The patient should be placed in an airy and uncrowded room, and on a narrow bed, to make assistance easy. 'I have many times seen men rise to stool', he wrote, 'and after a copious gush of watery evacuation from the bowels; to fall on the floor, sometimes apparently fainting, at other times convulsed: some of these have died within five minutes after rising to stool, who had not been 12 hours ill, and who had some degree of warmth of surface at the time of getting out of bed; having just before that been speaking rationally, through in a state of anxiety and restlessness'. Cholera was almost always fatal for European children, particularly those aged 2 or younger, for their symptoms were often not obvious, and parents overlooked the possibility of cholera until it was too late.

Despite all this common-sense, treatment saved some lives, and took several. One example of the latter is the case of William Griffiths, a gunner aged 28, who had lost an arm, and had been invalided home. He was taken ill soon after midnight on 26 December 1829 at Fort William, where he was awaiting embarkation to Europe. Griffiths did not report sick until daylight, thereby losing critical hours. 'On admission, he was quite cold', Twining recalled, 'the fingers shrivelled, pulse imperceptible ; tongue cold, moist, clammy, and nearly clean ; the face livid; eyes sunk in the orbits ; and there was much venous congestion of the eyes, giving the scleroticae and conjunctivae a lurid appearance'. Griffiths tossed about the bed, suffering from severe cramps. He also had difficulty in breathing. Given 20 grains of calomel with 2 grains of opium, he vomited it out promptly, following which a bizarre mode of treatment began. 'A free incision was made into a vein in the arm', recorded Twining, 'but not a tea-spoonful of blood obtained; the jugular vein was then opened, and only a trivial oozing of thick black blood, like treacle, issued slowly from thence'. Next, Griffiths was again given 20 grains of calomel and some opium mixed in sugared water flavoured with cinnamon, which he again vomited out. On this, his body was directed to be rubbed down by 4 men with the spirit of turpentine, while the radial artery was opened at the wrist 'by an oblique incision with a lancet; the integuments being first divided down to that vessel, with a small scalpel'. 13 ounces flowed from this incision, in 'a languid stream, and of dark purple colour', after which 'the blood came in a jet with arterial impulse, its colour was rather brighter red, yet not like the arterial blood of a healthy person'. Naturally, this gave no relief, and Griffiths felt weaker. He was given some brandy and hot water to drink, which he threw up and thereafter refused to have anything other than cold water; 'in fact', Twining added, 'he was totally unmanageable, and deaf to argument or entreaty of his friends'. 3 minutes later, the blood was allowed to flow once more from the same incision, and 'it came freely with a smart jet'. Griffiths' restlessness caused much of this blood to splash on to the bed. This stream of blood soon became feeble and stopped, due to clotting at the site of the incision. Remarkably, Twining commented, with some surprise, that after this round of venesection, 'the man seemed weaker and more exhausted'. The bleeding was therefore paused for 5 minutes. Unsurprisingly, 'The patient was now evidently more purple in the face, his breathing more laborious, and he appeared more feeble in tossing about in bed: the voice remained pectoral, but much weaker than on his arrival at the Hospital about one hour and a quarter ago'. Twining obtusely concluded that Griffiths' suffering seemed at this point to be due to 'the stagnation of venous blood, and the imperfect action of the lungs'. Astonishingly, bleeding was recommenced, despite the patient being at this stage of collapse, and 3 ounces more were extracted. Griffiths seems to have been bled around 50 ounces, or 38% of the total blood volume. This huge loss of blood hastened his demise, for he died 1 hour and 37 minutes after the last venesection. Similarly, Pierre Louis, a French sailor aged 18, was admitted to the hospital at 5 pm on 21 March 1830 with fever of 5 days' standing. Treatment was commenced for suspected cholera and, like Griffiths, he was bled over 50 ounces by 10 pm. Again, unsurprisingly, Louis died at 12.15 am. These huge and, by the standards of today, appalling depletions, always successfully hurried the patients to the grave.

Another interesting case was that of a doctor, aged 26, 'of slight make and delicate constitution', and recently arrived from England, who had been sick with 'Spasmodic Colic'. Suffering severe constipation, he had been bled copiously on 2 occasions. This failed to resolve the problem, and so 'the obstruction of the bowels was removed by large enemas given with the pump'. He recovered slowly, and it was only on the evening of 26

October 1830 that he remarked to some friends that he felt an increase in strength. At 9 pm the next day, 'he was affected with a purging, the stools copious, watery, and of a pale-yellow bilious tinge'. Despite his medical training, he did not suspect cholera, and so wasted critical hours waiting for daylight. He died in the afternoon of 28 October 1830. He realised that he was mortally ill with cholera only at noon, "when he desired his servant to bring him a small looking glass, and the instant it was brought, he said, 'I see I have got Cholera, which I did not even suspect before: there can be but little hope of my recovery'".

Joseph Cocket, aged 19, a dark-complexioned sailor aboard a French ship, fell ill on 13 December 1829. He was admitted to hospital at 12.15 pm the following day, in a state of collapse. 'Torpor and death were evidently approaching', Twining wrote, 'but we were unwilling to abandon the man while he was breathing'. Calomel, opium, and enemas were administered in vain. Then, 'the galvanic pile' was readied, and 'when it was acting so strongly as to have a powerful effect on several healthy persons, who with myself tried it; shocks were passed through the patient's arms, chest, diaphragm and liver; and the galvanism was directed so as to pass through the situation of the great solar plexus of nerves; but he showed not the least symptom of feeling its influence'. Cocket died at 8.30 pm.

Of equally sinister nature were fevers, variously classified as Remittent, Intermittent, and Insidious Congestive Fevers, among others. While most cases recounted by Twining recovered, he painfully recollected the fatalities, which he was certain had occurred 'in consequence of my most precise instructions being neglected'. In particular, he considered any delay in leeching as fatal, stating that 'The cause of delay in applying the leeches in these cases was generally the difficulty of procuring them promptly; and the friends considered it better to apply them late than altogether to omit them'. The case of a 'stout young man' is demonstrative of this. He had suffered a severe bout of remittent fever, and was 'considered by his friends nearly convalescent'. His fever used to peak at 7 am, so Twining would visit him at home once at that hour, and again in the afternoon. On 15 July 1826, Twining went to see him in the morning and found the fever coming on. Despite a hot forehead, 'the patient was walking about the room and hardly feeling any illness'. Twining urged him to go to bed and apply 12 leeches to his forehead. The patient agreed to obey. However, after Twining had left, the patient sat down and wrote letters until nearly 11 am. By this time the fever had subsided and, typically, the patient was perspiring heavily. At this critical stage, he ordered the application of leeches to his forehead. In response to an urgent summons, Twining went to see him an hour later, only to learn what had transpired, 'but all interference was useless, the patient was insensible on my arrival at his house, and died in ten minutes after'. Another illustrative case was that of Mr Phillips, aged 36, 'a stout, bloated, and fat man of dark complexion, born at Madras', who became feverish on 13 July 1830. The fever subsided in the evening, and he disregarded the matter. The next day, fever came at 2 pm, and subsided during the night. On 15 July, Phillips walked 2 miles to consult a doctor, who gave him a dose of jalap and advised admission to hospital. Mr Phillips does not seem to have had much confidence in hospitals, since he chose instead to be bled a 'few' ounces, and to be leeched from the left side. That same day the fever returned with increased violence. On 16 July, Mr Phillips walked a mile to attend to some business, and took no medical measures. That day the fever came with still greater violence, and it left him short of breath. He then decided to go to hospital the following day unless he felt better. The paroxysm of 17 July was worse, and it left Phillips delirious. Soon he became insensible, and was admitted to hospital at 5 pm 'in a state of muttering delirium'. Though the usual medicines, calomel and colocynth, were administered, Phillips's condition worsened. He died at 8 pm.

The final section of Twining's book records the details of a local fever, called 'Nakra or Nassa' by Bengalis, 'which literally means, the nose disease'. This ailment had not been studied by any other European doctor. 'It usually commences', Twining recorded, 'with a sensation of pain and distension within the nose, attended by extreme pain in the back of the neck, a hot forehead, and excessive weariness and pain in the loins, and in all the joints'. Soon the pain in the sinuses and nose would increase, the eyes redden, and the patient would complain of great thirst. 'The disease is said to be induced by irregular habits of living', he goes on, 'such as attending to business and going about in the sun, at hours which infringe on the usual periods of bathing, and of taking food and repose: sitting up late at night in earnest conversation on subjects inducing mental anxiety, is also supposed occasionally to bring on the disease'. This fever was usually seen to occur to persons between the ages of 10 and 45, and it was not fatal. Hence no medicines were used by locals, who only waited for the fever to resolve on its own, which it normally did in 4 to 5 days' time. However, 'They have a custom of drawing some blood from the nose, which is done by thrusting pieces of rough-edged sharp grass up the nostrils; or by puncturing the schneiderian membrane with a sort of awl or needle'. The amount of blood thus removed amounted to less than an ounce, but it gave immense relief to the sufferer. Strangely, Nakra did not seem to affect Europeans, though Twining noted that 'some of its characters very closely resemble the Fever which was epidemic in Calcutta in June, July, and August, 1824, and affected almost every Native as well as European in the place: but on questioning Natives subject to Nakra, and who suffered the Epidemic of 1824, I have always been told that the diseases are very different as far as relates to the feelings of the patient, and that the suffering under an attack of Nakra is much more severe'.

Had Twining lived to issue other editions of his textbook, or even to write more books on the diseases of Bengal, we would have obtained more information about prevalent ailments of the time. Twining's grave has no identifying plaque, and is located at the far left corner of South Park Street cemetery. The huge marble memorial slab dedicated to him, in St John's Church, is proof of his professional and personal reputation.

CHAPTER TEN

FREDERICK HARRINGTON BRETT AND EUROPEAN SURGERY IN BENGAL

Frederick Harrington Brett was appointed to the Company's Bengal Army as Assistant Surgeon on 22 September 1825. He was an MRCS, London. We next read about him through the notice of his daughter's birth on 2 March 1832 at Shahjahanpur, Oudh, where he was posted as Civil Assistant Surgeon. Then, on 6 January 1841, Brett was promoted Surgeon, in place of Dr George Baillie, retired, with his seniority from 16 December 1840. We get an idea of the rapidity with which illness struck, when we read that Baillie had been appointed in place of Dr Richard Laughton, who had been invalided. Laughton did not return to England. Instead, he sought, and was permitted to reside in the 'north-western hills', possibly Shimla, since he was to draw his pay from the Meerut pay office. Laughton had joined service at almost the same time as Brett, 18 September 1825. Brett's book, *A Practical Essay on Some of the Principal Surgical Diseases of India*, was published in 1840, in Calcutta. At that time, Brett was Assistant Surgeon to the Governor-General's Bodyguard. His work is unique in that it was one of the earliest and most thorough studies of surgery in India. Surgical hospitals were uncommon in India, and only one existed at Calcutta, until, as Brett writes, he had established similar institutions in the 'Upper Provinces of India, Lucknow, Cawnpore', and elsewhere, which had set an example of how surgery could be successfully conducted.

Brett begins his book by stating that in England surgeons popularly opined that, operations in India turn out 'unfavourably'. Against this view, which Brett dismisses as a 'decided error', he presents two arguments. The first has to do with 'The confidence of the natives of India, who resort to European hospitals being greatly increased by successful surgical operations', while the second states that 'Nothing can be more favourable, when the constitution has been well prepared, than the mild and genial season of an Indian spring during the months of February and March, or even the cold season', for 'serious operations, or the rapid healing of wounds'. Brett makes another point when he writes that 'A thorough acquaintance with the languages of India is most essential for a medical man', without which he will not be consulted, and 'he will very rarely be called upon to operate'. This Brett concluded from his own experience, 'during a number of years in all the populous cities he has had occasion to visit from Calcutta to Lahore'.

The European, on first landing in Bengal, 'is generally in the highest state of plethora', due to which he or she seldom escapes a severe attack of inflammation. Brett bemoans the lack of proper advice to the Company's officer cadets, who need an experienced medical man to 'act the part of a friend, I would almost say of a parent to them', and impress on them 'the necessity of adopting those habits which are so essential to the preservation of their health and lives in this country'. Interestingly, Brett touches upon the fact that the Company did not overpay their physicians and surgeons, when he emphasises that the cadets should have a medical superintendent, 'who should be adequately remunerated'.

'For the first few years of his residence in India', writes Brett, the European 'becomes in high condition, especially during the cold season'. However, danger lurked, for 'his system, both vascular and nervous, is under a constant state of excitement, from the continuing in-pouring of nutriment, stimulation and high temperature, and he labours under plethora from *repletion* as well as plethora from *diminished secretion*' [Brett's italics]. The European is thus 'on the precipice of disease', and if he survived, he did so with a feeble constitution, 'his appetite impaired, his energies diminished, the secretions and excretions scanty, and the skin dark, harsh, and dry'. Then follows some overt racism, for Brett writes that the European is 'no longer recognisable as the energetic active European', but, his 'muscular system is much reduced', and he becomes "the 'dried up Indian' with habits and constitution scarcely adapted for his native land'. Should the European not lapse into Indianness, he becomes 'gross, corpulent, and flabby'. Further, 'indolent habits' brought on by unwillingness to exertion, and 'confinement indoors' to escape the heat, rendered European particularly susceptible to inflammations. Brett recommended that 'If Europeans cannot adopt their mode of life to a tropical climate but must indulge in habits totally incompatible with such climate, they should at all events endeavour to convert their food into wholesome nutriment, and preserve the robustness of their frames by practicing athletic exercises, in the cool of the day, and wrestling in imitation of the Puhlwans'. Brett himself 'has long admired and practiced the calisthenic exercising of the Asiatics, and attributes a better state of health and stamina, and a capability for active pursuits, far superior to that enjoyed by him in England, to the systematic use of these exercises'. 'In the Governor General's Body Guard', he writes, 'there is a very good specimen of a gymnasium amongst the troopers, some of whom are very well developed athletics, among the old and most respectable hands'. As such, Brett was one of 'The few Europeans who have entered thoroughly into the spirit of these exercises'. Few in India have 'immunity from disease' like these Indian wrestlers or 'Puhlwans'. In fact, 'There are none whose constitutions resist the exciting causes of disease so well, although their blood is abundant and vascular system vigorous'. Those Europeans, who take up this bodily exercise, 'return to their native land with vigorous constitutions capable of really enjoying their native country'.

Brett felt 'it would be well for a young man to go through the whole system at first under a regular Puhlwan', before beginning specialised training using "The 'Moodgurs', the 'Dundh', and the 'Lezum'", in addition to 'Friction and shampooing'. Undoubtedly speaking from personal experience, Brett wrote, 'Nothing is so conducive to a perfect capillary circulation, to the healthy action of the liver and of all the secretions, the tone of the stomach, and the sthenic state of the nervous and muscular system, enabling us to bear up against a long and sultry day'. The European was advised to drink moderately, since 'Moderate stimulation is requisite to the European in India, water drinkers are not observed to be the healthiest people'. These good habits would go a long way in keeping the European from that singularly debilitating and 'exceedingly common inflammatory disease', hepatitis. Uncommon among the locals, this ailment derived from the action of the heat, which 'accelerates the circulation, therefore increases exertion; the greater the natural functions of the organ, and its importance in the economy [the liver], the more will it partake of the effects of high temperature acting on the general circulation'.

Another inflammatory ailment noted by Brett is scrofula, which he notes, 'is the disease of the Zunana, and populous cities of Hindostan in all its forms, especially the lymphatic glandular suppurations and sinuous ulcers of the cellular tissue under the skin of the neck (Kanthmala), ulceration of the spongy heads of the bones, suppuration of cartilages, and synovial membranes, and strumous ophthalmia'. The cause of this ailment 'would appear to depend on some peculiarity in the condition of the blood, especially in its disposition to the formation of tubercles in the various tissues, and the constitutions favouring their formation are probably an unusual serosity of blood, and its languid motion in numerous small capillaries'.

Ozoena was presented as another disease endemic among the locals, who called it "'peenus kee beemari'". Characterised by a profuse discharge from both nostrils, 'Its ravages are such as to extend to the destruction of the septum, the inferior turbinated bones, the cartilaginous alae, and the dorsum of the nose, of the superior turbinated bones, and the floor of the nares and hard palate'. Sometimes the affected parts would heal with the conclusion of the disease. In such cases, Brett records that 'the Rhinoplastic operation' was carried out 'where the parts had quite healed', in order to restore normal appearance. The treatment included washing the ulceration with warm water, touching it with silver nitrate, applying a poultice of bread and water, the poultice to be replaced every three hours, the nitrate every sixth day, and the whole supplemented by mercurial pills and other laxatives, with advice for a change of air.

Next is the malignant ulcer of the nails, 'most painful and distressing', which affected both locals and Europeans in India. Possibly 'modified by a syphilitic or pseudo-syphilitic taint of constitution in the natives', this ulcer caused so much pain as to keep the patient from exertion of any kind. Beginning as an inflammation at the root of the nail of the thumb or big toe, it proceeded to destroy the nail, which fell off, 'leaving a red, unequal, sensible surface, with an inflamed irritable border, which bleeds on the movement of the member'. It caused fever that increased with the night, and pain, which prevented sleep. The two available and tested treatments included the application of the 'lunar caustic' and 'honey of borax'. Ulcers also resulted from in-growing toenails, where Brett chose to use his plan, 'to slit up the nail suddenly using a sharp scalpel', rather than follow the usual method of lifting up the nail, and applying fomentations. In his method, Brett said, 'The pain is momentary and the source of irritation is at once removed'.

One of the most feared inflammations of the time was 'chronic mortification', 'to be seen in the toes of old persons, in whom the action of the heart is feeble and the arteries ossified'. For this dread disease 'The slightest exciting cause' such as 'the cutting of a corn, or the paring of the nails' was enough. Soon inflammation would be seen, followed within days by the appearance of 'Red streaks marking the course of inflamed absorbents', from the foot towards the leg. The glands of the groin were inflamed, and gangrene struck. In all such cases, if the cause of the disease could not be removed, or the progress of the disease stopped, it remained for the surgeon to 'promote the separation of the mortified from the living parts'. The surgeon would try to use 'scarifications, leeches, and other antiphlogistic measures', keeping in mind the age and constitution of the patient, considering the shock to the body that these treatments entailed.

Ominously, the 'undeniable principle' was that 'in all cases of traumatic gangrene where the constitution is sound', including gunshot wounds, amputation would have to follow 'after the first few hours have been allowed to elapse', during which the system had recovered from 'the first shock'. Indeed, 'the latest period within which the operation can be accomplished with any prospect of success is within 36 hours from the accident'. The same rule applied to all other cases of gangrene. To keep the disease from spreading, the application of nitric acid lotion, poultice of charcoal and linseed, and camphorated fomentations, was advised. The patient was also prescribed to take quinine with opium, ammonium carbonate with laudanum, and to take nourishing food and wine.

Of equal seriousness was 'Hospital gangrene', to be seen 'Wherever the combination of crowded hospitals and impure atmosphere together with high temperature and moisture exist, aggravated by inattention to cleanliness'. A 'full and sharp pulse', followed by 'rigors succeeded by heat, but no perspiration', anorexia, a tongue covered 'with a thick white mucus', characterise this ailment. Soon the pain 'becomes excessively severe and burning, and the most alarming symptoms of collapse often terminate the scene'. Another form of this was erysipelas seen in infants 'in lying in hospitals, commencing at the umbilicus, extending to the pudenda, and terminating fatally in gangrene'.

Recounting his own experience with parasitic tumours, Brett recalled how in Delhi he had seen 'an adult native', whose 'body was covered with, I had almost said, *countless* adipose tumours, varying from the size of a pumpkin to that of a pea' [his emphasis]. Of these, Brett removed one 'from the spinous processes of the dorsal vertebrae weighing about 3 lbs'. This made him conclude that these tumours 'undoubtedly originate in the effusion of lymph, and in such instances, are traced to inflammation'. Occasionally, he thought, they were congenital, as in the case of the man he had seen in Delhi. The simplest form of the local tumour 'is that produced by the infiltration of lymph, the *ordinary vascular sarcoma*' [his emphasis]. This was commonly seen in Bengal, and which Brett called '*hypertrophy* of the *scrotum* and *cellular tissue*' [his emphasis]. In these cases the tumours grew to a 'considerable extent'. Brett and other surgeons in Bengal recorded that patients suffered pain and heat in the affected part, 'often ushered in by a smart paroxysm of fever'. In the earliest stages, this growth could be controlled by using 'purgatives, issues, alteratives, local friction, and a careful avoidance of the weather particularly when combined with the local application of cold and moisture'. Since most locals neglected the growth at this stage, it would grow painlessly, to 'an enormous bulk'. The first corrective surgical operation for such a tumour carried out in Calcutta, was on a local aged 36, who walked 'in a slow swinging manner, the tumour hanging down to the calves of his leg'. The patient 'was in great misery and alarm at his unsightly appearance, and the great inconvenience he experienced from its weight'. After the operation, and the draining of the fluid in it, the tumour was found to weigh 56 lbs, and was 55 inches in circumference. Brett wrote that similar operations should begin with the patient being given a large dose of laudanum, 'not less than 90 or 100 drops'. He then goes on to describe the surgical procedure to be followed in cutting out the growth, which he describes as 'a yellowish hard substance of fibrous consistence and creaking beneath the cutting instrument'. In 1837, Brett records that this procedure was carried out on 7 persons, of whom 2 died 'of mortification of the wound', which he states was the consequence of operating 'during most sultry weather in a Bengal climate, and in a very crowded hospital'. Of the remaining 5 who were released fit, 1 died three and a half months later of dysentery. Brett carried out 7 such operations at Calcutta, in which the aggregate weight of the tumours, minus their fluid, was 280 lbs. By 1840 this procedure had become well established, and many surgeons were practising it. Brett felt that the disease was endemic to 'damp and warm climates, the relaxing effects of which doubtless favour their greater development'. Further, 'They do not appear to be confined more to the sedentary than the laborious classes of individuals'.

From the hypertrophy of the scrotum Brett moves to that of the pudenda, which he says is as common among 'females in Hindostan' as it is among men. Hypertrophied prepuces are 'so very common in the lower extremities of the Bengalis as to be seen almost daily on visiting any part of the city'. This disorder, Brett states, has been wrongly called '*Elephantiasis*' [his emphasis], 'but has no connection with that tubercular disease'. Rather, 'It is a pure vascular sarcoma, with hydroceles, and is evidently the same disease with that which occurs in the West Indies, Africa, Ceylon, and occasionally in Europe'.

The '*Bronchochele*' [his emphasis; he later calls it goitre] was presented as a very common tumour 'at various localities throughout the range of the Himalayan Mountains', so much so that Brett wrote, 'At Almorah I have usually observed one out of every ten affected'. He had come across it in the Terai as well. 'The disease', he writes, 'commences early in life, affecting both sexes indiscriminately, and may attain to very considerable dimensions without greatly incommoding respiration or deglutition'. Following popular medical thought of his time, especially the findings of Sir John McClelland (1805-83) in the same regions, Brett concludes that 'those villages, in which goitre exists, are always erected on, or in close vicinity to, great limestone formations; and that the water is always furnished, for the use of the inhabitant of such villages, by springs which are derived from limestone rocks'. This, he says, was remarked on by McClelland, through a survey that extended across 1000 square miles. Repeating McClelland's findings, Brett states that the 'morbid principle' in the water from these springs is 'removed or modified' by the distance the water travels, and that 'The lowest caste of persons in the Himalayan mountains are more subject to the affection than the higher orders, owing to the poverty of the former compelling them to use more water, and less milk, than their superiors'. Having reached this conclusion, Brett states that the best treatment for goitre is iodine, which may be' administered in solution, or the tincture diluted, the dose being gradually increased'. In cases where the goitre interferes with respiration, radical surgery was recommended, while the equally popular treatment involving the introduction of a seton stitch was dismissed as risky and 'slow and uncertain'. The surgical procedure to be followed is that pronounced best by Dr Robert Liston (1794-1847), who is probably best known for his reckless speed in operative procedures.

Another of Brett's patients in Calcutta was 'an interesting young female of 17 years of age', who had developed an inflammation in the region of the parotid gland 5 years earlier, which burst and discharged for some time through the meatus auditorius. When this ceased, the abscess grew again, and drained once more, this time through the parotid duct. Then the abscess grew for the third time, 'until it acquired such a size as to occasion great deformity and to impede the functions of deglutition and voice, and was attended with considerable pain'. Brett's operation to remove this growth began well enough, 'until the dissection was carried to the deep attachments at the base where it encircles the [carotid] artery'. When this happened, 'the patient was deluged in a torrent of blood chiefly from the external carotid'. The consequence is obvious, for as Brett relates, 'She swooned and an involuntary discharge of urine and faeces took place'. Meanwhile, Brett ligatured the artery, and haemorrhage stopped immediately. The girl recovered consciousness, and over time, the wound healed, 'chiefly by adhesion, and partly by cicatrisation'. Some months later, the girl had recovered, except that during the operation, Brett had 'unavoidably wounded' branches of the portio dura of the seventh pair of nerves, due to which portions of her face were paralysed forever. Brett recounted how reputed surgeons in Europe had not been successful in similar operations, while he had followed, once more, the directions of 'that truly able surgeon, Mr Liston'.

Brett next relates an incident from October 1830, of how when he was returning from Almorah, 'a native of the hills, named Khoondooa' sought his surgical assistance. Khoondooa was then 27, and since the age of 10 he had been troubled by a scratching and irritation at the chin, 'but no pain'. However, 'A swelling at the chin and inside of the mouth slowly formed', which had increased to such proportions during the intervening period that 'the mouth was much distorted and stretched; the lips could not be closed; some of the teeth had fallen out, and others were displaced in various directions', and since the growth filled most of the mouth, the tongue had been pushed backwards. Brett found 'a tumour investing the alveolar process of the lower jaw, at the symphysis'. It was of the size of an orange, and of a bony hardness, causing, in addition to deformity, difficulty in chewing and speech. An apt pupil of Robert Liston, Brett took 15 minutes to excise the tumour, during which there was 'free bleeding, followed by syncope'. The patient luckily revived, and the wound was sutured, bound with adhesive plaster, and bandaged into place with the help of pasteboard, since Brett had sawn through the lower jaw. No more dressings were required after the fourth day, and the patient was declared cured. In order to numb the senses as far as possible, in this case, as in others, Brett would have habitually administered 80 to 100 drops of laudanum.

Brett renamed elephantiasis '*lepra tuberculata virulenta*' [his emphasis]. To his mind, this disease, 'very common in the valley of the Dhoon and in Bengal', especially among the poorer people, who lived on 'very unwholesome grain', was a kind of leprosy, which in turn derived from syphilis, whose symptoms resemble those of leprosy. Uncertain of his premises, Brett presents us with two anecdotal cases. The first is that of a Brahmin, who had lost several joints to leprosy, which he had suffered for 4 years. Nonetheless, he lived with his wife and child, neither of whom caught the disease, especially the child, whom the man 'constantly nursed'. The second relates the plight of a havildar of the Governor-General's Body Guard, Moosahib Khan, who was afflicted with 'incipient disease in its most distinct form', and was certain that he had contracted it while sharing a hookah with another man from the same regiment, 'who had been invalided for a very inveterate and advanced case of leprosy'.

For the treatment of leprosy, Brett wrote that 'We are indebted to the Hindoos for almost every efficacious remedy in this disease', and proceeded to select the ones that were best, premising that 'almost every one of them have been tried by many able European practitioners in this country'. Their efficacy, therefore, 'rests on the most unquestionable authority'. The first of these is 'mudarr', which in Brett's time was erroneously listed as *Asclepias gigantea*, later renamed *Calotropis gigantea*. This plant has medicinal properties, and Brett, following others, prescribes its roots mixed in powdered form with 'Protoxide of Arsenic' and black pepper, as a certain cure for leprosy 'in the incipient stage'. Other such formulae include mixtures of 'Junglee Neel' [*Indigofera mimosides*?] 'Sahar Punkha' [*Galega officinalis*?], 'Shah Tara' [*Fumaria parviflora*], 'Burree hurh' [*Terminalia chebula*], and 'Moonghee chirayta' [*Gentiana chirata*], pounded and mixed with water, fermented, and finally reduced over a fire. The diet prescribed by 'Hindoo physicians' includes game of all kinds, including deer, and birds, 'Sushtika rice' or 'rice of sixty days growth raised during the rains in the months of August and September', and 'Moong' [*Vigna radiata? Phaseolus aureus?*] Brett writes 'Phaseolus moong'], with 'urhur' [*Cajanus cajan*], mixed as a porridge. Brett goes on to compile a long list of other medicinal plants used by local physicians. 'Some Fakeers', he writes, 'are said to be able to cure the disease by administering a root procured from Nipal [*sic*], which causes copious salivation, putting the patient at the same time on a regimen and prohibiting salt, and sexual intercourse'. Another cure, which worked in the case of Moosahib Khan 'after other remedies had apparently checked the spread of the disease', was the 'ioduret of arsenic'. However, this was hard to prepare, and Brett found that a substitute compound, made of 'Hydriodate of Potass', 'Arsenous acid', and rose water, worked equally well.

'Lepra albida' or' leucopathia' was similar to leprosy. Brett wrote that he knew it could be cured by 'Stimulating the affected part with sulphur *douches*, and with sulphur ointment and volatile liniments'. In fact, the locals considered it incurable, and Brett particularly noted that 'It is exceedingly common, and many would give a large sum of money to any medical man who would cure them'.

'Urinary calculi' were commoner among those living in the western provinces of India than in Bengal, since 'the moister and more equable climate of Bengal' along with the common diet of rice and lentils, removed the main cause of this ailment. Due to this, lithotomies were frequent. Brett writes, 'I have had occasion to operate on four patients in one day, all residing in the same village or its immediate neighbourhood, and upwards of one hundred cases have occurred to myself during my abode in India'. The largest calculus he had removed, weighed 'about four ounces'. Once he had removed '221 calculi of small size from the interior of the prepuce in a case of phymosis with complete closure'. Using the fact that chemical analysis of calculi extracted in India showed the same composition as those from Europe, Brett dismissed the theory that a diet of animal flesh caused them. In the case of almost all the locals, diet 'with scarcely any exception, has been vegetable and farinaceous'. 'Neither is there any foundation', he wrote, 'for attributing the supposed rarity of calculi in hot climates to the vegetable food, to which the inhabitants are habituated'. The children of dyspeptic and gouty parents were particularly prone to calculi, as also in persons who lead 'sedentary and luxurious' but declining lives, particularly 'old Indians who have suffered from hepatic affections and led irregular lives'. Europeans in India 'often induce a fit of the gravel by excess or irregularity whether as to the quantity, quality, and time, of receiving the ingesta'. Treatment mainly included the administration of alkaline carbonates 'in the form of effervescing draughts, with an excess of the alkali'.

Of the bladder stone, Brett noted how 'The natives of India have from time immemorial been in the habit of bringing down the calculus by pressure above the pubic region, moulding as it were the hypogastrium, and causing the stone to descend towards the outlet of the pelvis; with two fingers in the rectum they then not only seize but cause it to bulge in the perineum'. For the benefit of those who would not believe this, Brett added, 'This I have myself witnessed'. He noted that Indian patients went to European doctors 'with confidence in the superiority of European skill', and so seeking 'speedy relief from agonising pain'. In fact, 'The patient is infinitely more pleased by immediate operation, which when set about with the least possible ceremony is not looked upon at all seriously by him'. For his operations, Brett used 'a sharp scalpel, a straight staff, and forceps'. An hour before the operation, the patient, if an adult, was given 100 drops of laudanum.

To the modern reader, the procedure, as described by Brett, seems barbaric. The surgical instruments, including two scalpels, curved and straight forceps, a scoop, and a long, probe-pointed knife, along with bandage, lint, warm water, and oil, were placed on a chair to the right of the surgeon, and covered with a towel. The patient was laid 'on a firm table about two feet and a half high, with his head and shoulders well raised by pillars', while a low chair was readied for the surgeon, 'whose breast should be in a line with the patient's abdomen'. Next came the tying down of the patient: 'The hands and ankles being now secured by lithotomy garters of broad worsted tape, a bandage passed around the neck and under the hams, the thighs separated and pelvis fixed by able assistants'. The necessary 'free' and 'bold' incisions having been made, the surgeon carefully inserted his finger into the perineum, after which the finger guided further cutting, including the prostrate, which 'is completely divided on withdrawing the knife'. The stone having been located in the bladder, the forceps would be introduced to remove it. Sometimes the stone would have to be crushed. Following the operation, the wound was washed with warm water, and oiled lint pushed in, if desired by the surgeon. The patient was then shifted to a bed 'previously brought close at hand, for that purpose'. The patient's head and shoulders were laid higher than the rest of the body, the knees supported by bolsters, with the thighs slightly apart. The patient was given diluting drinks to produce urine, and probably told by the surgeon to enjoy 'Great tranquillity' on the successful completion of the procedure. As was usual then, the wound was kept open in order to drain, and 'to granulate from the bottom'. Despite all this, mortality does not seem to have been high. Brett, at least, claimed that the number of fatal cases was '1 in 15', and that his last 68 cases were all successful. Urine generally flowed from the 'natural passage' by the 8th day in adults, and 4th or 5th day in children. Sometimes in adults the process was delayed until the 15th or 20th day.

Children were not spared this horrific operation. In fact, as Brett wrote later, 'three-fourths of the patients who present themselves with the stone are children'. He introduced the case of James Diggs, who was 3 when his parents took him from Delhi to Meerut to consult with him. Deeming him too young for the operation, Brett advised his parents to wait until the following winter, when they took him to Kanpur, where Brett was stationed. The procedure was carried out, but the stone broke when extraction was attempted. Brett realised that a part of the stone was encysted, and rather than operate again, he chose to leave it 'to the effects of nature'. The entire operation had lasted 4 minutes. Brett recorded that 'The encysted portion dropped on the bed on the 3rd day, having been carried out by a jet of urine through the wound'. By the 8th day the child had fully recovered; Brett saw him several years later, and he was in good health. This case is comparable to another, of Jhoomloo, aged 7, on whom the second operation or, "'*La operation a deux temps*'", was performed. Jhoomloo had been suffering from bladder-stone since the age of 5, and he was brought to Brett in November 1834, in an emaciated state. At Jhoomloo's father's request, Brett agreed to operate 'as a last alternative'. The operation went well until the stone was seized with forceps. Brett recalled, 'the stone was repeatedly seized, and as often escaped from the grasp of the forceps, being evidently retained, either by the firm contraction of the bladder, or by a portion of it, being encysted'. Since these operations greatly tested the endurance of the patient, despite the high dose of laudanum, and Brett found 'the child becoming much exhausted', he stopped probing at once and ordered Jhoomloo 'a full dose of tincture of opium combined with aromatic spirit of ammonia' and sent him to bed. The following morning the operation was undertaken once more. This time, the child was placed in an assistant's lap, 'with his back towards him [the assistant], bent and raised the knees by placing his arms under his hams, the perineum being lowered as much as possible, and the body kept in the erect position, so that the stone might gravitate as much as possible towards the wound'. Brett again inserted his finger in the wound, felt the stone, and grasping it with forceps, drew it out in a moment. The stone had indeed been encysted in the wall of the bladder. Brett stated the salutary lesson he had learnt from this case: 'I have not the slightest doubt that had I persisted in my efforts to remove the stone, the child would have expired on the table, and the expediency of procrastination on the occasion is thus exemplified'. As he later noted, one of the greatest and necessarily fatal dangers of operating on children, was peritonitis. Dealing with this called for 'the most energetic measures'. However, the high rate of mortality from peritonitis is clarified by his statement that of those of his patient struck down by post-operative peritonitis, 'One or two of the cases have happily recovered'. Fomentations to the abdomen apparently helped keep peritonitis at bay, and 'young practitioners' were assured that 'One or two paroxysms of fever in children, without any other unfavourable symptom' was normal.

These operations had their still more horrific moments. In another case, 'the patient was deluged with blood', which stopped temporarily after the stone was drawn out. The wound was plugged, and 'the internal pubic artery was compressed with the finger for a long time'. This did not work, for severe haemorrhaging returned as soon as the finger was removed, followed by 'syncope, and alarming symptoms'. The patient's condition worsened through the night, and death followed. Brett explained this by positing that in this patient 'There was apparently an irregular distribution of the internal pudic'. This was merely a hypothesis, since the family did not allow post-mortem. In another similar case, 'a large branch given off close to the internal pudic' haemorrhaged severely, but Brett, and his assistant, Evans, managed to apply ligatures, after which the operation proceeded successfully.

More ominously, 2 of Brett's patients, on whom he had operated early in his career in India, succumbed to tetanus. Today, post-operative tetanus is considered appalling. Brett, given his times, blamed the weather: 'they occurred about the same time, during the unhealthy season of May, when the hot winds had subsided and easterly winds prevailed'. This season was 'unfavourable for operating', for 'The rains had not set in; the heat at that time was suffocatingly great'.

Comparing the benefits of lithotrity versus lithotomy, Brett felt that Indians opted for the operation more easily and oftener, because 'The feeling of fear is inconsiderable in uncivilised life'. 'Were I in England', he said, 'I should not hesitate to practice lithotrity on all favourable cases'. Despite all his willingness to learn from local medical traditions, Brett was imbued with a considerable degree of racism. This statement, however, is equally applicable to the fact that as a surgeon, Brett preferred lithotomies to lithotrities. Equally, he was aware that he was far less adept at lithotrity. In 2 cases, the patients wearied of lithotrity and though the stones had been broken, 'left me, though labouring under irritation'.

In females, lithotrity was the preferred method of extracting calculi. The danger lay in 'too hasty measures', which led to contusion and lacerations, the prime reasons for 'distressing incontinence'. 'Lithotomy is very easily accomplished in the female', Brett noted, but it carried the same danger of bringing on incontinence. He had carried out lithotrities but not lithotomies on females, 'as I have succeeded with dilatation whenever I have had occasion to remove the stone from the female bladder'.

Prostatic enlargement was often mistaken for abscess, as exemplified by the case of a colonel, posted in the 'Upper Provinces', who met Brett at Danapore while travelling downriver to Calcutta under medical certificate. The colonel's doctor, 'an eminent Surgeon of that Presidency', had written to him to return at the earliest to Calcutta since he suspected the colonel to have 'an abscess in the perineum'. 'On my introducing a large sized catheter', noted Brett, 'to which he was at first very reluctant to submit, it passed into the bladder without difficulty'. Brett thereupon diagnosed an enlarged prostate and assured the colonel that he did not have an abscess. In similar cases of chronic enlargement, there was no permanent treatment, besides 'Alleviation of suffering, and perhaps a check to the growth of diseased prostrate'. The usual limited pharmacopeia was applied, including 'Cupping on the loins, leeches on the perineum', laxatives, enemas, and suppositories. Relief was obtained by using catheters, which the patient would be taught to use by himself every 8 hours. This catheter would preferably be 'a silver prostatic catheter of considerable length, calibre, and curvature'. Surgical intervention was the last choice, to be applied if all other efforts 'for relief of retention from diseased prostrate' were fruitless. In such cases, 'it has been recommended to puncture the third or middle lobe of that gland'. Brett never undertook a prostatic operative procedure, and he felt 'It must be exceedingly rare if ever that such a measure is requisite'.

Another strange ailment listed by Brett is incontinence arising from 'irritability of the bladder'. 'Young men with irritability of the bladder in the society of ladies', he said, 'have from motives of delicacy restrained their desire of evacuating their urine for a long period, causing great agony at the time, and have led in consequence a miserable existence from irritable bladder for the remainder of their lives'.

Diseases of the eye often require surgical treatment. In all cases of ophthalmic inflammation, 'Bloodletting may be general or local —the former is indicated in all acute forms of the disease, the latter is of advantage in the milder degrees of inflammation, or after general depletion, often causing the irritation, the compression and the pain to cease rapidly'. The surgeon was cautioned that in most locals, 'especially the poorer and sedentary classes of Bengal, the powers of the system are greatly enfeebled under ophthalmic inflammation, in which cases general bleeding is altogether inadmissible and the local even must be used with caution'. Leeching was the best method, which was not free of its own dangers. Leeches, placed on inflamed eyelids often caused oedema from erysipelas. In all cases, leech bites caused local irritation. Brett declared means of exciting counter-irritation useful in cases of ophthalmia. 'Of this character are the foot bath, with mustard sinapisms to the extremities', he wrote, 'and the application of the emplast; resinos; cantharid; to the back of the neck, behind the ears, or between the shoulders, for the purpose of producing a temporary rubefaction of the skin'. Purgatives, too, were deemed essential to the treatment of these cases, especially in children, since they caused the evacuation of 'a large quantity of serous and fibro-albuminous matter'. Interestingly, Brett theorised that 'The second effect of purgatives consists in the transferring the irritation of the mucus membrane of the eye to another very extensive portion of the mucus system'. Emetics were not recommended since the act of vomiting caused a rush of blood to the head and eyes. A local ointment, composed of opium and other ingredients, helped to control pain and irritation of the eye.

The 'Catarrhal Inflammation of the Lids' was common in 'the unhealthy confined cities of India … especially among the females of zenanas'. 'The plumbago (Soorma) which they are in the habit of applying to improve the expression of the eye may have something to do with this', Brett thought, 'aided sometimes by neglect of cleanliness; it commences with soreness, smarting and burning; it is increased by employment of the eye, as in reading and writing'. The treatment involved fomentation, personal cleanliness, proper diet, and application of ointments of nitrate of mercury, zinc sulphate, and lead acetate. Cataracts were more easily extracted in inhabitants of the 'Upper Provinces' of India, than Bengal, because the latter suffered from 'deepness of the orbit, smallness of the anterior chamber, their weak constitutional powers (owing to the poorness of their diet) render the reparative effort so weak as to hazard the union of the incision of the cornea, making this operation peculiarly inapplicable to them'.

The most important local advancement lay in plastic surgery. 'It is singular that the principles on which are founded some of our capital surgical operations in the present day, should have been known and practiced by the Hindoos from a very remote period', Brett wrote, 'especially the operations for couching, cutting for the stone, and the method of restoring lost portions of the body'. In fact, the local method had proved superior to European techniques in rhinoplastic procedures. However, Brett felt that this advancement was due to 'The frequent mutilations of the body practiced by Eastern despots'. Nonetheless, there were lessons to be learnt: 'An interesting fact, which may be turned to much practical advantage, has been well illustrated in India, —viz. that mucous membrane not only becomes integument when everted and exposed to the atmosphere, but that it becomes black by the deposition of pigmentum, and that integument when inverted becomes mucous membrane, as is exhibited in the enormous tumours of the scrotum, where the extended prepuce becomes mucous membrane, a channel of considerable length for the passage of urine enabling us to form a covering to the penis after extirpation of these tumours'.

Brett does not seem to have obtained fame in the service, though he was a competent and scientifically curious surgeon. His later life is not of great interest. Brett returned to England at the end of 18 years' service, and due to his previous and extensive experience as Surgeon to the Government Eye Hospital in Calcutta, obtained an appointment at the Western Ophthalmic Institution, Portman Square, London. He became a Fellow of the Royal College of Surgeons, England, and amongst other things, wrote in 1852 a book titled *The Gems of Tuscany, Being a Fragment for the Invalid and the Tourist in Italy*. This book begins with an address to the Fellows and Members of the Royal College by Brett, who writes of his long sojourn in India, and the pleasure of meeting his colleagues in 'the groves of the Academy' on this return home. He had been a traveller 'on the shores of the Bosphorus; amongst the Arabs of the Desert, to the Sphinx and the Pyramids; the Isles of Greece; and in many other parts of the south; and studied in the schools of Vacca and of Scarpa, of Viussens, Cotunnius, and Vansalva', for the last 3 years, he wrote, which allows us to calculate that he left England in 1849. Now, after an adventurous life, 'which would furnish materials for the wildest romance', during which he had been robbed by the 'rapacious plunderers of the law' and by the 'Arabs of the Desert', he had returned to England 'to shake hands with many an old friend and good-hearted Fellow of the Profession'.

During his trip Brett had learnt that surgeons needed vacations. Surgeons, 'whose health and energies are incessantly devoted to the benefit of mankind, and whose self-devotion and industry are not always adequately appreciated by the public' ought, in Brett's view, save their lives by taking a month's trip to Italy, 'during these days of rapid communication'.

The *London Gazette*, 1 May 1855, informs us that 'Surgeon Frederick Harrington Brett, MD, of the East India Company's Service', was to have 'the local rank of Staff-Surgeon of the First Class while employed with the Army in the East, Dated 28th March 1855'. Brett does not seem to have served in the Crimea. In any case, he seems to have died in great obscurity, far away from home, in early December, 1859.

CHAPTER ELEVEN

MESMERISM AND SURGERY IN BENGAL: JAMES ESDAILE

I was astounded to learn that there was a Mesmeric Hospital in Calcutta. Nonetheless, it existed, most certainly for over a year, and many patients were successfully treated there. Brett's book on practical surgery in India revealed to us his technique of trying to deaden pain as far as possible, for the patient, by administering up to 100 drops of laudanum. Despite this, and the speed with which Brett, influenced by his role model, Robert Liston, operated, the patient must have felt considerable pain. We saw how Brett upbraided Europeans for choosing lithotrity over lithotomy, when in his surgical opinion the latter was many times more effective. His claim of having performed 68 successful lithotomies without a single fatality is no doubt impressive. However, the fact remains that contemporary medical practice was painful for the patient. Continuous doses of mercury affected the mouth, sometimes so severely that ulceration led to adhesions of parts of the mouth. The Peruvian bark caused gastritis, which was partially countered by the huge amounts of laxatives and emetics given to cleanse the system. Venesection, whether done by the conventional method of slitting a vein, or the concealed malevolence of the scarificator, was painful and frequently a direct cause of the patient's death. To us, today, these methods of medicine seem barbaric. To the English doctor battling local diseases in a foreign climate with his limited anatomical and physiological knowledge, as well as his inadequate medicine chest, it was a process of learning to which he himself often fell.

Mesmerism became a popular accompaniment to surgery because it apparently removed surgical pain. This in turn seemed to reduce shock in the patient. Next, it allowed the surgeon to operate slowly, and more confidently, so that operations were successful. Further, it was inexpensive, and did not necessitate the use of either opiates, or of tying down the patient, or of having assistants hold down the patient. However, the scientific relevance of mesmerism was far from being universally accepted. Initiated by James Esdaile at Hooghly, in Bengal, its relevance and authenticity was examined by a board of doctors who, as we shall see, recommended the establishment of the Mesmeric Hospital in Calcutta.

James Esdaile, born in Montrose in 1808, studied medicine at Edinburgh, graduating in 1830. Being sickly, he was prescribed life in a warm climate, and Esdaile was appointed to the Company's service as Assistant Surgeon. He reached Calcutta in July 1831, having lost his wife on the voyage. He worked in this capacity until 1835, when his health failed under the strain of field service, and he sailed for Europe under medical certificate. He went home, of course, and married Mary Ann, his second wife, on 2 July 1838 and of his travels, he wrote an interesting book, *Letters from the Red Sea, Egypt, and the Continent* (1839).

Esdaile returned to Calcutta in November 1838. He was posted as Civil Assistant Surgeon to the general hospital at Hooghly, which he called 'a country charity hospital'. Esdaile spent nearly 6 years there, and during that time, probably due to loneliness, for Mary Ann had succumbed to the climate, he became sufficiently influenced by mesmerism to begin practising it, albeit hesitantly at first. By 1845 Esdaile's mesmeric surgical practice gained considerable popularity among locals, and the Deputy Governor of Bengal, Sir Thomas Herbert Maddock (1792-1870), set up a committee of 7 members, including 4 doctors (one of them, the president of the committee, was a representative of the Medical Board, which had neglected Esdaile's official report on the successful use of mesmerism) to examine Esdaile's claims, which were then being hotly debated amongst the medical fraternity in Bengal. Esdaile, like all other army surgeons holding civil appointments, was ordered to active service with the Army of the Sutlej, in February 1846.

Meanwhile, committee studied the case-histories of the patients treated by Esdaile, and commended him to the notice of the Council, and suggested that facilities be made available to him in Calcutta to conduct his work on mesmerism. The Bengal Government thus granted Esdaile, on his return from active service, the use of a small hospital in Calcutta for one year, from November 1846 to December 1847. This hospital was located in Mott's Lane. Senior medical men were appointed to oversee it, and their reports, following inspection, were encouraging. Even Lord Dalhousie officially appreciated Esdaile's dedication and work by appointing him Presidency Surgeon of Bengal in 1848. Aged 40, Esdaile was the youngest doctor until then, to hold this prestigious post. However, Esdaile had never liked India, despite the adulation and popularity he attained there. One reason for this could be his personal sorrow, which was indelibly linked to India.

In the meantime, chloroform had become the common anaesthetic in England, with Robert Liston famously proclaiming, 'This Yankee dodge beats mesmerism hollow'. With the arrival and increasing use of ether in India, and despite the fact that many patients died due to its inexpert use, mesmerism was no longer in demand. Esdaile nevertheless persisted with his practice, declining to use his position for enlarging his private consultancy. He continued with mesmerism at his dispensary on Sookeas Street until he left India. In 1850, he became Marine Surgeon. The following year he completed the mandatory 20 years' service in the Company's employ, and qualified for retirement. James Esdaile departed from Calcutta in June, 1851, and never returned. He married his third wife, Eliza Weatherhead, later in the same year, and remained happily married to her until his death in 1859. Though he had initially settled in Scotland, he found that the cold climate exacerbated his chronic bronchitis and asthmatic tendency. Consequently, he moved to Sydenham, Kent, where he spent his final years.

For the present, we shall focus on 3 works related to Esdaile, his magnum opus, *Mesmerism in India, and its Practical Application in Surgery and Medicine* (1846), *The Introduction of Mesmerism (with the Sanction of the Government) into the Public Hospitals of India* (1852; second edition 1856), and *Records of Cases treated in the Mesmeric Hospital, from November 1846 to December 1847, with Reports of the Official Visitors. Printed by order of the Government* (1847).

At the beginning of the first book, Esdaile listed 73 surgical procedures painlessly and successfully carried out at Hooghly between August 1845 and January 1846. These range from the amputation of an arm to the removal of scrotal tumours. Esdaile described the appearance of the patient in the mesmerised state thus: 'The eyes are usually closed, but the eyelids are sometimes seen a little separated, or half open and tremulous, and the eye is even wide open, fixed, and insensible to light'. Further, blood circulation was not hindered during a trance; rather, it was like that 'of a sleeping person'. Recovery from entrancement is however, not always pleasant: 'They open their eyes, and at the same moment recover all their faculties; but it is seen that the pupil is insensible to the light: this they also become aware of; they know that their eyes are open and that they ought to see, but do not'. This causes great shock to the mind, and typically 'with a fearful cry they bury their faces in their hands, like persons struck blind by lightning ; but this soon passes off'. Nevertheless, it was 'a trial of the nerves which it would be very imprudent and even dangerous, to make with any but such singularly impassive subjects as my Indian patients'.

Who, then, was the ideal patient for mesmeric surgery? Esdaile wrote, “I am now able to say from experience, that debility of the nervous system predisposes to the easy reception of the mesmeric influence, and I augur well of a patient's powers of submission, when I recognize in him the listless dejected air, ‘L'air abattu,’ that usually accompanies functional debility of the nerves”. In fact, ‘Taking the population of Bengal generally, they are a feeble, ill-nourished race, remarkably deficient in nervous energy ; and natural debility of constitution being still further lowered by disease, will probably account for their being so readily subdued by the Mesmerist’. Contrasted to the disbelieving European, the ‘mental constitution’ of the locals is favourable to mesmerism. Europeans, on the other hand, are generally hampered by the ‘morbid irritability of the nerves’, and ‘the mental impatience of the civilised man’. On the other hand, Esdaile’s patients were the simple, unsophisticated children of nature; neither thinking, questioning, nor remonstrating, but passively submitting to my pleasure, without in the smallest degree understanding my object or intentions’. Further, ‘The process being a natural one, the more the parties are in a state of nature the better: the bodies of my patients being naked, and their heads generally shaved’ helped.

Inevitably, the greater part of the first chapter of Esdaile’s book on the practical application of mesmerism to surgery defends mesmerism from being disbelieved and dismissed as conjuring. Mesmerism was no quackery, for ‘the genuine medical quack is he who, professing to cure disease, yet allows his patients to suffer and perish, by ignorantly, or presumptuously, despising any promising or possible means of relief’. Esdaile argues for mesmerism by stating that ‘Instead of doubting and dogmatising about Mesmerism, I would earnestly entreat my medical brethren to put it to the test by personal experiment, for it is a thing to be done, and not talked of only’. The way to this is by explaining how a mesmeric trance may be induced in the patient. However, a warning precedes, ‘I beg leave to warn all who have not yet a practical knowledge of the subject, that to produce the phenomena of Mesmerism is by no means a thing so light and easy as some imagine’. To produce ‘the extreme degree of coma, so intense as to permit the performance of surgical operations, without awaking the patient’, it took a couple of hours’ hard work, ‘and the process often does not succeed till the second, or even fourteenth time’. Successful mesmerising required a good mesmeriser, for ‘If asked to select a natural Mesmeriser, I should be disposed to choose a person of a high organisation, in whom the nervous and circulating systems were equally active, with determined will, a resolution to do the thing if possible, and a love of truth and humanity’.

Besides this, the other needful qualities included 'Healthy young persons, who are tractable and patient, and who will give the necessary degree of attention, can be made to work out our intentions in the most efficient manner'. To this end, Esdaile wrote, 'Finding it impossible, after the first month, to prosecute the subject in my own person, owing to the great bodily and mental fatigue it caused,—for I spared neither,—I set to work my hospital attendants, young Hindoos and Mahomedans; and such has been my success, that everyone I have taught has become a skilful Mesmeriser'. This success had led to his not having to mesmerise patients any more. He could safely leave them to his assistants.

On 9 June 1845 Esdaile met a local magician, who enjoyed 'a high reputation for his successful treatment of hysteria'. This magician had been called in to treat a case, but 'came too late', for Esdaile had in the meantime applied mesmerism successfully. Nonetheless, in order to confirm his theory that mesmerism was superior to the practices of 'the Mumbo Jumbo men of Africa, the medicine men of America, and the charmers of this country', Esdaile requested the deputy magistrate of Hooghly, Baboo Essanchunder Ghosaul, 'to introduce me to him as a brother magician, who had studied the art of magic in different parts of the world'. After much persuasion, the local magician agreed to show Esdaile 'his process for assuaging pain'. The magician began by muttering charms over a brass pot containing water and a twig with a few leaves, sitting at some distance from the patient. Next, 'he dipped his fore-finger into the water, and, with the help of his thumb, flirted it into the patient's face; he then took the leaves, and commenced stroking the person from the crown of the head to the toes, with a slow drawing motion'. Esdaile noted that during this action, the magician's knuckles almost touched the patient, while the magician declared that the entire process would take an hour or more, which convinced Esdaile that this was similar to mesmerism. When his turn came, Esdaile told the magician that he would better understand Esdaile's charm 'if performed on his own person'. Again the magician was persuaded to agree, and he lay down while Esdaile "chanted, as an invocation, the chorus of the 'King of the Cannibal Islands!'" Then 'I desired him to shut his eyes, and he clenched his eyelids firmly, that I might find no entrance to the brain by that inlet'. Scarcely had 15 minutes passed, when 'he jumped up, and said he felt something disagreeable coming over him, and wished to make his escape'. 'Over-persuaded' to lie down again, the magician before long felt the impact of Esdaile's mesmerism for, as Esdaile wrote, 'I soon saw the muscles around the eye begin to relax, and his face became perfectly smooth and calm'. This did not last long, but the evidence that mesmerism had worked, came from the magician's response, who, on waking soon after, 'clapped his hands to his head, cried he felt drunk, and nothing could induce him to lie down again'. The following day Esdaile met the magician again, and regretted that he had failed to properly exercise his charm and put him to sleep. To this the magician replied that Esdaile did put him to sleep, but only because the magician had allowed it.

The first patient, on whom Esdaile practiced mesmeric surgery, was Madhab Kaura, a hog-dealer, who had been sentenced to 7 years' imprisonment, with hard labour in irons on the roads, for causing severe bodily injury to another man. Kaura, however, soon developed hydroceles, and was prescribed an operation at the 'charity hospital' where Esdaile worked. The operation proved too painful for Kaura, upon which Esdaile decided to use mesmerism to relieve him. To this end, Esdaile writes that he turned to his 'native sub-assistant surgeon', Budden Chunder Chowdaree, an alumnus of the medical college in Calcutta, if he had ever seen mesmerism applied to surgery. The assistant surgeon replied that 'he had seen it tried at the medical college, but without effect'. It was then 11 am, and only one side of the scrotal sac had been emptied of fluid. As he wrote later in his book, Esdaile had not read a single book on mesmerism: 'when I made my first experiment; and having succeeded In getting nature to speak, I determined to listen only to her for some time, and for months purposely refrained from reading on the subject, in order that my senses might not be predisposed to see things in any particular light, and that my judgment might be left unbiased by the opinions of others'.

Esdaile began mesmerism to calm Kaura. Due to the pain of his operation, Kaura had assumed a position in which 'he threw his head over the back of the chair, and pressed his hands along the course of the spermatic chords'. Esdaile recounts, 'The man continuing in the position described, I placed his knees between mine, and began to pass my hands slowly over his face, at the distance of an inch, and carried them down to the pit of his stomach'. This was continued for 30 minutes, at the end of which Esdaile was a bit dismayed to find Kaura's answers to questions 'quite sensible and coherent'. Nevertheless, the mesmerising continued for another 15 minutes.

The heat and the muscular and mental strength required for the passes tired Esdaile, and he 'gave it up in despair', when he noticed that the man's grimaces had lessened, and when asked to open his eyes, answered 'there was smoke in the room'. This encouraged Esdaile, and he resumed mesmerising Kaura: 'I now breathed on his head, and carried my hands from the back of his head over his face and down to the epigastrium, where I pressed them united'. After another hour of this, Kaura's eyes became lustreless and the eyelids grew heavy. He said he needed to sleep, and when ordered to open his eyes, again said he could only see smoke in the room. Soon 'his countenance showed the most perfect repose'. His hands no longer pressed on his groins, but were crossed on his chest. To questions he replied incoherently. Esdaile, now exhilarated, tested the trance by pinching Kaura, and pricking him with a needle in the small of the back, with his assistant watching Kaura's face closely for any expression of pain. Esdaile rushed to the district collector's office and the court, and asked Mr Russell, the district judge and Mr Money, the district collector, to return with him to see mesmerism at work, 'as I wanted the presence of intelligent witnesses in what remained to do'.

Russell and Money went with Esdaile to the hospital. Kaura was in the same state that Esdaile had left him in. Further experiments to test his level of consciousness were carried out. Esdaile hallooed in his ear, applied fire to his knee, exposed him to liquor ammonia (which brought tears into the observers' eyes though they were a little removed from it), and made him drink a very strong mixture of ammonia. None of these stimuli had any effect on Kaura. He did as he was bid and his eyes, though exposed to harsh light, continued to be lacklustre. To see how long the mesmeric trance lasted, Esdaile ordered Kaura to be laid upon a mattress and not moved until he returned. Esdaile was tired, and it was 1 pm. He went off, probably to lunch and rest.

When Esdaile returned to the hospital at 3 pm, he was chagrined to find Kaura gone. Interestingly, few of the locals seem to have caught the relevance of Kaura's trance and oblivion to pain. When the prison doctor, Kureem Ali, went to the hospital, presumably to see how Kaura was doing, he was told that the sahib, having failed to revive Kaura, had ordered him to rest on the mattress. On this, Ali 'set about doing so, and succeeded by throwing water on his face'. Disappointed but not defeated, Esdaile returned to Russell and Money, and with them went to the prison to interrogate Kaura on what he remembered of the trance.

Kaura remembered nothing. Rather, the interrogation so frightened him that he began to cry, fearing that he had done something wrong and would be punished for it. Esdaile contented himself with recording Kaura's statement, which was signed by Russell, Money, and Chowdaree. He also planned on a second operation, aimed at relieving the other side of the scrotum. He would use mesmerism again, and, this time, have witnesses to prove the painlessness of the operation to the entranced patient.

On 6 April 1845, at 11 am, Esdaile began mesmerising Kaura for the second time, on this occasion in the Jail Hospital. To Esdaile's satisfaction, Kaura was labouring under a fever, due to the inflammation of the hydrocele. “So”, he wrote, “turning to the native doctors [Chowdaree, Ali, and Noboo], I said that I would try the ‘Belatee Muntur’ (the Europe charm)”. With Kaura lying on a bed, the mesmeric ‘haze’ was established in 10 minutes. However, the inflamed scrotum still elicited a response when touched. After 45 minutes, Kaura was in a mesmeric coma, and squeezing the inflamed part like a bladder brought no response’. Leaving Kaura entranced and relieved of pain, Esdaile went to Chandernagore, 6 miles away, on business. In the meantime, to establish the genuineness of the mesmeric coma, he asked Rev Fisher and Mr Money, to visit the patient. This they did, and recorded their statements in writing. This time Kaura was not revived until Esdaile returned at 3 pm, when he used ‘transverse passes’ to awaken the patient. Revived, Kaura said that though dizzy, he was free of pain, and wanted to sleep some more.

The third experiment was on 11 April 1845, again at the Jail Hospital. This time Esdaile mesmerised Kaura confidently, ‘I leaned my elbows upon my knees, placed my mouth over the back of my joined hands, and breathed along their upper surface; the points of my fingers being pointed steadily at his eyes, nose, and forehead, in succession’. In about 35 minutes Kaura was in a mesmeric coma, and Esdaile announced to the sub-assistant surgeons that he would operate on Kaura if some European gentlemen could be procured to witness the proceeding. To this end, Esdaile, rather strangely, left the patient and went to Chinsurah, 2 miles distant, where he met ‘a considerable party, consisting of the Baron Law de Clapernou, Governor of Chandernagore, Mr. Russell, the judge, Mr. Wauchope, the magistrate, J. St. Pourcain, Esq., Mr. Clint, Principal of Hooghly College, and Mr. Clermont, head master of the Lower School’. All these persons accompanied him to the hospital. In their presence, a gong was sounded in Kaura’s ear, to no effect. Esdaile then carried out the planned surgical procedure, to which Kaura remained wholly insensible. He continued to sleep until midnight. Though Esdaile found the testicle ‘considerably enlarged’, he recorded this as having happened after the patient awoke from the trance. Further, Kaura had been suffering from chronic diarrhoea. During the trance, this too had ceased. It was a moment of revelation for Esdaile. He felt humbled, for he wrote: ‘I now know (and I deplore my long ignorance) that the battle was fought, and won, before I was born, by the truthful and benevolent Puysegur, Deleuze, and their companions, and that I, under the tropics, am only again demonstrating what they, on the banks of the Seine, had long ago established’.

Esdaile found mesmerising too exhausting a job for one practitioner, given that it could be successfully used on so many patients. Thus he taught his assistant surgeons and compounders the technique. In fact, the cook of his hospital was one of the best mesmerisers.

On 7 April, Janokee Singh, 'a hardy looking peon' came to hospital with an intensely painful and sloughing scrotum, the result to applying 'some acrid leaves' to it. The whole affected part sloughed off on 15 April, and the patient could not sleep until the compounder mesmerised him in 30 minutes around 11 am. Thereafter Janokee Singh slept until 7 pm the following day, the first sleep he had had since admission. Over the next few days it became easier to mesmerise him, requiring only a few minutes to induce sleep. On 20 April, Kowsoalla, 'aged forty, a peasant woman', was mesmerised. Soon it became possible to mesmerise her in a minute. Bissumber Chowdhry was admitted on 3 May for retention of urine, due to which he was in great discomfort, his bladder having swollen to such proportion that it was prominent at the navel. Mesmerised, the patient slept, and awoke the next day, when he voided urine freely and was completely relieved.

Rantoonee Bhuttachungie, a Brahmin aged 40, was presented to Esdaile on 5 May 1845, with a 'prodigious fungus haematodes protruding from the left elbow joint'. It had been growing since he was 5, but an attempt made 12 days previously by a local surgeon to excise the mass had resulted in the structure of the fungus having been broken up by the actual cautery applied to it all over, in order to stop the bleeding'. When Esdaile saw it, 'it was a frightful mass'. Ordering the patient to be 'carefully mesmerised', Esdaile went to Chinsurah to consult with Dr Elton, the army surgeon there, on how to proceed in the case. Elton returned with Esdaile to see Bhuttachungie for himself. They found him fully mesmerised, and Elton suggested immediate amputation of the left arm, which was done at once. Elton saw no change in the patient's features when the arm was taken off. By 17 May, Bhuttachungie was free of pain, and sleeping well.

On 7 May, Nazir, aged 20, reported to the hospital with the consequences of 2 months' ophthalmia, which had destroyed the left eye, and made the right eye lachrymal, its cornea was 'muddy coloured with superficial ulcerations', and with a pterygium or benign growth of the conjunctiva. Esdaile mesmerised him, until Nazir spoke of his desire to go to sleep. Stopping at once, Esdaile prescribed for Nazir, 'the eyes to be daily mesmerised for ten minutes, and then be put to sleep'. By 22 May, Nazir's right eye had cleared up, the lachrymal tendency was gone, and he could read some Bengali and Persian words.

One of Esdaile's visitors around this time was an English lady. Esdaile of course liked displaying the use of mesmerism to one and all. The visitor declared, 'It's impossible! It can't be! I won't believe it; it's all a trick!' Then, after witnessing a dental extraction and a minor but painful surgical operation performed, she congratulated Esdaile on his 'new powers of doing good'. Esdaile was not particularly delighted by this, since he hinted, 'in the most respectful manner, that there was something still more wonderful to me than Mesmerism; and that was, the extent of human incredulity on the subject'.

Esdaile went to visit his patient, Mr Clermont, 'Headmaster of Hooghly College', on 22 May. He found Mr Clermont out at work, and Mrs Clermont suffering one of her nervous headaches, which commence with a pain in the back of the neck, that spreads over the scalp, and around the eye-brows'. She had, Esdaile claimed, never heard of mesmerism. To remove her discomfort, he asked her to sit with her back towards him, and he soon put her into a mesmeric sleep, from which she awoke quite recovered.

Mesmeric surgery had its humorous moments too. We did not previously come across a similarly light mood in a heavy medical textbook. Sibehurn Singh, 'a young, robust man', had his thumb nearly cut off by a sword 14 days ago. The attempt to reunite it went wrong, and on 29 May he went to Esdaile, who realised that the top of the thumb would have to be removed. He was mesmerised, and the part was amputated. On his waking, Esdaile asked Sibehurn, 'Have you any pain?' The reply was 'No'. Then the doctor asked, 'Has anything hurt you today?' Again the same negative was received. Esdaile next queried, 'Do you wish your nail cut off?' 'Yes', was the reply. 'Look at it', said the doctor; 'It's gone!' Sibehurn exclaimed, and followed it up with 'Who did it?' 'God knows', the doctor said. "How did it happen, has it fallen off itself?' Sibehurn asked; the doctor remained evasive, 'I can't tell – I know nothing about it'.

A boy of 12, Modoomohun Ray, was taken to the hospital with a serious compound fracture of both bones of the forearm. Soon Esdaile concluded that the injury would have to be opened to let out the matter that was forming inside. The child was naturally scared of operations, and all previous attempts to mesmerise him had failed. Esdaile put a piece of wet cloth over the boy's eyes, and went off on his other work, 'telling him that it would cool his brain'. The others were dismissed, and Esdaile returned silently to mesmerise the boy, which he accomplished in 10 minutes. The operation was carried out, and the boy was left to sleep it out.

Early in June, Lokee, a woman aged 60, was admitted with an ulcerated tumour in the calf of her leg, infested with maggots. Simple mesmerism could not offer more than 'common sleep'. Thus Esdaile decided to operate on her on 12 June. She was put into a mesmeric coma 'after much trouble, first by one person, and then another', following which he operated in the presence of one Captain Elder, without her feeling a thing. On 24 October 1845, Lokee returned with the same complaint. She was mesmerised daily, for 2 hours, 'without effect', due to which Esdaile decided to operate on her 3 days later, without mesmerising her, since they could spend no more time and effort on her. During this, second, operation, 'The poor old woman screamed miserably the whole time, crying that I was murdering her'. This was an instructive case, for through it Esdaile learnt that the old woman's ardent wish for sleep had countered the mesmeric influence, the 'excitement of mind being destructive of the mesmeric influence for the production of coma'.

Similarly, in June there was the case of Kaloo, 'a Fuqueer', who had 'an excrescence, larger than a man's fist, at the end of his penis'. Ordinarily this would have been a surgical challenge and an excruciatingly painful procedure for the patient. However, Esdaile put Kaloo into a trance in a few minutes, and then, in the presence of several Europeans, carried out radical dissection, cutting out not only the tumour but also the glans, as it was a cartilaginous degeneration of all the structures of the part'. Kaloo woke once briefly during the amputation, then relapsed into sleep again.

On 3 June, Esdaile carried out one of his most serious surgical procedures on Teencowrie Paulit, 40, a peasant of Madra. 2 years ago, Paulit had 'a tumour in the antrum maxillare', which had since 'pushed upon the orbit of the eye, filled up the nose, passed into the throat, and caused an enlargement of the gland of the neck'. He had mostly been unable to sleep for the previous 5 months, and Esdaile's assistants had failed to mesmerise him over a fortnight. Esdaile then took over, seating Paulit on a chair and reducing him to insensibility. Then, Esdaile writes, 'I performed one of the most severe and protracted operations in surgery'. He excised the entire tumour, and Paulit only moaned occasionally, and coughed out blood that had entered his throat. By the time he awoke, the operation was finished and he was laid upon the floor to have his face sutured. The bandages were removed on 6 June, when it was seen that the wound had healed well, and Paulit was able to speak plainly, when he reported that he felt nothing, indeed recalled nothing until he had been laid on the floor.

The same day, 6 June, Esdaile was called at 8 pm to see the wife of the Deputy Magistrate of Hooghly, Essanchunder Ghosaul, whom we have already met as one of the witnesses to Esdaile's interaction with the local magician. In fact, the magician had been summoned for the same reason, and it is ironic that Esdaile and the magician should have been thus placed on equal footing, to treat Essanchunder's wife, who was 'in dreadful convulsions' that reminded Esdaile of tetanus and hydrophobia, for 'she was speechless, and suffering from a constriction in the throat, that threatened to suffocate her every minute; and she constantly beat, or pointed at the part'. Then, 'At one moment her body was perfectly rigid, and in another it was bent back like a bow'. Knowing conventional contemporary medicine to be useless in such a case, Esdaile decided to use his 'new solvent power', and after an hour's hard work, left her catalepsed. By 1 July, the lady had completely recovered. The fits never returned.

On 17 June Esdaile came across a still stranger case. He was being driven through Hooghly town, when he saw a crowd before the police station. On inquiry, he was told that a man had been caught kidnapping a boy. Esdaile entered the police station, and saw a boy aged 10 or 12, 'half stupid', with one eye bruised, sitting on the lap of his rescuer. Ordering the child to the hospital, Esdaile spoke to the kidnapper, who told him he was a barber, which was proved by the instruments with him. The boy later told Esdaile and, still later, the magistrate, that he had been to a field near his home early in the morning of 17 June, when he saw his kidnapper come down from the road to him, 'mutter some charms', and taking his hand, led him away, 'but without force'. He was a 'clever, well-behaved' boy, but he could recall nothing until he came to his senses at the gate to Chandernagore, 2 miles from his home. In fact the boy and his kidnapper had been accosted by a close acquaintance, who asked the child what he was doing there. The boy was unable to answer, and 'appeared to be idiotic'. The friend became worried and splashed water on the boy, which revived him. When questioned again, the boy replied, 'that he was obliged to follow that man, though he did not know him, and after saying this, he fell down, and bruised his eye on the ground'. The barber maintained that he had met the boy on the road, 'crying and looking stupid' and so had taken him along to hand him in at the nearest police station.

Esdaile felt that this was a new aspect to mesmerism, one which he had hitherto had no hint of. Further, he speculated that 'As accident had made me a witness in the case, I anticipated that I should be called upon to speak as to the possibility of such a mode of abduction; and as I was completely ignorant of the subject, I determined to make experiments, to satisfy myself'. He went to the Jail Hospital, sought out a patient on whom he had mesmerised for 'inflammation of the eye', and found that he could induce 'artificial somnambulism' through mesmerism in the same patient.

When called before the magistrate to depose, Esdaile declared that he considered such mesmeric somnambulism as described by the boy, quite possible. However, when the case went up to the judge 'it was found to be utterly impossible to convey even a glimpse of my meaning in the minds of the native law officers who had to try the case'. The judge asked Esdaile if he could demonstrate if 'it was possible for one person to make another follow him involuntarily'. Esdaile asked for 3 volunteers, whom he named. They were not to be told the reason for their summons. Two or three days later, in a court packed with curious Europeans and locals, Esdaile used his volunteers to demonstrate the way in which mesmerism could be used to induce 'artificial somnambulism'. 'Whether the barber stole the boy mesmerically or not, I will not pretend to decide', he wrote, 'but it gave me an opportunity of proving, in the most public manner, that the thing could be done, and no one has ventured to deny publicly that I stole the men; and, with the facilities of a native barber, I could almost engage to steal a man, woman, or child, daily'.

Esdaile was sure that the barber had kidnapped the boy, as were the magistrate, the local law officers, and the judge. Irrespective of mesmerism, the fact that the boy had been found accompanying the barber was enough for the judge to sentence him to labour in irons for 9 months. A higher court upheld the judgment. Nonetheless, the government sent for the papers, and concluded that Esdaile's dramatic experiments 'had made too deep an impression on the mind of the court'. On this ground, the barber was set free. This made Esdaile conclude that the abrupt and ignorant dismissal, 'as the offspring of deception, or delusion', of 'the unexpected exhibition of new and wonderful bodily, or mental phenomena', represented intellectual backwardness. It was better to study the phenomena diligently, as he had done.

So popular had mesmerism become, and so used were Esdaile and his assistants to applying it, they soon had a routine in place to treat patients. Esdaile gives us this routine: 'A person presents himself before me for the first time and I see he has a disease requiring an operation for its removal; he is desired to go into another room (which is dark,) and repose himself after his journey, not a word being said about an operation, as this would cause a mental excitement, destructive to the mesmeric influence. One of my assistants follows him; seats himself (if unperceived, so much the better,) at the head of the bed; and by using the process to be hereafter described, often reduces the patient to a state of coma by the end of my visit: I then do what is necessary, whether it be to take off, or straighten a limb, without his knowledge or consent'.

However, people were unwilling to really believe in the effectiveness of mesmerism in medicine, if only because of Esdaile's remoteness from Calcutta and its European population, whose testimony alone would make mesmerism respectable. Thus, Esdaile yearned to be in Calcutta, writing 'I would have preferred the plain of Calcutta for my theatre, and all the inhabitants for spectators, if it had been possible'. Esdaile certainly had spectators, whom he probably invited to see his experiments. He even called in colleagues to operate or perform normally terribly painful procedures on patients he had mesmerised. In one spectacular case, dated 13 August, one Dr Finch, with a Dr Bedford as witness, applied muriatic acid freely to the ulcerated right temple of a woman named Gendoo, who had been mesmerised by one of Esdaile's assistants. Muriatic acid would have caused intense pain in a conscious patient. Gendoo remained dangerously entranced, to the extent that Finch was unable to revive her, and Esdaile could do so only with much trouble, as 'the voluntary and semi-voluntary muscles of the chest' were 'completely paralysed' and she was in danger of dying. 5 days later, Dr Bedford, presumably sceptical of mesmerism, asked Esdaile if he could apply muriatic acid to the woman's ulcer without the help of mesmerism. Esdaile realised that this amounted to torturing his patient, but he agreed on the ground that 'it might not be said that I interfered to save my phenomena'.

Dr Bedford wetted the end of the stopper with muriatic acid and touched the ulcer with it. For a few seconds the woman did not react, enforcing Bedford's scepticism and Esdaile's embarrassment at his own 'thick-coming fancies'. Then the woman broke into screams and began walking about, distracted by great agony. Esdaile mesmerised her, and took the opportunity of her coma to cut out some tubercles from around the ulcer, which were hindering healing. Again she was woken with difficulty, and reported that she remembered no pain.

On 9 July, Mrs Clermont, whom Esdaile had cured of migraine, required a tooth extraction because half of one of her wisdom teeth had emerged, while the other half remained covered by 'indurated and ulcerated gum'. The following day Esdaile seated her on a chair and, having mesmerised her, removed the offending tooth. Mrs Clermont had no knowledge whatsoever of it, and on awaking yesterday, arose as if from common sleep, and went to adjust her hair in the glass, when she saw blood about her mouth, and this first attracted her attention to the tooth; she thought the gum had burst, and was still expecting me to call'. Mesmerism was no conjuring trick, Esdaile said, for 'this is the power trifled with, and made a show of for money'.

Esdaile's successes continued to be viewed most suspiciously by his colleagues. On 17 July, Esdaile mesmerised a patient, and removed his hypertrophied prepuce in the presence of Mr Davidson, commissioner of the district, and Mr Alexander, Registrar to the Board of Revenue. On seeing this, Davidson remarked that he wished a doctor who had been dismissive of Esdaile had been there, for he had said, 'you do this by opium'.

Esdaile was stopped on the road to Chinsurah and asked to go into a temple and see a sick 'Fuqueer'. He found within a man, aged about 60, who, though 'healthy-looking', was nearly blind from cataract, and had a scrotal tumour weighing 30 pounds. After medically examining the man, Esdaile remained noncommittal, and resumed his journey to Chinsurah, where he visited Dr Ross, his friend, the army surgeon. As always, craving European witnesses, Esdaile asked Ross if he would accompany him to a mesmeric surgical session. Ross agreed to, and picking up the 'Fuqueer' on the way back to the hospital, they set the best mesmeriser available, the cook, to work. The tumour was removed, as were the testes. Again, as always, Esdaile could not resist the triumphal joke he played on his patients. He asked the 'Fuqueer', woken from the trance, to show him the tumour again. The man felt for it and found it missing, with Esdaile delighting in his look of amazement', which 'was something not to be easily forgotten'.

On 17 September, in the presence of Rev Fisher and Dr Heathcote, Esdaile performed removed the cataract from a patient's eye so easily that Dr Heathcote asked him if the eye had been dilated using belladonna.

Esdaile met Mr Calder on 25 September. Calder had been in India for 20 years, and complained of general rheumatism, nervousness, and debility'. He could not walk without the help of a stick, could not climb stairs, or of late, drive a buggy. Additionally, 'his nerves were shattered', he had weak eyesight, tremulous hands, and felt the ground slipping from under him when he walked. During the last couple of years, 'he has gone a tour of doctors, and swallowed a dispensary of physic, to no good purpose'. Esdaile passed Calder's case to an assistant surgeon, who soon induced mesmeric trances that allowed the patient to get a good night's sleep, every night. Soon Calder was able to resume all his normal activities such that by 25 October he was able to inform Esdaile that not only was he climbing stairs, but walking over 4 miles every day.

'Fear and expectation' were ruinous of mesmerism, and so the technique was to hide the intention from the patient by calling it only a trial. The entire process would be long, for 'No trial under an hour should be reckoned a fair one; two hours are better; and the most perfect success will often follow frequent failures, but insensibility is sometimes induced in a few minutes'. After this, the patient should be told to lie down, and compose to sleep. Then the practitioner is asked to 'Bring the crown of the patient's head to the end of the bed, and seat yourself so as to be able to bring your face into contact with his, and extend your hands to the pit of the stomach, when it is wished; make the room dark, enjoin quiet, and then shutting your patient's eyes, begin to pass both your hands, in the shape of claws, slowly, within an inch of the surface, from the back of the head to the pit of the stomach; dwelling for several minutes over the eyes, nose, and mouth, and then passing down each side of the neck, go downwards to the pit of the stomach, keeping your hands suspended there for sometime'. This process was to be repeated for 15 minutes, 'breathing gently on the head and eyes all the time'. After this, 'the longitudinal passes' would be stopped, 'by placing both hands gently, but firmly, on the pit of the stomach and sides'. The comatose state may be tested not by questioning or speaking to the patient but by gently testing the 'cataleptic tendency' in the arms. It was not possible to tell the depth of the trance, which could sometimes be 'completely broken by the knife', though the process, if continued, could put the patient back to sleep. The patient could be revived using the means adopted by Esdaile, 'Blowing sharply in the eyes, rubbing the eye-lids, and eyebrows, and sprinkling cold water in the face, are the methods for de-mesmerising the brain, and when locally applied, are equally efficacious in de-catalepsing rigid limbs'.

On 26 November, Esdaile operated on Mahes Banergie, aged 40, who had 'an enlarged testis, the size of a child's head'. It was 'red, glistening, and very painful', and there was a scrotal hernia over it. Banergie was easily mesmerised, and Esdaile first dealt with the hernia, 'handling the inflamed part very rudely', despite which the patient did not wake. Next, in the presence of one Captain Richardson (for Esdaile was very sensitive of accusations that he was fudging, and so never passed up an audience of Europeans), he removed the offending organ. During the second part of the operation, Banergie moved, 'as in an uneasy dream' but awoke only when the arteries were being tied up.

Like Brett, Esdaile too came up against elephantiasis. 'Endemic sources of disease abound here to a dreadful extent', he wrote, adding that the government ought to clean up the 'Ragged old tanks, and offensive pools and holes of water', which formed a chain near towns and villages, and along the roadside, since these were the sources of the disease, being full of 'malarious exhalations'. Indeed, 'every cottage may be said to be built over a green putrefying pool, out of which the mud to build a house had been taken, and which is reckoned a domestic convenience'. In these pools the debris of the house and its locality gather, animals bathe, and the same water is later used for drinking, 'as it is conveniently near, and saves the trouble of going to the nearest large tank, or the river'. Consequently, 'The effects are as dreadful as might be anticipated in a debilitating climate, and among an ill-fed people, and are deeply written in the personal appearance of the natives of the country'. He continued, 'Ague, remittent fever, spleen, rheumatism, diarrhoea, dysentery, and cholera are inherited by the poor people along with their homes; and the general constitutional debility is evidenced by the incredible frequency of elephantiasis, diseases of the skin, and parasitic growths on the body'. This was not unique to Bengal, said Esdaile, since ague and splenetic inflammation was common in Scotland 50 years ago, when every home had its midden before the door.

We get a perfect idea of contemporary local living conditions through Esdaile's description of a family house in Bengal, to which he was called on 16 May 1845. This house belonged to one of the richest families, and there were 8 persons in it, suffering 'under different degrees of the same disease, and of which two men of the same party had died, shortly before'. 'In the worst cases' noted Esdaile, 'the feet were swollen, and hard as in elephantiasis, and a brick-red inflammation extended half way up the leg, and was still advancing'. The others were 'worn out with fever, and their bodies were generally or partially dropsical'. Since the affected all belonged only to one family and its servants, Esdaile suspected 'some local source of contamination', and asked to see their home. 'The house', he recorded, 'is a large two-storied pile, in which, as usual, all the family connections live'. The rooms occupied by the afflicted were alright, 'but, on looking out of the back windows, I saw that the house rose right over a large, ragged, neglected tank, covered with green filth, and smelling vilely, and that this was the only part of the house so situated'. Further examination revealed a state of nightmarish insanitation, 'I then examined below, and perceived that the water was led upon a brick platform to a passage in the lower story, to save the people from going out; numerous narrow lanes, the sides as high as the house, led from the tank to the different parts of the house, and all opened into the court around which this family exclusively lived in small ill-ventilated rooms'. This stagnant pool, into which the excreta of the family had been flowing, was the source of their ailment. Further, Esdaile, when asked about the prospects of the sick, regrettably concluded 'that there was little hope, except for one of them', and by 1 December he had been proved right. Elephantiasis, Esdaile theorised, 'was only an aggravated form of the malarious fever that usually ends in elephantiasis and dropsy; the stage of elephantiasis being only more acute than usual, from constitutional peculiarity, or the severity of the disease'.

In 6 years previous to his discovery of mesmerism, Esdaile had operated on 11 cases of scrotal and penile tumours caused by elephantiasis. Since April 1845, he had used mesmerism and operated 17 times. All his cases had concluded successfully and he had removed in all 28 tumours, varying in weight 'from a few pounds to eighty pounds'. Of these cases, in 9 cases the patient had to be castrated, and in 1 of these the penis too had to be removed. Esdaile, as usual, was busy fighting critics of mesmeric surgery, especially since he 'had every month more operations of this kind than take place in the native hospital in Calcutta in a year'. The reason behind his popularity could only be painless surgery, he added, for 'It ought to be added, that most of these persons were not paupers, but people in comfortable circumstances, whom no inducement short of painless operations could tempt to enter a charity, or any other hospital; and all who know the natives are aware of this'.

One unusual case was that of Gooroochuan Shah, a shopkeeper aged 40, who had a monstrous scrotal tumour. It weighed 80 pounds, and kept him from moving, so he had long used it 'for a writing-desk'. His feet were oedematous, and his pulse weak, which made surgery risky. Esdaile operated on him on 29 October, Shah having been admitted to hospital 4 days earlier and mesmerised daily. 2 men held up the tumour in a sheet, 'pulling it forward at the same time'. He operated quickly, with swift incisions, despite which there was considerable bleeding. The haemorrhage caused the patient to faint after he had been successfully revived from the trance. Nonetheless, Shah rallied, and was allowed to go home on 1 December.

Esdaile's one and only public display of mesmerism was on 29 July 1845, when, as a correspondent reported in a letter to the editor of *The Englishman* dated 30 July, European visitors from Barrackpore and Calcutta went to Hooghly in 2 steamers, while other Europeans and locals from Chinsurah and neighbouring areas gathered in huge numbers. Soon the small hospital was overcrowded. The audience included 6 doctors. Esdaile performed as usual, operating on an old man, who woke during the operation. Unfazed, Esdaile's assistants put him back to sleep, and the operation, noted only as an otherwise painful one, was carried out with the patient in a state of insensibility. Other feats of mesmerism were carried out, including one in the Jail Hospital, which was larger. Here a youth was placed against the wall of a room, while Esdaile mesmerised him from the opposite wall, 80 feet away. Esdaile yearned for recognition from his fellow Europeans and colleagues. Despite his claims of success, doubts seem to have remained, particularly in the medical community.

By July 1846, Esdaile had performed over 100 mesmeric operations. By then he had become famous and despite claims that he was not giving public performances, doctors from Calcutta frequently flocked to Hooghly to see him operate. Esdaile, presumably basking in newfound glory, allowed his colleagues free access to his patients, to check things for themselves. On 14 October 1846, even the Presidency Surgeon, Dr Stewart, attended a session and reported very favourably on the operation he witnessed. As had been said before, Esdaile's report to the Medical Board of Bengal was not acknowledged, following which he wrote directly to the government. In response to his letter, Sir Robert Maddock set up a committee, aptly named the Mesmeric Committee, of 3 doctors and 3 'unprofessional men', presided by a fourth doctor, who was also the representative of the Medical Board. Esdaile was asked to come to Calcutta and demonstrate his skill. Clearly, it was felt necessary to have Esdaile operate away from his usual stamping grounds. Esdaile was successful, and the committee, through its president, reported to the government that, 'The general result arrived at, then, on the question of pain during the mesmeric surgical operations we witnessed, amounts to this, that in three cases there is no proof whatever that any pain was suffered, and that in the three other cases the manifestations of pain during the operation are opposed by the positive statement of the patient that no pain was experienced'.

The government's response was guarded. On the one hand, it refused to introduce mesmeric surgery into general practice, saying that 'The Committee's Report has been ordered to be published, and the Deputy-Governor entirely concurs with the remark of the President in Council, that it is sufficient for the present that it should be allowed to work its own way towards producing conviction among the profession and the public ; and that, at this stage, any more direct encouragement on the part of Government to the general introduction of the mesmeric practice would be premature'. However, considering 'it incumbent on the Government to afford to the meritorious and zealous officer by whom the subject was first brought to its notice such assistance as may facilitate his investigations, and enable him to prosecute his interesting experiments under the most favourable and promising circumstances', it was agreed to place Esdaile 'for one year in charge of a small experimental' hospital in some favourable situation in Calcutta, in order that he may, as recommended by the Committee, extend his investigations to the applicability of this alleged agency to all descriptions of cases, medical as well as surgical, and all classes of patients, European as well as native'. Before further steps were taken, Esdaile was to prove his theories through this hospital, and was 'directed to encourage the resort to his hospital of all respectable persons, especially medical and scientific, whether in or out of the Service, who may be desirous of satisfying themselves of the nature and the effect of his experiments; and his Honour will nominate, from among the Medical

Officers of the Presidency, Visitors, whose duty it will be to visit the hospital from time to time, inspect Dr Esdaile's proceedings, without exercising any interference, and occasionally, or when called on, report upon them, through the Medical Board, for the information of Government'.

Lord Dalhousie, on taking over as Governor General, soon found time to go through reports on the Mesmeric Hospital on Mott's Lane. He sent for Esdaile, who offered to perform mesmeric surgery in his presence. Dalhousie refused the need for further evidence, apparently saying, 'That is perfectly superfluous – there can be no doubt about the matter'. `Soon thereafter, Esdaile was appointed Presidency Surgeon of Calcutta, and was invited to dinner with Dalhousie. On this occasion, which must have redeemed all the doubts and misgivings Esdaile had felt, and others had felt about him, Dalhousie, on being thanked for the appointment, replied, 'You have nothing to thank me for, Dr Esdaile – you have only to thank yourself; I have only done an act of justice'.

Esdaile's promotion meant that the hospital on Mott's Lane would be closed, and some of the principal local men petitioned the Governor General to prevent this. Dalhousie rejected the petition on the principle that the local would have to look their own resources for help. Hence, a subscription hospital was set up, this time in Sookeas Street, under Esdaile's superintendence. It lasted only 18 months, since at the end of that time Esdaile was promoted by Sir John Littler, Deputy Governor, to be Superintendent of one of the government hospitals, 'for the express purpose of enabling me to introduce mesmerism into regular hospital practice'. Sir John was keenly interested in mesmeric surgery, and often visited the hospital with friends and staff. By the time Esdaile left India, he had performed 261 operations using mesmerism, of which 84 had been carried out in the Subscription Hospital. When Esdaile retired, Dr Webb, Professor of Demonstrative Anatomy at the Medical College, took over the charge of conducting mesmeric surgery. A perusal of the Records of the Mesmeric Hospital shows that besides mesmerism, electromagnetism was also used.

Despite all this, there remains room for doubt. Dr O'Shaughnessy, Professor of Surgery at the Medical College, and a Visitor to the Mesmeric Hospital, reported to Dr Forsyth, Secretary of the Medical Board on an operation he performed at Dr Esdaile's request, on 13 December 1846. O'Shaughnessy first observed that 'there appeared to be so little uniformity in the proceedings of the Mesmerisers'. Then, as Dr Esdaile had a sore finger, he invited his colleague to remove a scrotal tumour from a patient who was perfectly mesmerised. In the operating room, other doctors were present. Esdaile proceeded to 'test' the depth of the patient's mesmeric trance by pricking him. No response being elicited, Esdaile placed a small piece of burning charcoal, first on his chest, and later on the back of his hand. In the latter case, O'Shaughnessy saw the patient move his hand a little but not otherwise react. Nonetheless, O'Shaughnessy remained sceptical of the depth of the patient's insensibility, for he remarked to his colleagues that there was 'constant varying of the pulse, and nervous-like throbbing of the carotid arteries'.

The operation commenced, and as soon as O'Shaughnessy had opened the left testicle, 'the man cried out most bitterly'. O'Shaughnessy spoke to him encouragingly but was interrupted by Esdaile, who told him that it was no use talking, for the man was fast asleep. O'Shaughnessy, however, proceeded with the operation as fast as he could and all the while the patient cried out as if in pain. As soon as the operation was done, and before any questions were put to him, or indeed before he was awoken from the trance, the patient said, 'I see nothing, I know nothing, I was sleeping, and felt no pain'. O'Shaughnessy did not examine the patient further, but he remained sceptical. Subsequent visits confirmed his doubts, for he reported, 'Its inapplicability to all cases attended with fever, much pain, or cough, or general disturbance of the system; and from its total failure to produce any effect upon two boys, who were admitted into the Mesmeric Hospital, one with fungus haematodes of the arm, and the other with disease of the thigh bone (they were labouring under that disturbance of the system usual in all such severe surgical cases, which was given as a reason by Dr Esdaile for his want of success with them) I am disposed to think it never can be made available for general surgical practice'.

O'Shaughnessy continued with his damning evidence on mesmerism by saying that in cases of curing stiff joints, 'I think from what I saw at Dr Esdaile's Hospital, the same amount of daily rubbing and working the affected part, would be equally successful, whether the patient was sleeping or awake during the process, and therefore I attach no value to mesmerism in such cases'. The medical cases in the Mesmeric Hospital were those of 'rheumatism, sciatica, epilepsy, and paralysis'. In these cases, there was no benchmark to judge the particular efficacy of mesmerism over conventional treatment, since only the patients could report on their state of health, and O'Shaughnessy, from long experience, knew that the 'patient is not always to be depended upon'. Similarly, he saw nothing spectacularly impressive in the treatment of epilepsy. 'Cases of paralysis', he wrote, 'are also unsatisfactory, as a change of diet, and better shelter from the weather, often produce effects on them, which medical men too frequently attribute to their treatment, and the same may be said where mesmerism is substituted for medicines'.

Dr Stewart, Presidency Surgeon and Professor of Midwifery, another Visitor, had a similar opinion to offer. "Little or no progress appears to have been made', he said in his report dated 23 June 1847, 'in the investigation of the efficient cause of mesmeric agency in producing 'insensibility to pain' in some cases, while it fails in others". Until proved by experiments, Stewart felt 'no theory of its action can be worth listening to, and no dependence placed by the Profession at large upon mesmerism as a therapeutical agent'.

Esdaile, however, was not as worried by these adverse reports as he was by a new development, the use of ether to render patients insensible during surgery. Unlike his colleagues, he addressed his dismissal of ether not to a fellow medical practitioner, but to one Mr Halliday, Secretary to the Government of Bengal. In his report to Halliday dated 21 June 1847, Esdaile recounted the reasons against using ether. Firstly, 'It is to disgusting, that it is utterly impossible to get many persons to inhale it at all'. Then, 'It often only produces intoxication in those who can persevere to the necessary degree'. Thirdly, 'The effects are very uncertain', being sometimes transient, and at other times alarmingly intense, making it hard to help the patient recover from it. Fourthly, fatalities resulting from the use of ether had already been reported, and that it 'altered the constitution of the blood'. Finally, it could not be used in cases where disease had led to general debility. Esdaile then proceeded to recount the advantages of mesmerism over ether, concluding that it was far safer.

Dr Hough, the Physician General, and Dr Lamb, Inspector General of Hospitals, wrote to Sir Robert Maddock on 27 December 1847 that Esdaile had refused to provide them with 'a Return of the number of cases which were not admitted to the Institution under his care in consequence of their being unfitted for treatment on the principles pursued there'. Such a Return would allow a comparison with 'similar Returns from other Public Medical Institutions at the Presidency', from which 'an estimate might be formed of the comparative success of treatment by Mesmeric Agency, and by ordinary medical practice'. Earlier in the year, in August, Dr Mouat had recorded his feelings on this shortcoming: 'Dr Esdaile has not recorded in his published report, nor has he entered in his Hospital Journals so far as I can ascertain, the number and nature of the cases which he is in the habit of dismissing as unfit for mesmeric treatment'. Mouat thought this was wrong of Esdaile, for 'To establish a fair and just comparison between the relative and absolute value of different plans of treatment, all these matters should be candidly and fairly recorded'. Mouat recorded one such case on

Friday, 13 August 1847, when 'A case of nervous headache, supposed to be dependent on the state of the stomach, was dismissed as unfit for mesmerism'.

Like O'Shaughnessy and Stewart, Mouat remained unimpressed by mesmerism. One of the mesmerisers had been taken with a stiff neck, and had been cast into a state of catalepsy. On Saturday, 14 August, Mouat, doing the rounds of the medical ward, noted that 'the stiff-necked mesmeriser was able to bend his head, and one of the rheumatic cases walked about tolerably well'. This was not be wondered at, for Mouat wrote, 'I have seen severer cases of both one and the other exhibit the same results from no treatment at all, in the same length of time'. 'I need scarcely add that', he continued, 'I consider them both particularly unsatisfactory examples of their kind'.

Mouat was similarly doubtful about a surgical case, which involved a middle-aged man with a scrotal tumour weighing 'probably about 80 lbs'. Despite entrancement, the patient appeared to Mouat to be quite conscious, though asleep. He pointed this out to Esdaile, who was ready to operate. Esdaile said that he was satisfied, and that 'he did not expect the man to lie quite quiet throughout the operation'. When the operation began, the patient soon 'uttered the usual cries of agony', saying that he was dying, and wanted to be taken to the Ganges so he could die in the proper manner. The operation was swiftly completed, but soon the patient had haemorrhaged much, and almost collapsed completely. When he discussed this with Esdaile, the explanation left poor Mouat still more bewildered, 'that the mesmeric alternated with the natural delirium, and that both were accompanied by intervals of complete consciousness and a rational state, and that all these conditions were followed by oblivion of each and all of their several occurrences upon the final waking of the patient'. 'There is something so contradictory and so incomprehensible in all this that I am unable to follow it', Mouat wrote.

In an especially telling statement, Mouat recorded of his visit to the medical ward on Monday, 20 September, 'The deaf man is as deaf as ever'. Bengalis were, he noted, prone to faith in supernaturalism, and locals thronged Esdaile's hospital 'are attracted by the fame which that gentleman's operations have obtained throughout Bengal, and all come to him, impressed with the fullest and firmest belief, in his supernatural powers'. 'In fact', he added, 'the common name under which the Mesmeric Hospital is known among the lower classes is that of the house of magic, or jadoo hospital'.

This was not all. Mouat discussed the matter with 'a distinguished Wrangler of Trinity College, Cambridge', then residing in Calcutta. It was clear that mesmerism was a matter of fooling the mind, 'That pure imagination or some such influence has produced much of the apparently curative result in many if not most of the medical cases which have derived any appreciable benefit'. This feeling was reinforced by a conversation with Sub-Assistant Surgeon Tameez Khan, a recent graduate of the Medical College, who had been placed under Dr Esdaile by order to study mesmerism. Khan informed Mouat that rather than bring a mesmeric trance upon their patients, 'the young mesmerisers were constantly in the habit of falling asleep as soon as the doors were closed, a result not much to be wondered at when the heat and quietude of the darkened chamber, with the powerfully soporific influence of the unvaried movements of the hands and arms are considered'. The doctors' visits became known to the mesmerisers from the movements in adjoining rooms, and they awoke from sleep, opened the doors, 'and appeared active and alert in their operations'.

At the end of his term as Visitor, which concluded on 9 November 1847, Dr Mouat presented a report to the Medical Board. In this report, he stated that 'In general the existence of any degree or amount of disease in the system, appeared to be regarded as an efficient contra-indicating and adverse agent' for mesmerism. It followed that mesmerism would have very limited applicability to chronic diseases, and would not be useful in acute cases requiring immediate 'amputation, excision, or dissection', since the patient could not be entranced at once, even as fever, which invariably accompanied these acute cases, rose, and made mesmerism still more impossible. In any case, Mouat's observations showed him that mesmerism was a long-drawn matter, requiring in some cases up to 8 days and in other cases as many weeks, before the patient could be rendered sufficiently insensible for an operation to take place. It followed that 'As a rapid, speedy, and certain agent for producing the insensibility requisite for perfectly painless operations, it does not appear to me, from the evidence afforded in the Mesmeric Hospital, to be entitled to any degree of confidence'. Mouat considered the general applicability of mesmerism to surgery as 'not merely doubtful, but chimerical and impracticable'.

Moving on to the operating cost of the Mesmeric Hospital, Mouat noted that a mesmeriser could at best, given the physically demanding nature of his work, 'continue his process for about six hours a day'. Considering that every patient needed an hour and a half of mesmerising, one mesmeriser would have to be employed for every 4 patients, which, in a hospital of 300 beds, meant an expense of 750 rupees per month, or 9000 rupees a year. This, he continued, would have been only a secondary consideration had mesmerism been able to effectively cure 'one-half only of the cases that present themselves'. Mouat followed this up with the most damning indictment of Esdaile's practice in Calcutta saying, 'our present Indian experience of the matter is in reality limited to one class of diseases (morbid enlargements of the scrotum) and that by no means the most frequent, formidable, or fatal, that occurs in the general practice of a Surgical hospital'.

Mesmerism did not prolong life, Mouat said, and Esdaile's returns of the sick at the Mesmeric Hospital were not reliable statistics, given that the most ill and debilitated were sent away, and no records kept of these rejections. Comparing the number of operations on scrotal tumours done at the Mesmeric Hospital with those carried out at the Medical College Hospital during the same period, Mouat noted that in the former, fatality was pegged at 1 in 15 cases, or, if the Hooghly cases were added to this total, at 1 in 20 1/3rd cases; in the latter, it stood at 1 in 18 ½, 'a difference in mortality which would not warrant or justify the supposition of the prophylactic influence of Mesmerism'.

Indeed, the first case operated on in the Mesmeric Hospital, 'the removal of a schirrous mamma', had been a failure. Esdaile recorded that 'two-thirds of the tumour was removed without her feeling it'. But Mouat had had his hand on the patient's pulse from the beginning of the operation, and he 'ascertained that she suffered from the very moment of the knife coming in contact with her skin'. Similarly, a case of fungus haematodes was unsuccessfully excised, leading to the amputation of the arm at the shoulder joint, without mesmerism, which led to the patient's death.

O'Shaughnessy's assessment of Esdaile's surgical operations echoes Mouat's. In O'Shaughnessy's view, like laudanum, which was most used to benumb the patient to surgical pain, and ether, whose use had only recently commenced, mesmerism 'could no longer claim the exclusive power of affecting' insensibility in the patient. Rather, the surgeon, fearing that 'the patient might wake up, and spoil the experiment before the operation was concluded' was forced into 'a hurry and want of precision in his proceedings'. To O'Shaughnessy, ether was an 'inestimable boon'.

Having dealt the death-blow to mesmerism in surgery, Mouat turned to the medical cases, particularly epilepsy. In this ailment, mesmerism had no especial claim to cure, since 'Charms, amulets, every imaginable variety of empiricism, most of the articles of the materia medica, superstition, credulity, castration, and the amputation of the big toe, have all been tried in turn, and each can boast of its miraculous cures'. Mouat was certain that cases of epilepsy' incurable by ordinary means, will be found equally unyielding to the mesmeric influence'.

Another medical man who found mesmerism of little use was Dr R M M Thomson, the Marine Surgeon. In a report dated 2 August 1847, he stated that many of Esdaile's cases, discharged fit by him went to Thomson. When asked why, these patients replied that they had not been mesmerised or put to sleep, nor were their ailments any better. In fact, they had informed Esdaile they were better, so that they would be discharged in order to allow them to seek medical advice elsewhere.

Dr J Jackson, Surgeon to the Native Hospital, submitted his report to the Medical Board on 16 November 1847. To him too mesmerism seemed to be of little effect, since 'With all the appearance of perfect consciousness at the commencement of the operation, some patients have been awoke at the first or second incision, and have then writhed and cried out in all the suffering of acute pain'. In cases in which the patient stated that he had felt nothing, Jackson had noted 'The writhing of the body and much inward groaning'. Like Dr Thomson, Jackson too noted that some patients possessed 'perfect insusceptibility, and after undergoing the mesmeric manipulations for a certain number of hours for a succession of days, have left the Mesmeric Hospital in disappointment, and have gone elsewhere for operation'. Echoing Mouat, Jackson called the first operation, on a woman for the removal of an ulcerated breast, 'most unsuccessful as a painless operation'. He went on to doubt the painlessness even of the operations on the scrota, saying 'in not one of these was the patient perfectly motionless, there was compression of the lips, distortion of the countenance, movements of the hands or feet, and inarticulate sounds, or groaning'. Nonetheless, unlike in ordinary operative procedures, the patients had not been restrained.

On 31 December 1847, the allotted year of the Mesmeric Hospital having been completed, Esdaile compiled his report to the government through Mr Halliday. Clearly the negative reports of O'Shaughnessy and Stewart had influenced the government, and Esdaile hurried to his own defence. None of the Visitors, other than Dr Mouat, had followed a medical case treated by mesmerism to its conclusion. Only Dr Stewart had 'spoken with confidence on both the medical and surgical branches of the subject'. Probably Esdaile was not made privy to O'Shaughnessy's report. Nonetheless, he felt it necessary, keeping in mind the government, which had funded the experiments, the public concerned, and his own subject, to defend his position. Since Dr Stewart knew that his report 'was to be printed for public information', it behove Esdaile to query whether Stewart had availed of the 'advantages of observation' that his position gave him.

Dr Stewart had written that all the operations he witnessed at the Hospital involved the excision of scrotal tumours caused by elephantiasis.

Esdaile wondered at this, stating that Dr Stewart had 'not witnessed a single operation in my hospital, since it was opened, a year ago'. Similarly, Stewart's allegation that Esdaile 'greatly deceives himself in the amount of good affected in these [medical] cases by Mesmerism' was dismissed by Esdaile on the same grounds.

Nevertheless, at the end of his report, Esdaile hoped that the government would not give up encouraging the use of mesmerism in medicine and surgery. He noted that 'all the nine passed students of the Medical College, who were ordered to attend my hospital for two months to learn practical mesmerism, got their certificates of proficiency in a month or six weeks; seven of them having succeeded in producing the mesmeric trance in their patients, and they have promised to carry their new knowledge into practice'.

One does not know how mesmerism fared at the hands of these new surgeons, or indeed how far Dr Webb, who succeeded Esdaile, was able to continue with teaching mesmerism at the Medical College. However, it is impossible to arrive at any conclusion regarding Esdaile and his mesmeric surgery. There seem to have been no positive reports of mesmerism amongst the European population of Calcutta. On the other hand, the locals had, as Mouat pointed out, immense faith in Esdaile, who, nonetheless, found it necessary to turn a number of them away. To compare Esdaile's experiences with those of mesmerisers elsewhere in the world is futile since, on the one hand, Esdaile claimed he had read no book on mesmerism, and, on the other hand, his surgical feats were indeed confined to one specific kind of surgery in Calcutta. Why was he not able to take on other surgical cases successfully in Calcutta? We shall never know. That mesmerism requires susceptibility is true. Today we are aware of psychosomatic disorders, pain thresholds, and indeed have some idea of how pain may be reduced, though temporarily, by analgesics. In Esdaile's time, surgery meant intense pain and, often, death from either haemorrhage, or post-operative shock. If nothing else, Esdaile's unique contribution to surgery lay in that he provided some sufferers with the hope that they could undergo operations and survive. If he managed to help them overcome their fear of pain through hypnotism, it did not, and does not, matter, given that most of his operations were successful.

BIBLIOGRAPHY

Alphabetical List of the Medical Officers of the Indian Army, with the Dates of their Appointment, Promotion, Retirement, Resignation, or Death whether in India or in Europe; From the Year 1764 to the Year 1838. Compiled and edited by Dowell and Miles. London: 1839.

Balfour, Francis. *A Collection of Treatises on the Effects of Sol-Lunar Influence in Fevers; with an Improved Method of Curing them.* London and Edinburgh: 1815.

Bernier, Francois. *Travels in the Mogul Empire, 1656-1668.* Trans Archibald Constable (1891), second edition edited by Vincent A Smith. OUP: 1916.

Brett, FH. *A Practical Essay on some of the Principal Surgical Diseases of India.* W Thacker and Company: Calcutta. 1840.

Calendar of State Papers, Colonial Series, East Indies, China and Japan, 1617-1621. Edited by W Noel Sainsbury. Longman and Company: London. 1870.

Cust, Robert Needham. *Memoirs of Past Years of a Septuagenarian.* Privately printed. 1899.

Doss, Ramchunder. *A General Register of the Hon'ble East India Company's Civil Servants of the Bengal Establishment, from 1790 to 1842*. Baptist Mission Press: Calcutta. 1844.

Early Travels in India, 1583-1619. Edited by William Foster. OUP: 1921.

Esdaile, James. *The Introduction of Mesmerism (with the sanction of the Government) into the Public Hospitals of India.* Second Edition. W Kent and Company: London. 1856.

Falck, ND. *A Treatise on the Medical Qualities of Mercury.* London: 1776

Gregory, G. *A New and Complete Dictionary of Arts and Sciences.* Volume I. Collins and Company: London. 1819.

Holwell, Joseph Zephaniah, and friends. *India Tracts.* Third edition. London: 1774.

Holwell, Joseph Zephaniah. *An Account of the Manner of Inoculating for the Small Pox in the East Indies, with some Observations on the Practice and Mode of Treating that Disease in those Parts.* London: 1767.

James, SP. *Smallpox and Vaccination in British India*. Thacker, Spink and Company: Calcutta. 1909.

Johnson, James. *The Influence of Tropical Climates on European Constitutions: Being a Treatise on the Principal Diseases incidental to Europeans in East and West Indies, Mediterranean, and the Coast of Africa*. From the third London edition. W E Dean: New York. 1826.

Lewis, William. *The New Dispensatory*. Fourth edition. Dublin: 1778.

Lind, James. *An Essay on Diseases Incidental to Europeans in Hot Climates, with the Method of Preventing their Fatal Consequences; to which is added an Appendix concerning Intermittent Fevers*. First American from the sixth London edition. Philadelphia: 1811

Long, Revd. James. *Selections from the Unpublished Records of Government for the Years 1748 to 1767 Inclusive relating mainly to the Social Condition of Bengal*. Volume I. Government Press: Calcutta. 1869.

Lushington, Mrs Charles. *Narrative of a Journey from Calcutta to Europe, by way of Egypt, in the years 1827 and 1828*. Second edition. John Murray: London. 1829.

Marshman, John. *The History of India*. Part I. Serampore Press: Serampore. 1863.

Martin, Sir James Ranald. *Influence of Tropical Climates in Procuring the Acute Endemic Diseases of Europeans*. Second Edition. John Churchill: London. 1861.

Memoirs of William Hickey. Edited by Alfred Spencer. Volume III (1782-1790). Hurst and Blackett: London. No date.

Pettigrew, Thomas Joseph. *Biographical Memoirs of the Most Celebrated Physicians, Surgeons, Etc, Etc, who have contributed to the Advancement of Medical Science*. Volume I. Fisher and Son: London. No date.

Record of Cases Treated in the Mesmeric Hospital from November 1846 to May 1847 with Reports of the Official Visitors. Printed by order of Government. Military Orphan Press: Calcutta. 1847.

Reece, Richard. *The Medical Guide for Tropical Climates, Particularly the British Settlements in the East and West Indies and the Coast of Africa*. London: 1814.

Stewart, Charles. *The History of Bengal*. Black, Parry, and Company: London. 1813.

Supplement to' Some Facts in the History of the Twining Family'. Bennett Brothers: Salisbury. 1893.

The Annals of the Barber Surgeons, Compiled from Their Records and other Sources, by Sidney Young, one of the Court of Assistants of the

Worshipful Company of Barbers of London, with illustrations by Austin T Young. London: 1890.

The Diaries of Three Surgeons of Patna 1763. Edited by Walter K Firminger. Calcutta Historical Society: Calcutta. 1909.

The East India Sketchbook, comprising an account of the present state of society in Calcutta, Bombay, & c. Volume II. Richard Bentley: London. 1832.

The Gems of Tuscany, being a Fragment for the Invalid and the Tourist in Italy, by a Fellow of the Royal College of Surgeons. Ackerman and Company: London. 1852.

The Twining Family: Descendants of William Twining, Sr, of Eastham, Massachusetts, where he died 1659; with notes of English, Welsh, and Nova Scotia families of the name. Revised edition. Fort Wayne, Indiana: 1905.

Twining, William. *Clinical Illustrations of the more important diseases of Bengal, with the result of an Inquiry into their Pathology and Treatment*. Calcutta: 1832.

Wade, John Peter. *A Paper on the Prevention and Treatment of the Disorders of Seamen and Soldiers in Bengal, Presented to the Honourable Court of East India Directors, in the Year 1791.* John Murray: London. 1793.

Wade, John Peter. *Select Evidences of a successful Method of Treating Fever and Dysentery in Bengal.* No further details available.

Wilson, CR. *Early Annals of the English in Bengal, being the Bengal Public Consultations for the First Half of the Eighteenth Century.* Volume I. Thacker, Spink and Company: Calcutta and London. 1895.

Wilson, CR. *Early Annals of the English in Bengal, being the Bengal Public Consultations for the First Half of the Eighteenth Century.* Volume II, Part I. Thacker, Spink and Company: Calcutta and London. 1900.

Wilson, CR. *Early Annals of the English in Bengal, being the Bengal Public Consultations for the First Half of the Eighteenth Century.* Volume II, Part II. Thacker, Spink and Company: Calcutta and London. 1911.

Woodall, John. *The Surgeon's Mate, or A Treatise Discovering Faithfully and Plainly the due contents of the Surgeon's Chest, the Uses of the Instruments, the virtues and operations of the Medicines, the Cures of the most frequent diseases at Sea.* London: 1617.

Yates, William, and Charles Maclean. *A View of the Science of Life; on the Principles established in the Elements of Medicine of the Late Celebrated John Brown, MD, with an attempt to correct some important errors of that Work, and Cases in Illustration, chiefly selected from the records of their practice, at the General Hospital, at Calcutta*. Dover: 1801.